Basic and Clinical Aspects of Immunity to Insulin

Basic and Clinical Aspects of Immunity to Insulin

Proceedings
International Workshop
September 28 – October 1, 1980,
Konstanz, Germany

Editors
K. Keck · P. Erb

W DE G

Walter de Gruyter · Berlin · New York 1981

Editors:

Klaus Keck, Priv.-Doz., Dr. rer. nat.
Fakultät für Biologie
Universität Konstanz
D-7750 Konstanz

Peter Erb, Priv.-Doz., Dr. phil.
Institut für Mikrobiologie und Hygiene der
Universität Basel
CH-4003 Basel
Petersplatz 10

CIP-Kurztitelaufnahme der Deutschen Bibliothek

Basic and clinical aspects of immunity to insulin / ed. K. Keck ;
P. Erb. – Berlin ; New York : de Gruyter, 1981.
ISBN 3-11-008440-6
NE: Keck, Klaus [Hrsg.]

Library of Congress Cataloging in Publication Data

Main entry under title:
Basic and clinical aspects of immunity to insulin.
Bibliography: p.
Includes index.
1. Insulin–Congresses. 2. Insulin antibodies–Congresses.
3. Insulin resistance–Congresses. 4. Immunogenetics–Congresses. I. Keck, K. (Klaus), 1932– . II. Erb, P. (Peter), 1942– .
QP572.I5B37 612'.396 81-5393
ISBN 3-11-008440-6 AACR2

Printing: Karl Gerike, Berlin. – Binding: Dieter Mikolai, Berlin.
Printed in Germany.

PREFACE

Sixty years have passed since the discovery of the natural hormone insulin by Banting and Best. As a result of that discovery, diabetes is a disease which can be controlled, though it cannot be cured. Since that time, insulin has attracted the interest of a variety of people in different scientific disciplines. Chemically, insulin has been studied in great detail. The complete amino acid sequences are known for several varieties of insulin. The three-dimensional structure of insulin and pro-insulin has been worked out. The mechanism of activation of insulin from its inactive precursor provides an interesting model system for regulating biological activity of hormones and enzymes. More recently, studies on the interaction of insulin with its receptor have begun to show promising results in elucidating mechanisms of hormone activity. Clinically, these studies have also proved beneficial. With improved methods of purification and characterization of insulin, some of the complications evoked by its therapeutic use in diabetics have been diminished.

Insulin has also attracted the interest of immunologists for many reasons. Because it is a small molecule and it is chemically well-defined, it is an excellent immunological probe. As an antigen, insulin shows a pattern of immune response gene control linked to the major histocompatibility locus in both mice and guinea pigs. Insulin is one of the few antigens for which the fine specificity of Ir gene control can be mapped to specific immunogenic regions of the molecule. Furthermore, the immunological aspects of insulin resistance and the possible autoimmune component of juvenile diabetes in humans lend an aspect of immediate relevance to the study of insulin immunology.

In order to integrate the large quantities of information available regarding the chemistry and immunology of insulin as well as the clinical aspects of diabetes and its control, it is necessary to establish interdisciplinary lines of communication between specialists in these various fields. It was the intention of a Symposium held in Konstanz, FRG, from September 28 to October 1, 1980, to bring together clinicians, immunologists and chemists active in insulin research, to provide an open forum to exchange ideas and experience, to establish contacts and to intensify cooperation between these groups. Forty participants from the USA, Canada and Europe reported their current research activities. The rather intimate atmosphere allowed for lively discussion and, to a certain extent, overcame the interdisciplinary language barrier. The result was a very up-to-date picture of the current state of insulin research. The papers presented in this book are, in so far as is possible, a complete compilation of the data that were presented at this Symposium.

We are most grateful to the participants whose contributions made the Symposium a success.
A very special acknowledgement must go to our Symposium Secretary, Mrs Brigitte Bergmann, for her excellent organizational work and to Dr. Yvan-Jeanne Weiler for her invaluable help in the preparation of this book.
We most gratefully appreciate the generous financial support given by the Deutsche Forschungsgemeinschaft which made this Symposium possible.
We are also indebted to the following contributors: Merck Sharp & Dohme, USA; Farbwerke Hoechst AG, FRG and Novo Research Institute, Denmark.
Last but not least, we thank Walter de Gruyter & Co. for agreeing to publish the book.

Peter Erb
Klaus Keck

LIST OF PARTICIPANTS

Arquilla, E.R.
Dept. of Pathology, 101 City Drive South, Orange, California 92668, U.S.A.

Bertrams, J.
Abt. für Laboratoriumsmedizin, Elisabeth-Krankenhaus, Moltkestr. 61, D-4300 Essen 1, BRD.

Bösing-Schneider, R.
Faculty of Biology, University of Konstanz, D-7750 Konstanz, FRG.

Brandenburg, D.
Deutsches Wollforschungsinstitut, Veltmanplatz 8, D-5100 Aachen, BRD.

Büllesbach, E.E.
Deutsches Wollforschungsinstitut, Veltmanplatz 8, D-5100 Aachen, BRD.

Cecka, J.M.
Dept. of Zoology, University College London, London WC1E 6BT England.

Cohen, I.R.
Dept. of Cell Biology, Weizmann Institute, Rehovot, Israel.

Danho, W.
Hoffman-La Roche Inc., Nutley, N.J. 07110 U.S.A.

Erb, P.
Institute for Microbiology, University of Basel, Petersplatz 10, CH-4003 Basel, Switzerland.

Federlin, K.
III. Med. Klinik und Poliklinik der Universität, D-6300 Giessen, BRD.

Frenkel, A.
Dept. of Cell Biology, Weizmann Institute, Rehovot, Israel.

Freytag, G.
Dept. Pathol. University of Münster, Westring 17, D-4400 Münster, FRG.

Gattner, H.-G.
Deutsches Wollforschungsinstitut, Veltmanplatz 8, D-5100 Aachen, BRD.

Geiger, R.
Hoechst AG., G 838, Postfach, D-6230 F-Hoechst, BRD.

Hansen, B.
Hagedorn Research Laboratory, Niels Steensensvej 6, DK-2820 Gentofte, Denmark.

Kallenberger, I.
Faculty of Biology, University of Konstanz, D-7750 Konstanz, FRG.

Kapp, J.A.
Dept. of Pathology, Jewish Hospital of St. Louis, 216 S. Kingshighway, St. Louis, MO 63110, U.S.A.

Keck, K.
Faculty of Biology, University of Konstanz, D-7750 Konstanz, FRG.

Kontiainen, S.
Dept. of Bacteriology and Immunology, University of Helsinki, Haartmanink. 3, 00290 Helsinki 29, Finland.

Kruse, V.
Novo Research Institute, Novo Alle, DK-2880 Bagsvaerd, Denmark

Leeman-Abromsom, S.
Division of Tumor Immunology, S.Farber Cancer Center, 44 Binney Street, Boston, MA 02115, U.S.A.

Mann D.
National Institutes of Health, Bld. 10 Rm 4BM, Bethesda, Maryland 20205, U.S.A.

Markussen, J.
Novo Research Institute, Novo Alle, DK-2880 Bagsvaerd, Denmark

Momayezi, M.
Faculty of Biology, University of Konstanz, D-7750 Konstanz, FRG.

Neubauer, H.P.
Am Eichkopf 12, D-6240 Königstein/Ts. BRD.

Petersen, K.G.
Mediz. Univ. Klinik, Abtl. für Endokrinologie, Hugstetter Str. 55, D-7800 Freiburg.

Ramila, G.
Institute for Microbiology, University of Basel, Petersplatz 10, CH-4003 Basel, Switzerland.

Reeves, W.G.
Dept. of Immunology, University Hospital, Nottingham, England.

Rosenthal, A.S.
Dept. of Immunology and Inflammmation Research, Merck Sharp and Dohme Research Laboratories, P.O. Box 2000, Rahway, N.J. 07065, U.S.A.

Rosenwasser, L.J.
Tufts University School of Medicine, New England Medical Center Hospital, Boston, MA 02111, U.S.A.

Ruede, E.
Institut für Immunologie, Hochhaus am Augustusplatz, D-6500 Mainz, BRD.

Schernthaner, G.
2nd Dept. of Internal Medicine, University of Vienna, Garnisongasse 13, 1090 Vienna, Austria.

Schroer, J.A.
Lab. of Clinical Investigation NIAID, National Institutes of Health, Bethesda, Maryland, U.S.A.

Sørensen, E.
Novo Research Institute, Novo Alle, DK-2880 Bagsvaerd, Denmark

Shin, S.
Dept. of Genetics, Diabetes Research and Training Center, Albert Einstein College of Medicine, Bronx, New York 10461, U.S.A.

Singh, B.
Department of Immunology, University of Alberta, Edmonton, Alberta, Canada

Sklenar, I.
Institute for Microbiology, University of Basel, Petersplatz 10, CH-4003 Basel, Switzerland.

Spaeth, E.
Institut für Immunologie, Hochhaus am Augustusplatz, D-6500 Mainz, BRD.

Thomas, J.W.
202 Yalem Research, Jewish Hospital, 216 S. Kingshighway, St. Louis, Mo. 63110, U.S.A.

Velcovsky, H.-G.
Med. Poliklinik, Rodthohl 6, D-6300 Giessen, BRD.

CONTENTS

SECTION I. BASIC ASPECTS OF IMMUNITY TO INSULIN

Section I

Basic Aspects of Immunity to Insulin

INTRODUCTION:

INSULIN AS A TOOL FOR THE STUDY OF IMMUNOLOGICAL PROBLEMS

K. Keck
University of Konstanz, Faculty of Biology, D-7550 Konstanz, FRG

When we started our work with insulin we did not expect that it would become a subject of much interest among immunologists. Indeed, we were not the first to use insulin for basic immunological research. Arquilla and Finn demonstrated, in 1965 (1), that the response of guinea pigs to insulin is genetically controlled. If I am right the next group was Little and Counts in 1969 (2). They used insulin dinitrophenylated at Lysine B29. The rationale behind their experiments was the following: If an antigen is used that has the DNP-group at a single position, a restricted antibody response to this group could be expected. The results were discouraging, the antibodies were heterogenous.

During my stay at the Roswell Park Memorial Institute in 1972 we used the same approach, but with better techniques which became available at that time (3). We purified DNP-B29-insulin by electrofocussing and used this derivative for the immunization of rabbits. Electrofocussing of these antibodies showed the presence of 1 to 3 antibody clones. The index of heterogeneity was about 1. Unfortunately our rabbits in Konstanz did not cooperate: the antibodies were as heterogeneous as with other antigens. When we repeated this kind of experiments with mice, we observed that the response was under genetic control. And furthermore, we realized that for the

Basic and Clinical Aspects of Immunity to Insulin

study of this type of control the insulin was an excellent choice of antigen, for the following reasons: Insulins of different species, for example pig, cattle, sheep and horse, differ by only one to three aminoacids within the region of the A-chain loop, so the effect of small sequence difference on the immune response can be studied.

When immunologists deal with structural components of antigens they call them determinants. Two types of determinants play a role in the immune response: Immunogenic determinants or carrier determinants are those areas of the antigen or immunogen which render a molecule immunogenic. Haptenic determinants are structures on the surface of the antigen to which the antibodies bind, they determine the specificity of the antibody. One should avoid using the term antigenic determinants without defining which type of determinants is meant.

This raises two important questions: (1) Are carrier determinants and haptenic determinants really different structures? (2) Are there two sets of specific "recognition units" or receptors, one set for carrier determinants and another set for haptenic determinants?

I want to stress the point, that distinguishing between carrier determinants and haptenic determinants does not necessarily mean, that both must be different structures. They may be identical in some cases, but certainly they are processed differently, by different cell types and at different steps during the initiation of an immune response.

As to the second question: The binding sites of the antibody have been intensively investigated, but very little is known about the receptors for carrier determinants. Some experiments seem to indicate that the same V-regions might be involved as those found in the heavy chains of antibody. Possibly they are not associated with the same light chains as in antibody.

During the initiation steps of an immune response lymphocytes and macrophages first make contact with the antigen and a decission is made if an immune response (antibody production) or cellular reaction) is going to take place. If the antigen is recognized by these cells as "foreign", that is different from the bodys own molecules, it is handled as an immunogen. If the differences between the antigen and an homologous protein of the body are very small, the organism may be unable to see these differences, and hence may not produce antibody to this antigen. The specificity of this recognition process is the major area in which work with insulin has been uniquely successful.

In addition to sequence differences, insulin has some properties which makes it attractive for immunologists:
(1) Insulin is a rather stable molecule, it can be easily purified and is even commercially available in preparations of high purity. (2) Chemists have worked very hard on insulin. It is one of the best known polypeptide molecules. Its tertiary structure is well known. (3) Since insulin has only three primary amino groups, derivatives with defined structures can be made. (4) A great number of modified insulins is available, insulins with shortened or elongated chains and with artificially exchanged amino acids (See section III of this symposium).

However, as previously mentioned, the most important feature of the insulin is that it can be obtained in different forms which differ by only a few amino acid exchanges. The sequence differences between some of the insulins are listed in Fig 1. In contrast to most other animals the mouse, which is the most important animal for immunologists, has two insulins which differ from one another by two amino acids in the B-chain (4). Assuming, that the mouse is tolerant towards its own insulins, we have 5 sequence differences between mouse and bovine insulin, which may constitute prospective immunogenic determinants, if we immunize mice with bovine insulin.

A-Chain

		4		8 9 10	
Mouse I+II	- - -	ASP	- - -	THR-SER-JLE	- - -
Pig	- - -	GLU	- - -	THR-SER-JLE	- - -
Cattle	- - -	GLU	- - -	ALA-SER-VAL	- - -
Sheep	- - -	GLU	- - -	ALA-GLY-VAL	- - -
Horse	- - -	GLU	- - -	THR-GLY-JLE	- - -

B-Chain

		3		9		29 30
Mouse I	- - -	LYS	- - -	PRO	- - - -	LYS-SER
Mouse II	- - -	LYS	- - -	SER	- - - -	MET-SER
Pig, Cattle, Sheep, Horse	- - -	ASN	- - -	SER	- - - -	LYS-ALA

Fig 1. Sequence differences between insulins of different species.

Pig insulin has the same A-chain loop as mouse insulin, hence there are only 3 sequence differences as compared to mouse insulin (A4, B3, B30).

Table 1 shows the response of a number of inbred strains of mice to various insulins. The date clearly demonstrate that the insulins of pig, cattle, sheep and horse are differently immunogenic in different mouse strains, therefore the A-chain loops of some insulins constitute strong carrier determinants. (5,6). For example, the strain B10. needs the A-chain loop of bovine insulin for the production of antibody. Strain C3H.He cannot produce antibody if immunized with bovine insulin, however sheep insulin is immunogenic in this strain, demonstrating the important role of the sheep insulin A-chain loop

Table 1: Response of inbred strains of mice to Insulins of different species and Pig-Pro Insulin [1)]

Strain	H-2-haplotype	Response to Insulin of Pig	Cattle	Sheep	Horse	Response to Pig-Pro Ins.
Balb/c	d	+	+	+	+	+
B10	b	-	+	±	-	+
C3H/SW	b	-	+	±	n.d.	n.d.
B10.BR	k	-	-	+	+	+
C3H/He	k	-	-	+	+	+
SJL	s	-	-	-	-	-
SM/J	v	+	+	n.d.	n.d.	±
B10M	f	n.d.	-	+	+	-
C3H.NB	p	-	+	-	-	+
DBA/1J	q	n.d.	-	-	n.d.	-
PL/J	u	-	-	-	-	-
RIII/2J	r	n.d.	-	-	n.d.	±
C3H/HK	j	n.d.	-	-	-	+

1) 20 µg of the Insulin in CFA was injected i.p. on day 0, the same dose in saline was given on day 21. Mice were bled on day 30. IgG antibody was measured by the Farr technique.

sequence in the initiation process in this strain. All B10. strains have the same background; the same is true for the C3H-strains (for detailed discussion of genetic implications see 7,8). Comparison of the response of these strains clearly shows that the H-2 haplotype determins the responsiveness of mice to the insulins. As expected pig insulin is the least immunogenic of all the four insulins tested.

Table 1 also shows that the C-peptide of pig proinsulin which has probably about 18 sequence differences as compared to the mouse C-peptide can also act as a carrier determinant in a number of mouse strains (9).

Experiments of this kind have been carried out by others with synthetic polypeptides and also with enzymes of different species (see 10 -13). Both groups of antigens have disadvantages. Synthetic polypeptides in most cases have no definite sequence and tertiary structure, though some recent developments in this field have been encouraging (14). Enzymes of different species usually have more sequence differences than the insulins and importantly, they have no area like the A-chain loop which has a number of sequence differences within only 3 adjacent amino acids. This A-chain loop has a rather invariant tertiary structure because of the 3 cysteins which stabilize this area of the molecule by disulfide bonds.

The data in Table 1 suggest that some mouse strains need a certain sequence in the A-chain loop in order to respond to an insulin. We may ask the question, whether the A-chain loop is a carrier determinant, or whether residues adjacent to the loop may be a part of such a determinant or whether even the intact conformation of the molecule is necessary for the induction process which leads to antibody production.

Experiments carried out by Bagira Singh (this symposium page 45) will show that the isolated loop can act as a carrier determinant. Even more surprising are the data shown by Iron

Cohen who demonstrates that the tripeptide comprising amino acids 8 to 10 of the bovine insulin can constitute a complete carrier determinant (this symposium page 157).This is in good agreement with other data which suggest that carrier determinants may be preferentially sequence determinants and not conformational determinants (15). Allan Rosenthal (16) has shown that in in-vitro experiments T-cells from guinea-pigs of strain 13 can be stimulated with isolated oxidized B-chains. Also in this case a small peptide of the B-chain can act as a carrier determinant (see this symposium page 17).

Table 2: Crossreaction between Insulin and oxidized B-Chain at the carrier level[1)]

Strain	Immunogen	Coimmunogen	Antibody to			
			Insulin	DNP	OVA	BSA
BALB/c	DNP-Bov.Ins.	-	85,1	76,0	-	-
"	"	A-Chain(ox.)	91,3	94,8	-	-
"	"	B-Chain(ox.)	78,5	63,5	-	-
C57/BL	"	-	85,3	94,0	-	-
"	"	A-Chain(ox.)	82,1	98,2	-	-
"	"	B-Chain(ox.)	29,2	16,3	-	-
C57/BL	Ovalbumin	-	-		94,4	-
"	"	B-Chain(ox.)	-		92,1	-
C57/BL	BSA	-	-		-	89,2
"	"	B-Chain(ox.)	-		-	5,1

1) 20 ug of immunogen were injected together with 100 ug of the coimmunogen in CFA on day 0, boosted with the same dose in saline on day 21. Mice were bled on day 30. Antibody titer presented as per cent binding of ^{125}J labeled antigen.

Our own experiments with mice point to the same direction

(Table 2). C57BL mice respond to DNP-B29-bovine insulin. If a 5-fold excess of the isolated, oxidized B-chain is given simultaneously with the DNP-insulin the response is reduced dramatically suggesting that there might be competition between the insulin and the B-chain loop for a receptor which binds to both molecules. Such an effective crossreaction is not observed at the level of the antibody produced. When we carried out a specificity control, we were surprised by observing that the response to bovine serum albumin but not to ovalbumin is suppressed simultaneously and even more effectively by the B-chain co-immunization. This could mean that this strain recognizes a carrier determinant which is present on both molecules insulin and bovine serum albumin. If the assumption that carrier determinants are small sequence determinants is correct than it can be considered more likely to find crossreactions between non related molecules at the carrier level than at the level of the antibody. This would also provide a simple explanation for the often observed phenomenon of "antigenic competition".

The data presented in Table 1 further indicate that immune response genes (Ir-genes) located within the H-2 region control the response of mice to the insulins. This region, on chromosome 17, is the major histocompatibility region (MHC), which is analogous to the human HLA locus.

Ir-genes are usually inherited dominantly, as demonstrated in Fig 2A. This is not true for all hybrids. B10.BR mice respond to sheep insulin. The hybrids (B10.S x B10.BR) do not respond to this insulin (Fig 2B). In this case we have a recessive inheritance of responsiveness. Fig 2C shows an example of a complementation. Both parental strains C3H.SWX and C3H/He are nonresponder to pig insulin. However the hybrid strain is a high responder to this insulin. We have interpreted this data as suggesting that there may be a set of Ir-genes that control the recognition of a set of immunogenic determinants.

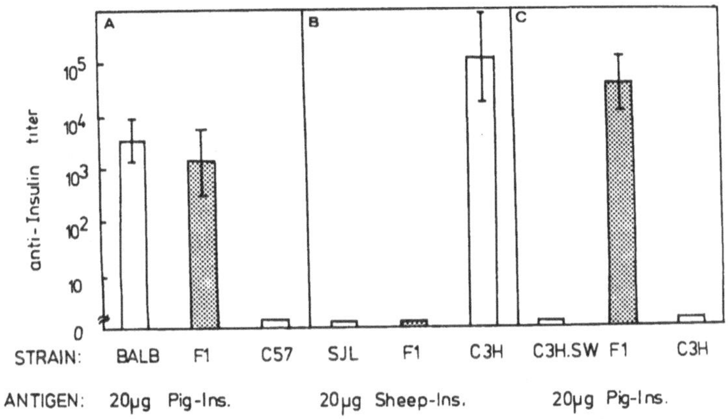

Fig 2. Inheritance of responsiveness to insulins. Dominant inheritance A, recessive inheritance B, complementation C.

Recognition in this sense means that these determinants are processed in a way that finally leads to antibody production. If we assume that the recognition of two or more carrier determinants are necessary for an immune response to be triggered, complementation can be explained in terms of complementary recognition of carrier determinants by each strain (for details see 17). One of these carrier determinants may be processed by an amplifier cell as proposed by Judith Kapp (this symposium page 71).

Recombinant strains allow the localization of Ir-genes within subregions of the H-2 locus. We have measured the response of several recombinant strains to some of the insulins (Table 3). Comparison of strain B10.A(5R) (which responds to bovine insulin) with strain B10.A(4R) shows that the gene necessary for the response to bovine insulin must be localized left to the A/B crossover. Similarly a gene controlling the response

Table 3. Response of mice with recombinant haplotypes to insulins of different species

Strain	H-2 Subregions									IgG-Response		
	K	A	B	J	E	C	S	G	D	Pig[x]	Bov[x]	Sheep[xx]
B10.BR	k	k	k	k	k	k	k	k	k	-	-	++
B10.A	k	k	k	k	k |	d	d	d	d	-	-	++
B10.A(2R)	k	k	k	k	k |	d	d	d	b	-	-	n.d.
B10.A(4R)	k	k |	b	b	b	b	b	b	b	-	-	-[xxx]
B10.A(5R)	b	b	b	k	k |	d	d	d	d	-	++	n.d.
D2.GD	d	d	d |	b	b	b	b	b	b	++	++	++
B10.	b	b	b	b	b	b	b	b	b	-	++	++

[x] 20 µg in CFA
[xx] 40 µg in CFA
[xxx] 100 µg in CFA

to pig insulin can be localized to the left of the B/J crossover in strain D2.GD. It is surprising that B10.A(4R) mice are unable to respond to sheep insulin even if given in high doses (up to 100 µg), since both haplotypes b and k should unable a response to this insulin. One possible explanation would be that a gene needed for this response may be impaired by the crossover event. Alternatively one may consider that two genes of the same haplotype are necessary in different subregions.

Besides the Ir-genes located in the H-2 region, other genes contribute to the regulation of antibody production. Certain background genes are necessary for complementation (17), allotype linked genes (genes linked to the genes which code for the immunoglobulin heavy chains) control the production of IgM antibody in strains which are non-responders with respect to IgG antibody (18,19,20). The same genes control the induction of tolerance by pig insulin (Fig 3). C3H.He mice do not respond to pig and bovine insulin, they respond however to sheep and horse insulin and to pig proinsulin. Preimmunization with pig insulin renders the animals tolerant to a successive immunization with one of the immunogenic insulins (19,21).

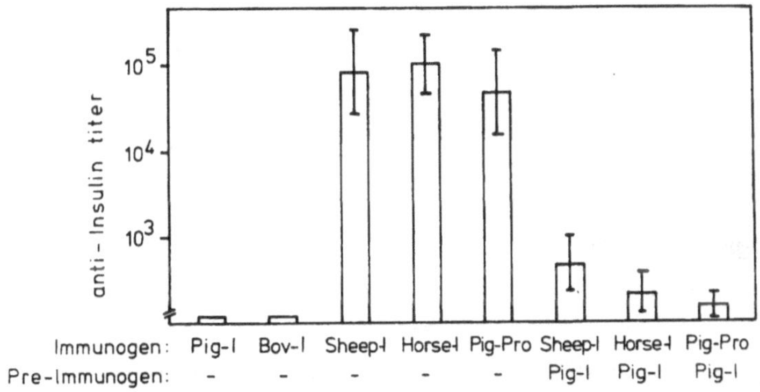

Fig 3. Suppression of IgG production to various insulins by preimmunisation with pig insulin in C3H.He mice

Massoud Momayezi has demonstrated (this symposium page 115) that insulin specific suppressor cells are generated under these conditions. The immunogen and the tolerogen may differ by only one amino acid (pig as compared to horse insulin). This raises the question whether there may be two types of carrier determinants on the antigen, immunogenic determinants and suppressor determinants, or whether the lack of a potent immunogenic determinant shifts the dose response to higher doses, low zone tolerance occuring with doses that in other cases would be immunogenic.

Others used different approaches to clarify the role of carrier determinants during the induction of an immune response. Rosenthal et.al. (22) have shown by in vitro experiments, that only the macrophages of responder parental strains are able to present insulin to F_1 (responder x nonresponder) T-cells. Erb (23) used in vitro cultures for the stimulation of insulin specific B-cells. It can be supposed that insulin will be a very useful antigen for answering the following questions: What kind of antigen specific factors are involved in T- and B-cell triggering, to which part (determinant) on the surface of the antigen do they bind.

Acknowledgments:
The expert technical assistance of Mrs. Bergmann is gratefully acknowledged. This work was supported by the Deutsche Forschungsgemeinschaft, Sonderforschungsbereich 138, "Biologische Grenzflächen und Spezifität".

Literatur

1) Arquilla, E. and Finn, I: J. exp. Med 122, 771 (1965)
2) Little, J.R. and Counts, R.B.: Biochemistry 8 2729 (1969)
3) Keck, K., Grossberg, A.L. and Pressman, D.: Immunochem. 10 331 (1973)

4) Markussen, J.: Int. J. Peptide Res. 3 149 (1971)
5) Keck, K.: Nature 254 5495 (1975)
6) Keck, K.: Eur. J. Immunol. 5 801 (1975)
7) Schreffler, D.C. and David, C.S.: Adv. Immunology 20 125-195 (1975)
8) Klein, J.: Biology of the Mouse Histocompatibility-2 complex, Springer-Verlag Berlin, Heidelberg, New York (1975)
9) Keck, K.: 2. Immun.-Forsch. (Immunobiology) 155 32 (1978)
10) McDevitt, H.O. and Benacerraf, B.: Advances in Immunol. 11 31 (1976)
11) Benacerraf, B. and Dorf, M.E.: Cold Spring Harbor Symp. Quart. Biol. 41 465 (1976)
12) Berzofsky, J.A., Richman, L.K. and Killion, D.J.: Poc. Nat. Acad. Sci. 76 4046 (1979)
13) Adorini, L., Miller, A. and Sercarz, E.E.: J. of Immunol. 122 (1979)
14) Singh, B., Fraga, E. and Barton, M.A.: J. Immunol. 124 784 (1978)
15) Singh, B., Lee, K., Fraga, A., Wilkinson, A., Wong, M. and Barton, M.: J. Immunol. 124 1336 (1980)
16) Rosenthal, A.S.: Immunological Rev. 40 136 (1978)
17) Keck, K.: Eur. J. Immunonol. 7 812 (1977)
18) Momayezi, M., Keck, K. and Kolb, H.: 2. Immun.-Forsch. (Immunobiology), 155 44 (1978)
19) Keck, K. and Momayezi, M.: In Brandenburg, D. and Woldmer, A. (Eds.), Chemistry, Structure and Function of Insulin and Related Hormons, Berlin 1980
20) Momayezi, M.: Dissertation, 1980, University Konstanz (FRG)
21) Keck, K.: Diabetologia 13 407 (1977)
22) Rosenthal, A.S., Barcinsky, M.A. and Blake, J.T.: Nature 267 156 (1977)
23) Erb, P.: Immunology 40 385-394 (1980)

GENETIC CONTROL OF THE IMMUNE RESPONSE TO INSULIN

A.S. Rosenthal, C.S. Lin, T. Hansen

Department of Immunology
Merck Institute for Therapeutic Research
Rahway, New Jersey

J.W. Thomas

Department of Pathology
Jewish Hospital of St. Louis
St. Louis, Missouri

W. Danho, E. Bullesbach, J. Föhles

Deutsches Wollforschingsinstitut
Aachen, West Germany

Introduction

The immune response to protein and peptide antigens is controlled by genes (Ir) linked to the major histocompatibility complex (MHC) of mammals (1). The I region of the murine major histocompatibility complex is comprised of a series of loci which controls a diverse array of immunologic functions, including the Ir genes which control the immune response to a variety of protein antigens (2) and the genes which encode the Ia cell surface glycoproteins (3). The relationship of Ir products and Ia molecules is not precisely defined since the total number of I-region gene products and each of their individual functions is still unclear. In addition to Ir genes and Ia specificities, several other immunologic phenomenon are controlled by I region loci. These determinants include: histocompatibility antigens (4), the antigens recognized in MLR (5) and GVH responses (6) and the cell membrane antigens which determine the successful interactions between macrophage and T-cells (7) and limit the cooperation between T and B-cells in the immune response (8). Several studies suggest that the above listed membrane structures are all determinants on Ia molecules and that they interact with antigen during antigen presentation.

Basic and Clinical Aspects of Immunity to Insulin

Species variants of insulin with limited amino acid differences were previously used to map the intramolecular sights recognized by T and B cells from inbred strains of guinea pigs and mice (9, 10, 11). Both the T cell proliferative and T helper responses were found to be under the control of Ir genes linked respectively to the guinea pig and mouse major histocompatibility complex. T cells from strain 2 guinea pig and $H\text{-}2^b$ mice respond to a well defined area on the A chain of insulin (A8-A9-A10). In strain 13 guinea pigs and $H\text{-}2^d$ mice the T cell response was not defined but was believed to be dependent upon or directed at some as yet undefined determinant(s) on the B chain of insulin. Antibody specificity has not been correspondingly shown to be restricted to the same intramolecular regions as T cell responsiveness (9).

This manuscript will review recent findings localizing more precisely the intramolecular site regulating the recognition of insulin in strain 13 guinea pigs and also describing a selective deletion of A loop responsiveness in a mutant $H\text{-}2^b$ mouse, the $B6^{bm12}$. Both types of data can be interpreted as indicating that Ia and antigen interact in a selective manner dependent upon the respective amino acid sequences of each.

Materials and Methods

Animals. Inbred strain 2, strain 13 and F_1 (2x13) guinea pigs were obtained from the Division of Research Services, NIH. Adult animals weighing 300-500 g were used as sources of all cells and antisera in this study.

Media. Cell cultures were performed in medium RPMI 1640 (Grand Island Biological Co., Grand Island, NY) supplemented with fresh L-glutamine (0.3 mg/ml), gentamicin (10 µg/ml), penicillin (200 U/ml), 2-mercaptoethanol (2.5×10^{-5}M; Eastman Kodak Co., Rochester, NY) and 5% fetal calf serum (FCS; Industrial Biological Laboratories, Rockville, MD). Hank's balanced salt solution (HBSS) was used for all washing procedures.

Antigens. Single component beef and pork insulin (Eli Lilly and Co., Indianapolis, Ind.) was used throughout these studies for either priming animals or for *in vitro* proliferation studies. (TG)A-L (L-tyrosine-glutamine, alanine-lysine) random polymers was purchased from Miles Yeda.

Synthesis of B chain fragments. The peptides used in this study were synthesized by the solution method of peptide chemistry using the strategy of fragment condensation and the tactic of acid-labile protecting groups (trityl for SH function; t-butyl esters for the α-carboxyl functions; t-butyl ethers for the hydroxyl functions and the t-butyloxycarbonyl- and 2-(4-biphenyl)-2-propyloxy carbonyl groups for the α-amino functions). The protected peptides fragments were purified on Sephadex LH 20 in dimethylformamide. Characterization was achieved by:

1. Thin layer chromatography on silica gel/60 sheets, using two solvent systems SBA (sec. butanol/formic acid/water (15/13.4/11.5) V/V, and SBN (sec. butanol/10% ammonia (85/15)V/V.
2. Elementary analysis, melting point, optical rotation.
3. Amino acid anaylsis.

The peptides proved to be homogenous. Deprotection to the S-tritylated peptides was achieved by treating with trifluor acetic acid in the presence of tritylcarbinol and anisole for 30 min. at room temperature followed by ether precipitation. Purification was accomplished by gel filtration on Sephadex G-15 in 30% acetic acid.

The purity of these S-tritylated peptides were checked by:

1. Thin layer chromatography on cellulose sheets in the system n-butanol/pyridine/acetic acid/water (15/10/3/12).
2. Electrophoresis at pH 1.9.
3. Amino acid anaylsis.

Figure 1 and Table I show the peptides used in these studies with their corresponding amino acid analyses.

Immunization. For the T cell proliferation assay, mice and guinea pigs were immunized with antigen in saline emulsified with an equal volume of complete Freund's adjuvant (CFA) containing 0.5 mg/ml of killed Mycobacterium tuberculosis, H37Ra (Difco Laboratories, Detroit Michigan). Each animal received 0.1 ml emulsion containing 50-100 μg of antigen in each footpad. Cells for culture and primary serum were collected 2-4 weeks after immunization.

Cell Cultures. Peritoneal exudate cells (PECs) were obtained by lavaging the peritoneal cavity of mice or immune guinea pigs, 4 days after the injection of

TABLE I.

Compound	Abbreviation	Amino Acid Analysis
AcOH Trt AcOH AcOH•His-Leu-Cys-Gly-Ser-His-Leu-Val-Glu-Ala-Leu-Tyr-OH	B_{5-16}-OH	Ser 0.90, Glu 1.08, Gly 1.23, Ala 1.02, Val 1.05, Leu 3.00 Tyr 1.00, His 2.00
AcOH Trt AcOH AcOH•His-Leu-Cys-Gly-Ser-His-Leu-Val-Glu-Ala-Leu-Tyr-OMe	B_{5-16}-OMe	"
AcOH Trt AcOH Ac-His-Leu-Cys-Ser-His-Leu-Val-Glu-Ala-Leu-Tyr-OH	Ac-5-16-OH	"
AcOH Trt AcOH Ac-His-Leu-Cys-Gly-Ser-His-Leu-Val-Glu-Ala-Leu-Tyr-OMe	Ac-5-16-OMe	"
AcOH $Z(Lys)_6$-Ser-His-Leu-Val-Glu-Ala-Leu-Tyr-OH	$Z(Lys)_6$-9-16-OH	Ser 0.91, Glu 0.91, Ala 1.00, Val 1.04, Leu 2.00, Tyr 0.96, Lys 5.90, His 0.96
AcOH Trt AcOH $Z(Lys)_6$-His-Leu-Cys-Gly-Ser-His-Leu-Val-Glu-Ala-Leu-Tyr-OH	$Z(Lys)_6$-5-16-OH	Ser 0.92, Glu 1.07, Gly 1.20, Ala 1.13, Val 1.10, Leu 1.00, Tyr 1.00, Lys 5.39, His 2.00
AcOH Trt AcOH•His-Leu-Cys-Gly-Ser-Asn-Leu-Val-Glu-Ala-Leu-Tyr-OH 10	[Asn_{10}]B_{5-16}OH	Asp 1.00, Ser 0.80, Glu 0.98, Gly 0.94, Ala 1.00, Val 1.02, Leu 2.78, Tyr 1.00, His 0.84
AcOH Trt AcOH AcOH•His-Leu-Cys-Gly-Ser-His-Leu-Val-Glu-Thr-Leu-Tyr-OH 14	[Thr_{14}]B_{5-16}-OH	Thr 0.80, Ser 0.95, Clu 1.00, Gly 0.91, Val 1.00, Leu 2.66 Tyr 1.00, His 1.68
AcOH Trt AcOH•His-Leu-Cys-Gly-Ser-Asn-Leu-Val-Glu-Thr-Leu-Tyr-OH 10 14	[Asn_{10}], [Thr_{14}] B_{5-16}-OH	Asp 1.02, Thr 1.00, Ser 0.83, Glu 1.00, Gly 0.97, Val 0.98 Leu 2.45, Tyr 0.97, His 0.83

Figure 1.

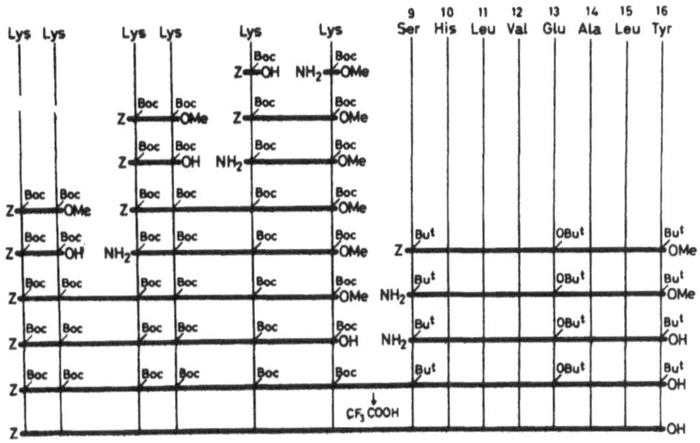

25 ml of sterile oil (Marcol 52; Humbel Oil and Refining Co., Houston, Texas) from non-immunized mice or guinea pigs twice in HBSS and treated with mitomycin C (40 µg/ml; Sigma Chemical Co., St. Louis, Mo.) for 60 min at 37°C at a concentration of 5-15x10^6 cells/ml. After four washes with HBSS, this cell population was used as a source of macrophages.

Populations of highly enriched antigen reactive T cells (PELs) were obtained after passage through a nylon wool adherence column (12) and were used to assess T cell proliferation by incorporation of radiolabeled thymidine into DNA. PELs resuspended in RPMI 1640 with 5% FCS were cultured in microtiter plates with round-bottom wells (Cooke Laboratory Products Div., Dynatch Laboratories Inc., Alexandria, Va.) for 72 hours in a 5% CO_2 humidified atmosphere at 37°C at a concentration of 1.2x10^6 PELs and 0.3x10^6 PECs/ml in the presence of continuous antigen. Tritiated thymidine (6.7Ci/m mol; New England Nuclear Corp., Boston, Mass.) 1 µCi/well was added 18 hours prior to termination. The cells were harvested onto glass filter paper by the use of a semiautomated microharvesting device. Tritiated thymidine incorporation was determined by liquid scintillation spectrometry and the results reported as number of counts above the control (counts per minute) unless otherwise stated.

Results and Discussion

The data presented in Tables II and III demonstrate that only a limited number of epitopes on a globular protein need be recognized for generation of cellular

TABLE II. DNA Synthesis can be Induced in Strain 13 Guinea Pigs Immune to Insulin by Molar Excess of N-Terminal Peptides Contained in the B(1-16) Fragment

Antigen	Peak ^{3}H-Thymidine incorporation (Δcpm x 10^{-3})	Moles Peptide/ Moles Insulin	% Stimulation
Insulin	31.6 ± 0.4	--	--
B(1-16)	35.6 ± 2.0	1.0	100+
B(1-10)	17.2 ± 0.6	3.0	54
B(1-13)	15.9 ± 0.6	3.0	50
B(5-13)	8.1 ± 3.7	5.5	26
B(5-16)	29.3 ± 1.9	8.0	93

TABLE III. Position Ten of Insulin B Chain is Critical for T Cell Activation of Insulin Immune Strain 13 Guinea Pigs

Antigen (10 ug/ml)	Δ cpm x 10^{-3}
Beef insulin	63.4 ± .42*
B chain	50.5 ± .31
B(1-16)	54.4 ± .45
B(5-16)	41.0 ± .41
B(5-16) [Ala → Thr]+	49.9 ± .35
B(5-16) [His → Asn]+	3.2 ± .03
B(5-16) [Ala → Thr + His → Asn]+,**	1.6 ± .02

*Mean ± SEM of two experiments

+Brackets indicate substitution(s) made from original sequence.

**Guinea pig sequence.

immunity as well as T helper cell activity. This study extends previous observations that denatured proteins can retain the ability to induce delayed hypersensitivity but loose antibody reactivity (13) and more recently that denatured antigen can elicit specific helper cells (14). The peptide sequence composed of the first sixteen amino acids of the insulin B chain (Figure 2) clearly contains all of the immunogenic information present in the native molecule as reflected in the generation of T cell proliferation and in the expression of T cell helper activity. B(5-16) is as active as B(1-16) and contains all of the immunologically important determinants. Synthetic sequences of the region B(5-16) having the amino acid sequences present in guinea pig insulin, or possessing only the B14 alanine of beef insulin but not the histidine 10th position, are not stimulatory. Using the (1-16) peptide, this reactivity was found to be reciprocal in that either peptide or whole molecule could be used as the immunogen. These observations support the concept that T cell responses are specific for a primary amino acid sequence on the antigen, and also emphasize the restricted nature of the T cell recognition process.

Several smaller peptides from the same region were also found to stimulate T cell proliferation, albeit less effectively than B(1-16). All of the peptides which activate T cells contain a common amino acid variation at the 10th position. This histidine for asparagine exchange makes guinea pig insulin unique among mammalian insulins--being unable to form heximeres with zinc (15). Using a computer generated space filling model developed by Mr. Richard Feldman of the NIH, we have located this residue as residing on the surface of the molecule. The other amino acid exchange (14th residue) within the B(5-16) peptide is not available on the surface of the molecule. If one considers variations from "self" to be a key in the recognition process, then the B-10 position assumes a critical role for T cell activation. A single amino acid has recently been shown to be critical for immune response to another peptide--human fibrin peptide (15). However, the failure of peptide B(9-16) to induce T cell proliferation emphasizes that the presence of this exchange alone is not sufficient for T cell activation. Moreover, a synthetic fragment consisting of B(1-4)-(9-16) also fails to activate insulin immune T cells, indicating that more than fragment size is important. Possibly another residue(s) important for Ir gene product interaction is contained within the 5-9 region. A requirement for recognition of two specificities--one for Ir and another for T cell--within even such a limited peptide sequence as the

Figure 2. Amino Acid Sequence of N-Terminal Sixteen Residues of Insulin B Chain

	1	2	3	4	5	6	7	8	9	10	11	12	13	14	15	16
Guinea Pig	Phe	Val	Ser	Arg	His	Leu	Cys	Gly	Ser	Asn	Leu	Val	Glu	Thr	Leu	Tyr
Pork/Beef	—	—	Asn	Gln	—	—	—	—	—	His	—	—	—	Ala	—	—

5th thru 16th amino acid of the B chain is not inconsistent with recent hypotheses for the mechanism of Ir gene function (16, 17).

While primary structure is of key importance in T cell activation, the role of conformation in orienting an amino acid sequence for recognition should not be overlooked. For example, the B(5-13) peptide is the smallest found to stimulate insulin immune T cells; however, slightly larger peptides B(1-13) and B(5-16) are more powerful stimulators of T cell proliferation. These additional residues may in some way sustain a propensity to reform the alpha helix found in this region of the native molecule (15). Helical regions tend to be important sites of immunological determinants in at least two other proteins, nuclease (18) and cytochrome c (19). Though transient in solution, such conformation may be essential for activation on the cell surface. Reasonably, both recognition events taking place during antigen presentation and the physiochemical nature of the antigen are important in achieving maximum T cell activation. Such a mechanism could conformationally approximate two non-sequential amino acids (e.g. B-5 and B-10) to create a single topographical determinant as suggested by Schwartz et al. for cytochrome c (20). Currently, we are attempting to resolve the extent to which recognition of specific residues and conformational integrity are necessary for T cell activation by the synthesis of pseudopeptide analogues.

The antibody specificity of the response to insulin and its fragments in inbred guinea pigs does not reflect the same characteristics as that of the T cell. Using radiolabeled species variants of insulin and isoelectrically focused sera, determinant specific antibody spectrotypes could not be detected in strain 2 sera (21). When radiolabeled fragment for which strain 13 T cells are highly specific, we could not detect significant binding in either strain 2 or strain 13 serum with high anti-insulin titers (in press). Even though immunizing with the B(1-16) fragment will produce antibodies which bind the fragment, they did not appear to bind the native molecule. The determinants recognized by these antibodies are probably not available on the surface of the insulin molecule. These results may be somewhat analogous to the data obtained in mice hyperimmunized with nuclease in which the antibody titer in low responders reached the same level as seen in high responders. However, when these hyperimmune sera were examined for binding of the nuclease fragment (99-146), the pattern of response was similar to that noted in the primary (18) suggesting that the failure to find determinant restriction of antibody specificity in the guinea pig is due to the magnitude of the response in the primary. Thus, shared specificity between antibody and T cell could be present but not detectable because it represents such a small percent of the total anti-insulin response. This has been recently emphasized in H-2^{b} mice where hybridoma antibodies have been produced which bind the same A chain loop region seen by strain 2 guinea T cells (22). More importantly, the fragment studied here is quite small in comparison to the nuclease fragment which is about the same size as the whole insulin molecule. Nonetheless, in our present studies of insulin where the T cell response is directed at a limited epitope, an antibody population with identical specificity to the T cell does not constitute a detectable portion of the antibody response.

Another recent finding of considerable importance both to our understanding of how the Ia molecules mediate Ir gene control of antigen recognition as well as to the nature of antigen processing itself is indicated by our finding of a selective deletion of immune responsiveness to beef insulin in B6.C^{bm12} mice.

B6-H-2^{bm12} and B6 mice were compared for their ability to respond to these same five soluble protein antigens. The data in Table IV indicate that both the MHC linkage of the immune response to beef insulin and mutant mice respond comparably with the wild-type to (TG)A-L, DNP-OVA, PPD and pork insulin. However, these same mutant mice failed to respond to beef insulin as did the wild-type mice, thus indicating that in the B6.C-H-2^{bm12} mutation there is a selective loss of the I-A^{b} region-controlled recognition of only a single protein antigen. Data from another experiment (data not shown) indicated that at all antigen concentrations tested, B6.C-H-2^{bm12} mice failed to respond to beef insulin, but generated a response to (TG)A-L similar to the wild-type, B6 mice.

TABLE IV. Mapping of Genes Controlling Proliferative Response to Beef Insulin and (TG)A-L

Strain	H-2	MHC Alleles K A B J E C S G D	Δ cpm thymidine incorporation[1] Beef insulin 100 μg/ml	(TG)A-L 100 μg/ml	DNP-OVA 10 μg/ml	PPD 10 μg/ml	Δcpm Medium
B10	b	b b b b b b b b b	10,425	12,301	35,609	54,337	7,491
B10.A (4R)	h4	k k b b b b b b b	1,635	0	61,800	81,267	20,323
B10.MBR	bq1	b k k k k k k k q	1,043	0	64,570	66,189	9,406
B10.AKM	m	k k k k k k k k q	1,712	42	35,602	42,234	6,127
B10.A	a	k k k k k d d d d	943	0	36,807	46,297	9,063
B10.D2	d	d d d d d d d d d	10,639	1,671	40,728	58,511	15,339
B6	b	b b b b b b b b b	20,370	20,772	48,281	65,861	25,468
B6.C-H-2[bm12]	bm	b b*b b b b b b b	0	9,058	34,994	36,227	11,705

[1]The Δcpm was derived by subtracting the values of medium only (right hand column) from antigen stimulated cultures.

Each experimental point represents the average of triplicates.

Summary and Conclusions

Synthetic polymers and peptides have provided information on the role of a few amino acids in determining the response to these antigens (23) and insight into the complexity of cellular interactions (24). The inexact nature of the sequence and conformation of these polymers encouraged the study of highly defined but often more complex protein antigens (25, 26, 27). Major conclusions drawn from our present observations as well as the work of others is first that the specificity of humoral and cellular responses can be spacially separated (28), individual determinants within the same molecule may be under the control of separate Ir genes (29), and lastly, that non-sequential amino acids may form conformational determinants for both antibody and T cells (30, 20). Many of the studies with defined antigens have concentrated on the specificity of T cell proliferation (31, 32) but, as recently emphasized, this specificity may not be identical to that of the Ir gene product (33).

Our findings show that both T helper and proliferative responses can be induced by a polypeptide fragment representing a highly restricted region of the native insulin consisting of a minimum of 8 amino acids around the histidine at the 10th position of the B chain. The existence in the I-region recombinants expressing selective loss of immune responsiveness to antigens of restricted heterogeneity strongly implies a loss of appropriate molecular interaction between a restricted region on the mutant Ia molecule and selected amino acid sequences on the antigen. These data also provide support for the concept that a potential degradation product(s) of antigen, in the form of a peptide, contains all of the necessary information for mediation of an Ia-Ir gene controlled T cell dependent immune responses to the native antigen. By extension the antigenic determinant "seen" by the antigen specific T cell receptor likely consists of an associative complex of Ia and a limited molecular sequence derived from the nominal antigen. Such events are likely to occur at the level of the antigen presenting cell (17).

References

1. McDevitt, H.O., Benacerraf, B.: Adv. Immunol. 11, 31-74 (1969).
2. Benacerraf, B., McDevitt, H.O.: Science 175, 273-279 (1972).

3. Shreffler, D.C., David, C.S.: Adv. Immunol. 20, 125-195 (1974).

4. Klein, J., Geib, R., Chiang, C.-Z., Hauptfeld, V.: J. Exp. Med. 143, 1439-1452 (1976).

5. Meo, T., David, C.S., Nabholz, M., Miggiano, U., Shreffler, D.C.: Transplant. Proc. 5, 1507-1510 (1973).

6. Livnat, S., Klein, J., Bach, F.H.: Nature New Biol. 243, 42-44 (1973).

7. Rosenthal, A.S., Shevach, E.M.: J. Exp. Med. 138, 1194-1212 (1973).

8. Katz, D.H., Benacerraf, B.: The Role of Products of the Histocompatibility Complex in Immune Response (D.H. Katz and B. Benacerraf, eds.), Academic Press, New York, pp. 355-389 1976.

9. Barcinski, M.A, Rosenthal, A.S.: J. Exp. Med. 145, 726 (1977).

10. Keck, K.: Nature 254, 78-79 (1975).

11. Rosenwasser, L.J., Barcinski, M.A., Schwartz, R.H., Rosenthal, A.S.: J. Immunol. 123, 471-476 (1979).

12. Lipsky, P.E., Ellner, J.J., Rosenthal, A.S.: J. Immunol. 116, 868-875 (1976).

13. Gell, P.G.H., Benacerraf, B.: Immunol. 2, 64-70 (1959).

14. Ishizaka, K., Kishimoto, T., Delespesse, G., King, T.P.: J. Immunol. 113, 70-77 (1974).

15. Blundell, T., Dodson, G., Hodgkin, D., Mercola, D.: Adv. Protein. Chem. 26, 279-402 (1972).

16. Benacerraf, B.: J. Immunol. 120, 1809-1812 (1978).

17. Rosenthal, A.S.: Immunol. Rev. 40, 136-152 (1978).

18. Sachs, D.H., Berzofsky, J.A., Pisetsky, D.S., Schwartz, R.H. Springer-Seminars in Immunopathol. 1, 51-83 (1978).

19. Corradin, G., Chiller, J.M.: J. Exp. Med. 149, 436-447 (1979).

20. Schwartz, R.H., Yano, A., Solinger, A.M., Ultee, M.E., Margoliash, E., Paul, W.E.: J. Supramolec. Struc. Suppl. 1, 237 (1979).

21. Thomas, J.W., Schroer, J., Rosenthal, A.S.: Macrophage Regulation of Immunity, (E. Unanue and A.S. Rosenthal, eds.), Academic Press, New York pp. 3-14, 1980.

22. Loblay, R.H., Schroer, J., Rosenthal, A.S.: Macrophage Regulation of Immunity, (E. Unanue and A.S. Rosenthal, eds.), Academic Press, New York pp. 87-94, 1980.

23. Benacerraf, B., Dorf, M.E.: Proceedings of the Cold Spring Harbor Symposium on Quantitative Biology 41, 465-475 (1977).

24. Katz, D.H., Hamaoka, T., Dorf, M.E., Maurer, P.H., Benacerraf, B.: J. Exp. Med. 138, 734-739 (1973).

25. Crumpton, M.J.: The Antigens (M. Sela, ed.) Academic Press, New York 2, 1-78 (1974).

26. DeWeck, A.L.: The Antigens (M. Sela, ed.) Academic Press, 2:141-248 (1974).

27. Reichlin, M.: Adv. Immunol. 20, 71-123 (1975).

28. Senyk, G., Williams, E.B., Nitecki, D.E., Goodman, J.W.: J. Exp. Med. 133, 1294-1308 (1971).

29. Schwartz, R.H., Solinger, A.M., Ultee, M., Margoliash, E.: Immunobiol. of Proteins and Peptides I. (M.Z. Atassi, A.B. Stavitsky, eds.) Plenum Publish. Corp, New York, 371-386 (1978).

30. Atassi, M.Z.: Immunochemistry 15, 909-936 (1978).

31. Berzofsky, J.A., Schwartz, R.H., Schechter, A.N., Sachs, D.H.: J. Supramolec. Struc. 179 (1977).

32. Corradin, G., Chiller, J.M.: J. Exp. Med. 149, 436-447 (1979).

33. Benacerraf, B.: J. Immunol. 120, 1809-1812 (1978).

ANALYSIS OF THE IN VITRO INDUCTION OF INSULIN-SPECIFIC HELPER T CELLS[1]

G. Ramila, I. Sklenar, P. Vogt, S. Studer, E. Zoumbou and P. Erb
Institute for Microbiology, University of Basel, Petersplatz 10, CH-4003 Basel, Switzerland

Introduction

Genes of the major histocompatibility complex (MHC) control and regulate a multitude of immunologically related functions, such as the immune response to certain antigens (these are the MHC-linked Ir genes), cell-interactions and their soluble mediators as well as the expression of histocompatibility antigens and I region associated antigens (Ia). These functions are controlled by multiple linked loci, each with a high degree of polymorphism. In the mouse, Ir gene function has been most clearly demonstrated with a number of antigens including the natural hormone insulin [1-3]. In man, while direct evidence for Ir gene function is still rather poor, the large number of diseases which have HLA associations is usually accepted as indirect evidence. Juvenile Diabetes is one of the diseases associated with the HLA-D region [4,5] which is the analogue to the I region of the H-2 complex of the mouse. Thus HLA association of diabetes suggests an immunological involvement in the aetiology, with the possibility of an autoimmune process [6].
Insulin treatment of diabetic individuals sometimes induces

[1] supported by the Juvenile Diabetes Foundation (grant no. 80R058)

Basic and Clinical Aspects of Immunity to Insulin

insulin resistance or other complications. A likely reason is that insulin which is used for treatment is obtained from animal sources and thus may evoke an immune response in humans due to differences in amino acid sequences and structure.
It is therefore important to study the mechanism and genetics of the immune response to insulin and their implications to diabetes and insulin complications. The basic knowledge for that task can be more easily accomplished in an animal model (eg. the mouse) than in man.
In this communication we present our current view about the mechanism of helper T cell (T_{HC}) induction to bovine and porcine insulin as well as provide preliminary data about our attempts to grow and maintain insulin-specific T cell long term cultures which express helper activity.

Materials and Methods

The in vitro induction and assay of insulin-specific T_{HC} has been described in detail elsewhere [7]. In brief, nylonwool purified T cells from spleen of unprimed mice are incubated in a Mini-Marbrook system with insulin and macrophages (MØ) obtained from the peritoneal exudate (PE) of starch-induced mice. After 4 days a small number of viable cells ($2,5 \times 10^4$ to 5×10^4) from each culture is added to normal spleen cells (5×10^5) and incubated with DNP-insulin in the wells of Microtiter plates. Four days later the antibody forming ability of these B cells is measured in the Cunningham plaque assay using DNP-coated sheep red blood cells (DNP-SRBC) as antigen. T cell long term cultures (LTC) are made in two ways: 1) in vitro induced T_{HC} are cultured with MØ (10^4) and with or without insulin in the wells of a Costar plate (2×10^6 cells/well). After 7 days the cells are redistributed with or without insulin into new Costar plates and cultured in the presence of fresh MØ and T cell growth factor (TCGF 10%) which is the purified (by ammoniumsulfate-precipitation and Sephadex G-100 gelfiltration) 24h supernatant of Con A activated spleen cells [8]. Every fourth day half of the medium is replaced by fresh medium containing 10% TCGF but no insulin.

2) BALB/c mice are immunized once i.p. with 20µg bovine insulin in CFA. Two weeks later spleens are taken and the T cells purified by nylonwool filtration. Some of these T cells were treated with anti-Ly 2 (monoclonal rat anti-mouse Ly 2, which has to be used with an anti-rat enhancing serum, both reagents were kindly provided by Drs. Phil Lake and Marc Feldmann, University College London) and complement (C') before setting up cultures. T cells are plated into the wells of Microtiter plates ($1x10^6$/well) or Costar plates ($2x10^6$/well) and incubated with MØ (10^3 respectively 10^4/well) and insulin(0,1µg/ml). After 7 days the T cells are redistributed as described above.

The medium used for culturing LTC is MEM (Gibco F-15) containing 2,2mg/ml sodium bicarbonate, 0,5% fetal calf serum and 0,5% fresh mouse serum. The cultures are kept in an atmosphere of 7% CO_2.

Further details of culturing and maintaining LTC will be given elsewhere (manuscript in preparation).

Results and Discussion

1) <u>Induction of insulin-specific T_{HC}</u>. The in vitro induction of purified T cells of certain mouse strains (eg. BALB/c, C57BL/10 = B10) with appropriate insulin variants (eg. bovine/porcine-insulin) and non-lymphoid accessory cells leads to the generation of insulin-specific T_{HC} [7]. The activity of these T_{HC} is measured by their ability to provide help to B cells to form anti-DNP antibodies after a 4 day incubation with normal

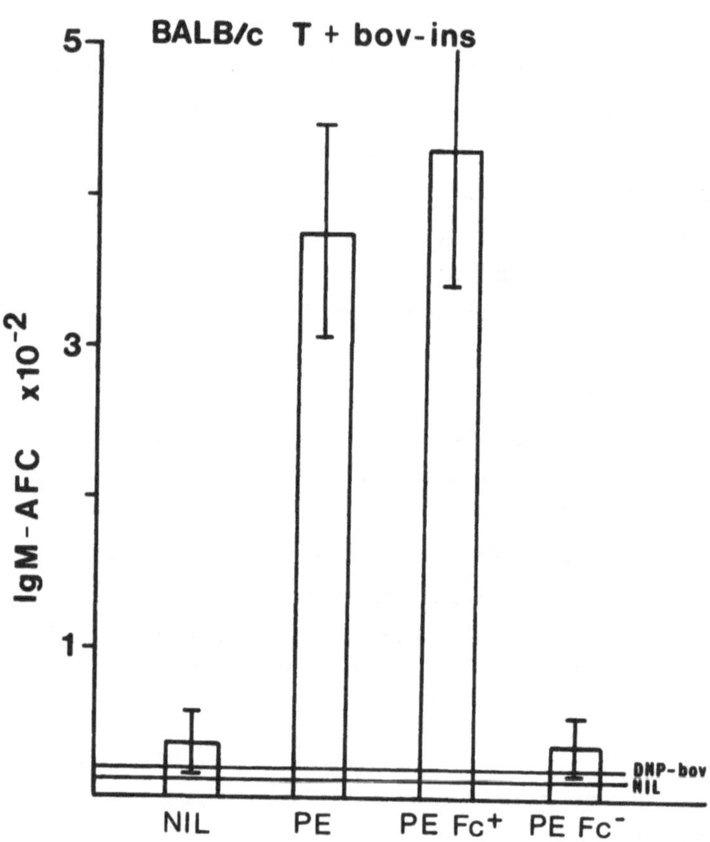

Fig. 1: Induction of insulin-specific T_{HC} requires Fc^+ PEC. $3x10^6$ nylonwool purified normal BALB/c T cells from spleen were incubated with bovine-insulin (0,1µg/culture) and with or without PEC ($5x10^4$) obtained from BALB/c mice injected i.p. with a 2% solution of starch 3 days previously. Before use some PEC were incubated with anti-SRBC IgG coated SRBC [9] for 30min on ice, spun for 10min at 600x g and the pelletted cells were carefully resuspended in the supernatant. The suspension was layered on top of Ficoll-Paque and spun at 600x g for 15 min at 4°C. The interface cells which contained the non-rosetting cells (PE Fc^-) and the pellet containing rosettes (PE Fc^+) were harvested and the red cells lysed with Tris-ammoniumchloride [9]. T_{HC} induction cultures were done using the Mini-Marbrook system. After 4 days the cells were harvested, counted and $5x10^4$ viable cells were added to $5x10^5$ normal BALB/c spleen cells as source of B cells and incubated with DNP-bovine insulin (0,01µg/culture) in Microtiter plates (Falcon II , 3040). Four days later the direct anti-DNP plaque

response of 3-4 independent cultures was determined using DNP-coupled SRBC as antigen. As controls, $5x10^5$ normal spleen cells were incubated without (NIL) or with DNP-bovine insulin alone (DNP-bov).

spleen cells (which contain B cells) and DNP-insulin [7]. The generation of such insulin-specific T_{HC} which is only possible by using a special culture system, ie. a modified Marbrook-Diener system, is dependent on the dose of insulin as well as on the presence of accessory cells [7]. Thc latter is illustrated in Fig.1. Only Fc-receptor bearing PE cells induce T_{HC} in the presence of bovine insulin. Other characteristics of these accessory cells are: they are phagocytic, adherent, radioresistant and Ia positive [9],thus expressing typical markers of the MØ lineage.
The interaction of MØ and T cells required for T_{HC} induction is genetically restricted and the genes responsible are located in the I-A subregion of the H-2 complex [7,10]. Moreover, the helper cell response was found to be under Ir gene control eg. $H-2^d$ T cells became T_{HC} if incubated with bovine or porcine insulin and $H-2^d$ MØ, while $H-2^b$ T cells only became T_{HC} if incubated with bovine but not with porcine insulin and MØ [7]. This is in close analogy to observations made by other groups using different assay systems [2,11-13]. The Ir genes controlling helper cell responses to insulin were also mapped to the I-A subregion of the H-2 complex [7].

2) Sites of Ir gene control. It has been shown by Rosenthal et al. [3] measuring T cell proliferation to insulin in the guinea pig that MØ are one site where Ir genes function. This has been confirmed by other groups including ourselves using also different antigens under Ir gene control [7,14-17]. For example, we found that T cells of F_1(B10xCBA) hybrids, the B10 being a responder (R), the CBA a nonresponder (NR) to bovine insulin, only became helper cells if incubated with bovine

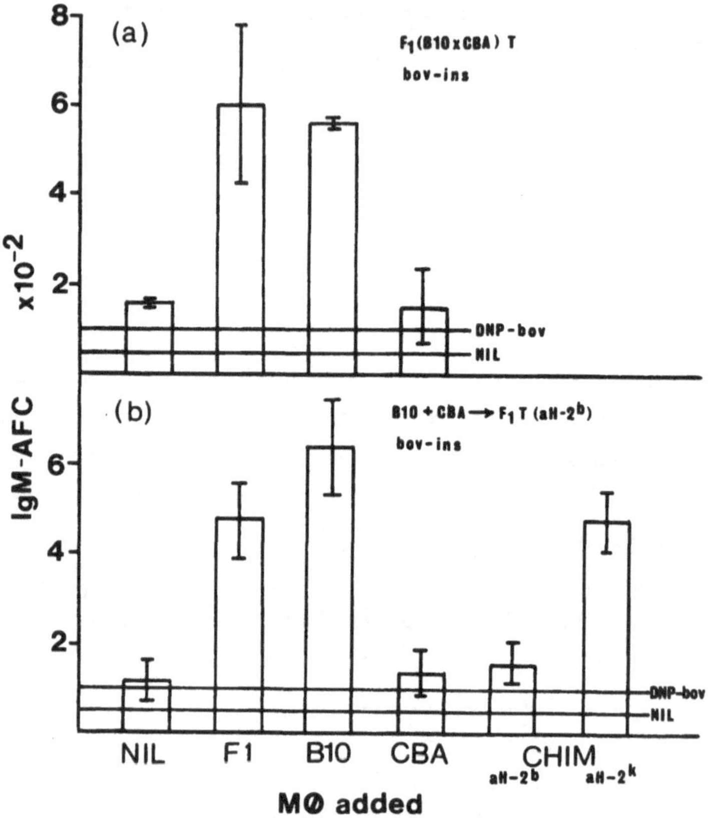

Fig. 2: Ir genes are expressed in MØ and in the environment where T stem cells differentiate.
(a) For T_{HC} induction F_1(B10xCBA) T cells were used, (b) nylonwool purified chimeric T cells of the type B10+CBA⟶ F_1(B10xCBA) were first incubated with anti-H-2^b (D-2) for 30min on ice, washed and then further incubated with rabbit C' (diluted 1:6) for 45min at 37°C. The resulting cells consisted entirely of H-2^k haplotype T cells.
The T cells were incubated with bovine insulin and with or without F_1, CBA, B10 or PEC from the chimeric mice. Some of the chimeric MØ were first treated with either anti-H-2^b (D-2) or anti-H-2^k (D-32) sera and C' as described above. The anti-H-2 sera were kindly provided by the Transplantation Immunology Branch, NIAID, NIH, Bethesda.
To test for helper activity F_1(B10xCBA) spleen cells treated with anti-Thy1.2 and C' were used. The monoclonal anti-Thy1 was a gift from Dr. Phil Lake, University College London.
For further technical details see legend to Fig.1 and ref.9,18.

insulin and F_1 or B10 but not CBA MØ though the F_1 T cells are of R haplotype (Fig.2a). Thus MØ of NR haplotypes are unable to activate responder T cells to become T_{HC}. However, these data do not exclude other sites of Ir gene expression, eg. T cells or the environment where T cells differentiate. To test that possibility chimeric mice of the type B10+CBA ⟶ F_1 (B10xCBA) were used, constructed by reconstituting lethally irradiated F_1 mice with anti-Thy1 and C' treated bone marrow cells of both parental haplotypes. Within a few months the haemopoietic system of the F_1 is entirely replaced by maturing haemopoietic cells of B10 and CBA origin. Purified T cells of such chimeric mice were treated with anti-H-2^b and C' to kill the H-2^b haplotype T cells. The remaining H-2^k (CBA) T cells which are tolerant to H-2^b were incubated with bovine insulin and either F_1, B10, CBA or chimeric MØ and after 4 days tested for helper activity in the usual way. Fig.2b demonstrates that F_1 and allogeneic B10 but not syngeneic CBA MØ were capable of inducing insulin-specific T_{HC}. This indicates that the T stem cells of CBA which is a NR to bovine insulin generated phenotypically responder cells by maturing in a responder F_1 environment. However, NR MØ (CBA) which also differentiated in a R environment did not become responders. Thus, chimeric MØ treated with anti-H-2^b and C' (to remove the H-2^b MØ of B10 origin) were unable to induce T_{HC} (Fig.2). In the reverse situation which is not shown here, where T cells of R mice differentiated in a NR host, eg. F_1(B10xCBA) ⟶ CBA, T_{HC} could not be generated from chimeric T cells even with MØ from R animals [18]. These data suggest that Ir genes are expressed in MØ and in the host (thymus?) where T stem cells differentiate and thus that both host and MØ, but not T cells and MØ must have identical Ir gene sets in order to allow the induction of T_{HC}. Two further predictions can be made, first, there is no need for Ir gene expression intrinsically at the level of T cells, and second, genetic control of T-MØ interaction and Ir gene regulation of the helper cell response are two phenomena with the same underlying mechanism. The role of the host's Ir gene set would be to instruct or select maturing T cells to respond to certain Ir gene products (Ia?), while the peripheral MØ might select out the appropriate antigen determinant for presentation to T cells. Ir gene defects at either site would result in nonresponsiveness of the animal. However, there is an alternative explanation, which so far is not supported by the evidence available. According to that hypothesis, Ir genes are solely expressed in T cells and the failure to generate T_{HC} would be due to lack of the appropriate recognition set on T cells. Further experimentation is required to resolve that problem.

3) Insulin-specific T cell long term cultures. According to the response pattern of R and NR mice and because of the limited amino acid sequence differences it is possible to determine the region of the insulin molecule recognized by T cells. Thus $H\text{-}2^b$ mice (R to bovine, NR to porcine insulin) respond to a determinant of the A chain loop region of the bovine insulin molecule, possibly A8 and A10 as this is the only difference from porcine insulin [2,11]. $H\text{-}2^d$ mice which are responders to porcine and bovine insulins probably recognize a different portion of the molecule, as the A loop region of mouse and porcine insulin is identical [11-13]. They most likely respond to a B chain determinant [19] though a configurational or structural influence of the A chain cannot be excluded. To get more information about the recognition potential of the T cells in terms of the immunological moieties of the insulin molecule it is necessary to work with T cells which express specificity for a single determinant. One approach to do that is to enrich insulin-specific T cells in long term cultures (LTC) and then to select T cells with a single specificity by cloning.

The technique of producing and maintaining T cell long term cultures to various antigens is established, and is by now almost a standard procedure. It has been possible to obtain T cell clones with cytolytic activity [20-22], or helper activity to sheep or horse red cells [8]. It seems to be more difficult to obtain T cell clones or LTC with functional properties such as helper activity to soluble antigens. The activity of LTC usually measured is proliferation in the presence of the appropriate antigen. The requirements to obtain and maintain LTC are rather high doses of antigen and the presence of T cell growth factor (TCGF) [23-25].

Using a protocol as described in the literature [23-24] we tried to make T cell LTC with insulin. Though we got LTC they expressed very little or no helper activity. The experimental parameters were then varied, ie. mice were multiple primed in vivo with insulin in adjuvant to enrich for insulin-specific T cells before setting up LTC from spleen or lymph node T cells, various time intervals between priming and setting up LTC were tested and the doses of insulin for priming and for the cultures were varied. The results were always the same, the LTC we obtained expressed a marked specific and unspecific suppressive activity if tested in our standard cooperation assay or in a few instances were totally nonfunctional. However all these experiments suggested a very critical role of the dose of insulin used, as high doses induced suppression or even were toxic to T cells. Thus a different approach was chosen. LTC were set up either from in vitro generated insulin-specific T_{HC} or from T cells obtained from mice injected once with insulin in adjuvant. Some of the T cells were also treated with anti-Ly2 and C' to kill possible suppressor cells before setting up cultures. The T cells were then incubated with syngeneic MØ and a low dose of insulin (0,1µg/ml). After 7 days the dividing cells were redistributed into fresh culture plates and cultured with TCGF and with or without insulin

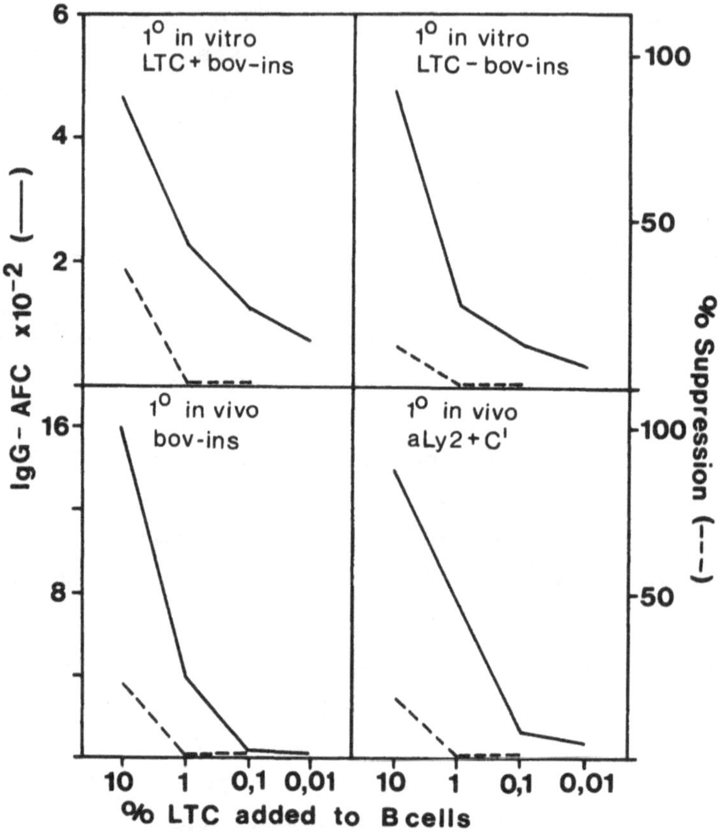

Fig. 3: T cell long term cultures with insulin-specific helper activity.
BALB/c T_{HC} were either generated in vitro (see legend Fig.1) (1°in vitro) or in vivo by a single i.p. injection of 20µg bovine insulin in CFA (1° in vivo) and 14 days later the splenic T cells were purified by nylonwool filtration. Some of these cells were treated with anti-Ly2 and C' before use and incubated with BALB/c MØ and bovine insulin (0,1µg/ml) as described in the text. In vitro generated T_{HC} were incubated with bovine insulin and MØ for 7 days, redistributed into Costar plates and incubated with MØ and with (LTC+bov-ins) or without insulin (LTC-bov-ins) as described in the text.
To test for helper activity graded numbers of LTC were added to $5x10^{5}$ DNP-CGG primed BALB/c spleen cells treated with anti-Thy1+C' and incubated with DNP-bovine insulin (0,05µg/culture) To test for suppressor activity graded numbers of LTC were added to $5x10^{5}$ DNP-CGG primed spleen cells and incubated with DNP-CGG (0,01µg/culture). Five days later the IgG anti-DNP response was measured. At the time of testing for helper

activity the LTC have been cultured for 5 weeks.

(o,o1µg/ml). After several weeks in culture the cells were tested for their insulin-specific helper activity. Fig. 3 demonstrates that both in vitro induced T_{HC} as well as in vivo primed T cells cultured for 5 weeks in vitro expressed insulin-specific helper activity. Anti-Ly2 and C' treatment of the original T cells slightly (in other experiments more) improved their helper capacity indicating that suppressor cells expressing the Ly2 marker were present in that population. However, even these LTC contained unspecific suppressive activity as demonstrated by the reduction of the number of plaque forming cells if added in high doses to DNP-primed B cells and the homologous antigen. It is likely that only by cloning it will be possible to separate T cells with helper and suppressor function entirely. Such attempts of cloning are now in progress.
Taken together, by following the protocol to make LTC to soluble antigens, as described in the literature [23-25], it was not possible to obtain T cell LTC expressing specific helper activity to insulin. Only by using very low amounts of insulin for the induction as well as maintainance of insulin-specific T cells, LTC with stable helper function were obtained.

Acknowledgments

Ivo Sklenar was supported by a fellowship of the SANDOZ-Stiftung zur Förderung der medizinisch-biologischen Wissenschaften

References

1. McDevitt, H.O.(ed.): Ir genes and Ia antigens. Academic Press, New York 1978.
2. Keck, K.: Nature 254, 78-79 (1975).
3. Rosenthal, A.S., Barcinski, M.A., Blake, J.T.: Nature 267, 156-158 (1977).
4. Solow, H., Hidalgo, R., Singal, D.P.: Diabetes 28, 1-4 (1979).
5. Farid, N.R., Sampson, L., Noel, P., Reich, T.: Diabetes 28, 552-557 (1979).
6. Nerup, J., Cathelineau, C., Seignalet, J., Thomson, M.: in 'HLA and Disease' (ed. Dausset, J. and Sveygaard, H.) Munksgaard, Copenhagen 1977.
7. Erb, P.: Immunology 40, 385-394 (1980).
8. Schreier, M.H., Iscove, N.N., Tees, R., Aarden L., von Boehmer, H.: Immunol. Rev. 51, 315-336 (1980).
9. Erb, P., Stern, A.C., Alkan, S., Studer, S., Zoumbou, E., Gisler, R.H.: J. Immunol., in press.
10. Erb, P., Feldmann, M.: J. Exp. Med. 142, 460-472 (1975).
11. Keck, K.: Eur . J. Immunol. 5, 801-807 (1975).
12. Rosenthal, A.S.: Immunol. Rev. 40, 136-152 (1978).
13. Cohen, T.R., Talmon, J., Lev-Ram, V., Ben-Nun, A.: Proc. Natl. Acad. Sci. USA 76, 4066-4070 (1979).
14. Marrack, P.C., Kappler, J.W.: J.Exp.Med. 147, 1596-1610 (1978).
15. Schwartz, R.H., Yano, A., Paul, W.E.: Immunol. Rev. 40, 153-180 (1978).
16. Singer, A., Cowing, C., Hatchcock, K.S., Dickler, H., Hodes, R.J.: J. Exp. Med. 147, 1611-1620 (1978).
17. Erb, P., Meier, B., Feldmann, M.: J. Immunol. 122, 1916-1919 (1979).
18. Erb, P., Vogt, P., Matsunaga, T., Rosenthal, A.S., Feldmann, M.: J. Immunol. 124, 2656-2664 (1980).
19. Rosenwasser, L.J., Barcinski, M.A., Schwartz, R.H., Rosenthal, A.S.: J. Immunol. 123, 471-476 (1979).
20. Gillis, S., Smith, K.A.: Nature 268, 154-156 (1977).
21. Nabholz, M., Engers, H.D., Collavo, D., North, M.: Curr. Top. Microbiol. 81, 176-187 (1978).

22. von Boehmer, H., Hengartner, H., Nabholz, M., Lernhardt, W., Schreier, M.H., Haas, W.: Eur. J. Immunol. 9, 592-597 (1979).

23. Augustin, A.A., Julius, M.H., Cosenza, H.: Eur. J. Immunol. 9, 665-670 (1979).

24. Schrier, R.D., Skidmore, B.J., Kurnick, J.T., Goldstine, S.N., Chiller, J.M.: J. Immunol. 123, 2525-2531 (1979).

25. Sredni, B., Tse, H.Y., Schwartz, R.H.: Nature 283, 581-583 (1980).

IMMUNOGENIC DETERMINANTS OF INSULIN: SYNTHESIS AND IMMUNOGENICITY OF THE A-CHAIN LOOP PEPTIDES OF BEEF INSULIN

B. Singh and E. Fraga

Department of Immunology & MRC Group on Immunoregulation
University of Alberta, Edmonton, Alberta, Canada T6G 2H7

Introduction

The immunogenic determinants on proteins with known sequence and conformation provide a simple and elegant way to answer a number of important questions in molecular immunology particularly related to the role of conformational vs. sequential determinants in the triggering of T and B cells. To this end, we have recently synthesised a number of peptide and polypeptide antigens of defined amino acid sequence and size and studied their immune response in mice and guinea pigs (1-4). The insulin molecule offers another model system for these studies because of the known amino acid sequences of insulins from various species (5), its highly conserved conformation (Fig.1) (6) and immunogenicity in mice (7,8), guinea pigs (9) and human diabetics (10). Earlier studies by Keck _et al_ (8) and Rosenthal _et al_ (9) have shown that immune responses to insulin in mice and guinea pigs are under Ir gene control. Beef insulin is immunogenic in both $H\text{-}2^b$ and $H\text{-}2^d$ mice whereas $H\text{-}2^d$ but not $H\text{-}2^b$ mice respond to pork insulin. These two molecules only differ in two amino acid residues, A8 & A10 in the A-chain loop region (Table 1). It was therefore concluded that $H\text{-}2^b$ mice recognise beef insulin by the A-chain loop determinants (7). Strain 2 guinea pigs also recognise some insulins by this route (11). However, the actual nature of this determinant remains unclear.

To define the molecular structure of this determinant and to

Basic and Clinical Aspects of Immunity to Insulin

Figure 1

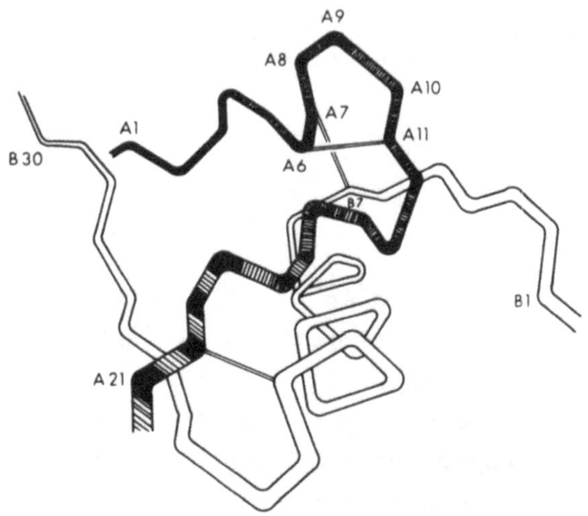

Fig. 1 Conformation of the peptide backbone of insulin molecule (6).

TABLE 1

AMINO ACID SEQUENCES IN THE A-CHAIN LOOP REGION OF INSULINS

Species	Sequence (positions 5 6 7 8 9 10 11)
Human, Pig, Rabbit, Monkey, Rat, Mouse, Whale (Sperm)	Gln-Cys-Cys-Thr-Ser-Ile-Cys (Cys 6–Cys 11 linked; Cys 7 linked to B7)
Horse	Thr-Gly-Ile
Beef	Ala-Ser-Val
Sheep	Ala-Gly-Val
Chicken	His-Asn-Thr
Fish	His-Lys-Pro
Guinea Pig	Thr-Gly-Thr
Whale (sei)	Ala-Ser-Thr

study the influence of other parts of the insulin molecule on immunogenicity of A-chain loop, we have synthesized the Ala-Ser-Val (A8-A10) tripeptide and the A-chain loop peptide (A5-A11) of beef insulin. The side chain of A7 Cys which

H-Gln-Cys-Cys(ACM)-Ala-Ser-Val-Cys-OH

ACL-Peptide

joins B7 was protected with a permanent acetamido (ACM) protecting group. We studied immunogenicity of these peptides in H-2^b mice for the triggering of beef insulin specific T-cells and found that Ala-Ser-Val is not the immunogenic determinant but the ACL-peptide with A6-A11 disulfide bridge is required for immunogenicity.

We have also studied the immunogenicity of Oxid. A and B-chains of beef insulin and the cross reactivity of the antibodies induced by these antigens in H-2^b mice.

Materials and Methods

Antigens: Beef insulin, oxid. A-chain and oxid. B-chain of beef insulin were purchased from Sigma Chemical Company, U.S.A. Sequential polypeptide Poly 18:Poly Glu-Tyr-Lys-$(Glu\text{-}Tyr\text{-}Ala)_5$ was synthesised as described earlier (1). Ala-Ser-Val and ACL peptide were synthesised as shown in (Fig. 2). Coupling of these peptides and glycine to Poly 18 was done by the glutaraldehyde method (12). The conjugates contained 0.5 peptide/ Poly 18 molecule.

Mice: Balb/c (H-2^d) and C3H.SW/SN(H-2^b) mice of 8-12 weeks of age were used for these experiments and were bred at the University of Alberta Animal Farm, Edmonton.

Immunization: Mice were immunized with 50 µg of priming antigen in complete Freunds' adjuvant (CFA) in the left foot pad and challenged 7 days later with 50 µg of beef insulin in

Figure 2

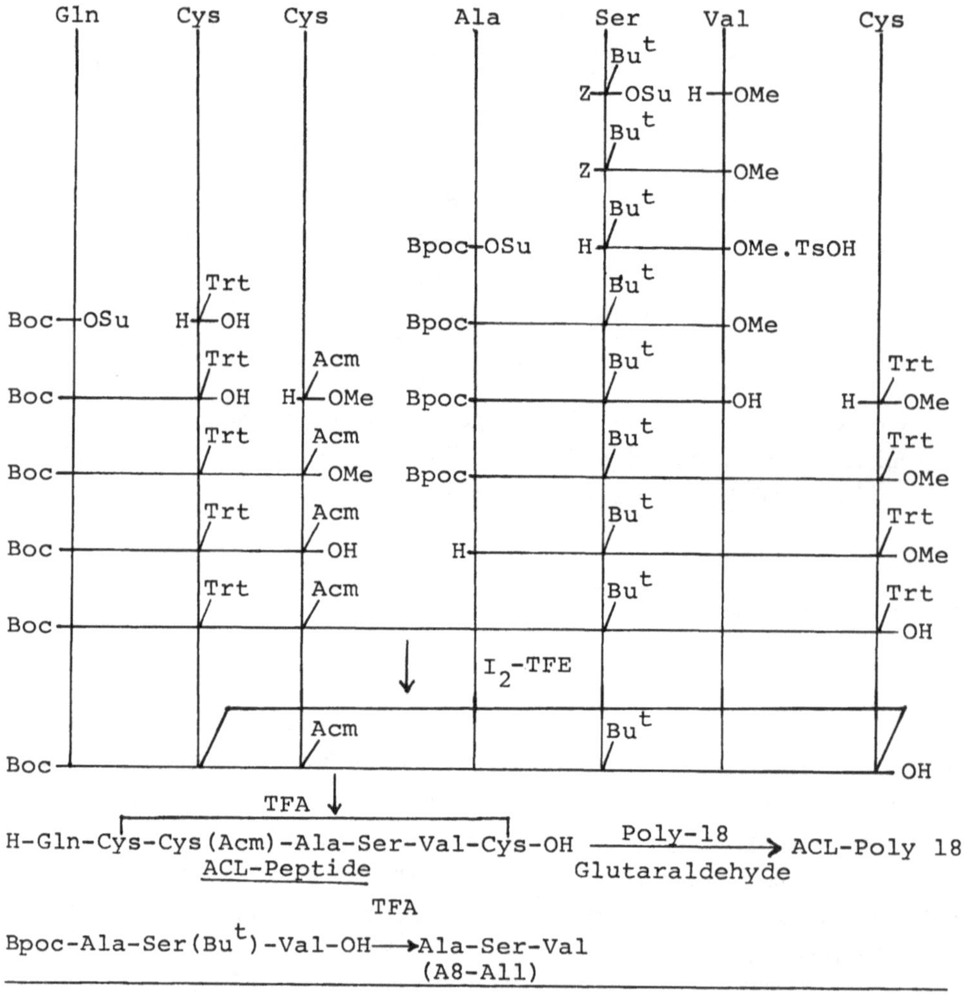

Fig. 2 Synthesis of Ala-Ser-Val, ACL peptide and ACL-Poly 18. Fragment couplings were done by using dicyclohexylcarbodiimide plus 1-hydoxybenztriazole (1).

Abbreviations: TFE: trifluroethanol, TFA: trifluroacetic acid, BOC: t-butyloxycarbonyl, Bu^t: t-butyl, Bpoc: biphenylisopropoxycarbonyl, Trt: trityl, TSOH: tosic acid, OMe: methyl ester, OSu: succinimide ester.

incomplete Freunds' adjuvant (IFA) in the right foot pad. Mice were bled one week later from the tail vein for antibody assay. Mice were primed with 25 μg of antigen in CFA per foot pad for the T cell proliferation assay. LN cells were harvested and cultured as described previously (13).

Solid phase radioimmunoassay (SPRIA): Beef insulin, Poly 18, Oxid. A and Oxid. B chains were coated on the wells of PVC microliter plates (Cooke Eng. #1-220-29) at 10 μg/ml in 0.2M Tris-HCl pH 7.2 buffer (0.1ml/well) overnight at 4°C. Wells were washed (3x) with 0.2 ml phosphate buffer (PBS) containing 0.05% Tween-20 (PBS-T) and incubated with 50 μl of antisera at appropriate dilution in PBS-T for 2 hrs. Plates were washed (3x) with 0.2 ml PBS-T. 50 μl of ^{125}I-goat anti mouse IgG (50,000 CPM) in PBS-T was added per well and incubated for 1 hr at room temperature. Wells were washed (3x) with 0.2 ml PBS and cut horizontally with a hot-wire cutter and counted in a gamma counter. The results are expressed as CPM bound/well or % response of a hyper immune serum.

T-Cell Proliferation assay: LN cells from primed mice were cultured with antigens as previously described (13) using RPMI 1640 medium containing 10% human serum. After 4 days cells were pulsed with (methyl-^{3}H) thymidine and harvested 24 hrs later onto glass filters using Titertek cell harvester which were then counted by liquid scintillation counter. The results are expressed as CMP±S.D. These assays were kindly performed by Dr. K.C. Lee of this Department.

Results

Induction of beef insulin specific helper T cells in H-2^{b} mice by synthetic A-chain loop peptide (ACL) using ACL-Poly 18 conjugate.

The synthetic A8-A10 tripeptide Ala-Ser-Val and the A-Chain

loop peptide (ACL), both failed to prime for the beef insulin specific responses in C3H.SW/SN ($H-2^b$) and Balb/c ($H-2^d$) mice. C3H.SW mice primed with the ACL-Poly 18 conjugate, and challenged with beef insulin produce antiinsulin antibodies (Table II). While Balb/c mice after the same treatment made no B cell response. ACL therefore is a immunogenic determinant in $H-2^b$ but not in $H-2^d$ mice. We have previously shown that Poly 18 itself is non-immunogenic in $H-2^b$ mice (2). Conjugates of Ala-Ser-Val with Poly 18 produced no response.

TABLE II

SYNTHETIC A-CHAIN LOOP PEPTIDE (ACL) CAN ACT AS HELPER DETERMINANT IN C3H.SW ($H-2^b$) BUT NOT IN BALB/C ($H-2^d$) MICE

Priming[1]	Challenge[1]	% Response[2]	
		C3H.Sw/Sn	BALB/c
Insulin/CFA	Insulin/IFA	90.6 ± 5.2	77.6 ± 6.8
ACL-Poly 18/CFA	Insulin/IFA	50.2 ± 5.5	1.9 ± 1.1
Poly 18/CFA	Insulin/IFA	10.75± 3.8	10.2 ± 5.2
ACL/CFA	Insulin/IFA	7.5 ± 1.5	N.D.
CFA	Insulin/IFA	4.6 ± 2.0	N.D.

1. 50 µg of antigen/mouse was injected in foot pads as described above.
2. The IgG response was measured on Day 7 after challenge by SPRIA on bovine insulin. The response of a hyperimmune C3H.SW sera was set as 100%.

In vitro T-cell proliferation of ACL-Poly 18 primed LN cells from $H-2^b$ mice by beef insulin: LN cells of C3H.SW/SN mice primed with Ala-Ser-Val tripeptide or the ACL peptide did not undergo in vitro proliferation on challenge with beef insulin. However, cells from ACL-Poly 18 primed mice gave a high level of proliferation (Table III). These results further confirm that ACL peptide is the T-cell activating determinant of beef insulin whereas the Ala-Ser-Val tripeptide is not.

A-Chain loop peptide (ACL) can act as an immunogeneic determinant for other antigens: Since poly 18 is non-immunogenic

TABLE III

IN VITRO T CELL PROLIFERATION INDUCED BY BEEF INSULIN IN 8×10^5 LN CELLS FROM ACL-POLY 18 PRIMED C3H-SW MICE[1]

Challenge Antigens	Concentration[2] (μg/ml)	CPM/Culture ± S.D.[3]
Medium	-	7040 ± 3241
PPD	50	24201 ± 4404
Bovine Insulin	1	36033 ± 4547
	3	22730 ± 6440
	10	30796 ± 10435
	30	28005 ± 12856
	100	36735 ± 6920

1. Mice were primed with 25 μg of ACL-Poly 18 in CFA per foot pad.
2. Concentration of antigens used for <u>in vitro</u> challenge.
3. Incorporation of (methyl-^{3}H) thymidine.

in H-2^b mice we chose it as a carrier for the ACL peptide. The non-responsiveness to Poly 18 could be due to a lack of helper T-cells. ACL in a link-associative manner (15) could provide the necessary help required to trigger poly 18 specific B cells in C3H.SW mice primed with ACL-Poly 18. Mice primed with ACL-Poly 18 produced high titer of anti Poly 18 antibodies whereas those primed with Gly-Poly 18 (as control) did not (Fig. 3). These results again confirmed the helper T-cell activating capability of the ACL determinant in H-2^b mice.

<u>Cross reactivity of antibodies produced by priming mice with beef insulin, Oxid. A-chain, Oxid. B-chain, ACL-Poly 18, Gly-Poly 18 and challenging with beef insulin</u>:

To determine the role of the priming antigen in the specificity of antibodies produced, Balb/c and C3H.SW mice were immunized with these antigens and 7 days later challenged with beef insulin. The binding of these antibodies to beef insulin, oxid A and B chains and Poly 18 was determined as shown in (Fig. 4). Priming with beef insulin produced antibodies which are exclusively directed at the B-chain in both the strains. ACL-Poly 18 and Gly-Poly 18 primed Balb/c (H-2^d) mice produced high titer of antipoly 18 antibodies since H-2^d are high responders to poly 18. No antiinsulin response was observed, which further confirmed that ACL is not an immunogenic determinant in H-2^d mice.

Figure 3

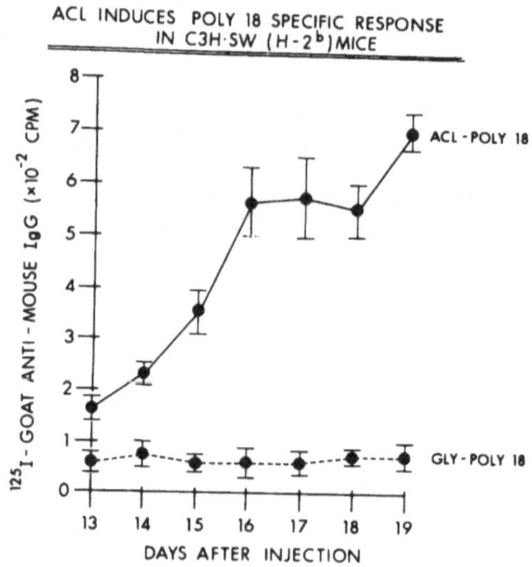

Fig. 3 Mice were immunized with antigens (50 μg) in CFA. Sera were tested for poly 18 specific antibodies at 1:20 dilution by solid phase radioimmunoassay on the days indicated.

Antibodies produced in ACL-Poly 18 primed C3H.SW (H-2^b) mice primarily bind beef insulin but not A or B chain. These antibodies then probably recognise a conformational determinant which is shared between A and B chains and is present on the intact insulin molecule. ACL-Poly 18 also induced Poly 18 specific antibodies in C3H.SW mice as described above. Gly-Poly 18 failed to produce any response. Antibodies from oxid. A

Figure 4

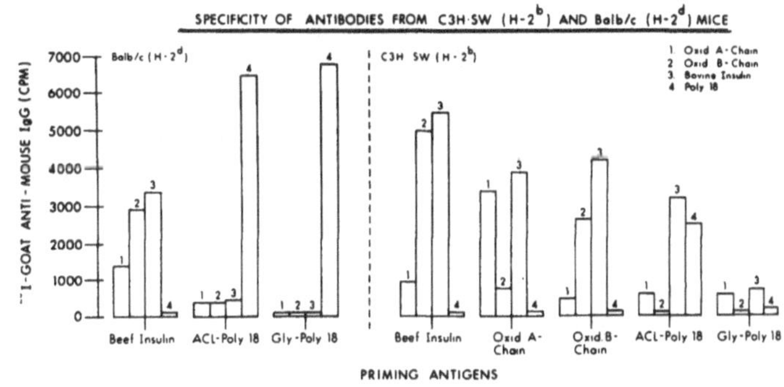

Fig. 4 Mice were primed with antigen (50 µg) in CFA in left footpad and 7 days later challenged with beef insulin (50 µg) in IFA in right footpad. 7 days following the challenge the sera were assayed at 1:20 dilution for binding to various antigens, as indicated using solid phase radioimmunoassay.

and oxid B chain primed C3H.SW mice bind insulin and only that chain which was used for priming. These results suggest that there are determinants other than ACL on beef insulin which can prime H-2^b mice.

<u>Time course of the development of the beef insulin specific antibody response in H-2^b mice</u>:
Influence of the priming determinants on the development of beef insulin specific antibodies in C3H.SW mice was investigated by immunizing mice with beef insulin, ACL-Poly 18, Gly-Poly 18 or CFA alone. Such antibodies could be detected in beef insulin and ACL-Poly 18 primed mice even at day 6 after challenge (Fig. 5). Mice primed with Gly-Poly 18 or CFA alone

Figure 5

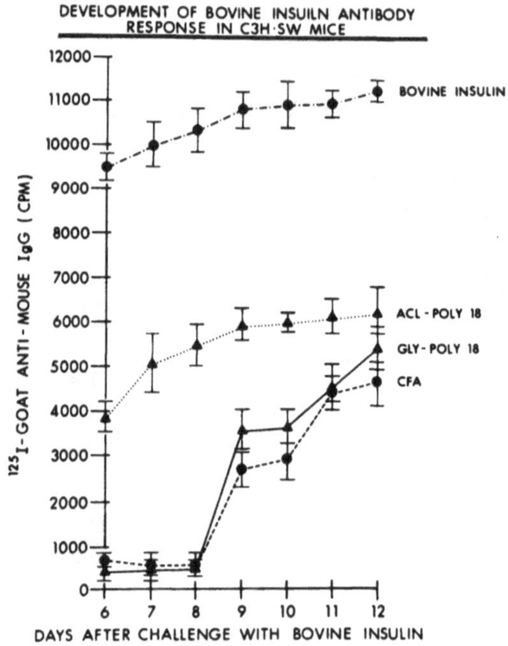

Fig. 5 Mice were injected with antigens (50 µg) in CFA in left footpad and 7 days later were challenged with bovine insulin (50 µg) in IFA in the right footpad. Sera were tested for bovine insulin specific antibodies at 1:20 dilution by solid phase radioimmunoassay on the days shown.

did not produce any antibodies until day 9 and thereafter the response increases rapidly but was never as high as in the beef insulin primed group. A single injection of insulin is therefore sufficient to induce antiinsulin antibodies.

Discussion

Amino acid residues A8, A9 and A10 on the A-chain of insulin have been implicated in antibody and T-cell proliferative responses both in mice (7) and guinea pigs (9). These residues are projected above the rest of the molecule (Fig. 1) and could therefore be a target for immune recognition. In a number of natural insulins, the major amino acid variation occurs in this region of the A-chain (Table I) but the overall conformation of the insulin molecule is highly conserved among the various species (6).

To define the nature of the immunogenic determinants in this region of insulins we have concentrated on the sequence of beef insulin. It is highly immunogenic both in $H-2^b$ and $H-2^d$ mice. The major immunogenic determinant for $H-2^b$ mice are located in the A-chain loop region (7). We first synthesised the A8-A10 tripeptide Ala-Ser-Val and found it to be non-immunogenic even after coupling to a carrier like Poly 18. A sequential polymer of Ala-Ser-Val was also non immunogenic in $H-2^b$ mice. It has been suggested that the determinants could involve the whole A-chain loop (ACL) peptide (A6-A11) and not just the A8-A10 residues (7,8). The disulfide bridge between Cys 6 and Cys 11 may also be required because such bond would provide conformational stability to the Ala-Ser-Val determinant. We therefore synthesised the heptapeptide (A5-A11) permanently blocking the Cys-7 side chain and then make a selective disulfide bond between Cys-6 and Cys-11 (14). This A-chain loop heptapeptide (ACL) induced beef insulin specific responses in $H-2^b$ mice but only if it was attached to a large carrier like Poly 18. We have recently shown that peptides containing at least 9 to 12 amino acid residues are required for immunogenicity in mice (3). Thus the ACL peptide on its own may be too small to be immunogenic. Poly 18 alone is non-immunogenic in $H-2^b$ mice but the ACL-Poly 18 conjugate triggers poly 18 specific antibodies in these mice. It appears, therefore that ACL can induce helper T cells which in a linked associative manner trigger Poly 18 specific B cells (15). Therefore, the ACL peptide is one of the major immunogenic determinants recognised by $H-2^b$ mice on beef insulin. It can also be concluded that this T-cell determinant is probably conformational in nature and not sequential. Similar conclusions were drawn for the immunogenic determinants on Cytochrome C in mice (16).

The antibodies induced by priming with beef insulin or ACL-Poly 18 differ in their binding to beef insulin, oxid. A. and oxid. B chains (Fig. 4). This may occur because helper T cells induced by the ACL determinant trigger specific B cells which produce antibodies against a conformational determinant shared between the A and B chains and is present only on the intact insulin molecule. Priming with oxid. A or B-chains leads to the production of antibodies which bind insulin and the chains used for priming. The differences in specificity of antibodies produced by priming with beef insulin, ACL, oxid. A and B chain in the same strain of mice suggest that apart from ACL these are other helper determinants on insulin. Probably, specific helper T-cells are induced by each determinant and these cells in turn cooperate only with specific B cells producing antibodies to a given region of insulin. In other words, the particular helper T-cells determine with which B-cells, out of all the possible antigen specific B cells they will cooperate and this process may involve another helper T cell population with idiotypic complementarity to the B cells (17,18).

The time course of the development of antibody specificity could also be linked to the determinant-specificity of the T-helper cells induced by priming with the antigen. The isolated ACL determinant can only induce a few T-cell specificities whereas the whole beef insulin molecule can trigger a number of them (see above). Therefore, the antibodies induced by beef insulin priming have a much higher affinity and specificity then those induced by ACL or oxid. A and B chains. Antibeef insulin IgG antibodies can be produced by $H-2^b$ mice, 9 days after a single injection in incomplete Freunds' adjuvant

(Fig. 5) without the need of a secondary immunisation. This would probably occur much more rapidly by using complete adjuvant.

We are now synthesising a number of amino acid substitutions in in the ACL at the A9 to study effects upon tolerance and immunity to insulins.

References

1. Barton, M., Singh, B., Fraga, E.: J. Am. Chem. Soc. 99, 8491-8498 (1977).
2. Singh, B., Fraga, E., Barton, M.: J. Immunol. 121, 784-789 (1978).
3. Singh, B., Lee, K.C., Fraga, E., Wilkinson, A., Wong, M., Barton, M.: J. Immunol. 124, 1336-1343 (1980).
4. Singh, B., Lee, K.C., Fraga, E., Wong, M.: Proc. Canadian Fed. Biol. Soc. 22, 95 (1979).
5. Dayhoff, M.O.: Atlas Protein Sequence Struct. 5, 3 (1978).
6. Bundell, T.L., Humbel, R.E.,: Nature 287, 781-787 (1980).
7. Keck, K.: Nature 254, 78-79 (1975).
8. Keck, K.: Eur. J. Immunol. 5, 801-807 (1975).
9. Barcinski, M.A., Rosenthal, A.S.: J. Exp. Med. 145, 726-742 (1977).
10. Reeves, W.G.: Recent Adv. Clinical Immunol. No. 2, p. 183-220, Churchill Livingstone, New York, 1980.
11. Rosenthal, A.S.: Immunol. Rev. 40, 135-152 (1978).
12. Avrameas, S.: Immunochemistry 6, 43-52 (1969).
13. Lee, K.C., Singh, B., Barton, M.A., Procyshyn, A., Wong, M:. J. Immunol. Methods 25, 159-170 (1979).
14. Sieber, P., Kamber, B., Eisler, K., Hartmann, A., Riniker, B., Rittel, W.: Helv. Chim. Acta 59, 1489-1497 (1976).
15. Mitchison, N.A.: Eur. J. Immunol. 1, 10-27 (1971).
16. Solinger, A.M., Ultee, M.E., Margoliash, E., Schwartz, R.H.: J. Exp. Med. 150, 830-848 (1979).
17. Adorini, L., Harvey, M., Sercarz, E.E.: Eur. J. Immunol. 9, 906-909 (1979).
18. Herzenberg, L.A., Black, S.J., Herzenberg, L.A.: Eur. J. Immunol. 10, 1-11 (1980).

ANALYSIS OF H-2 GENE REGULATION OF THE RESPONSE OF T LYMPHOCYTES TO INSULIN USING SYNTHETIC ANTIGENIC DETERMINANTS AND ANTI-IDIOTYPES*

Janet Talmon, Ruth Maron, Esther Gotlib and Irun R. Cohen
Department of Cell Biology, The Weizmann Institute of Science, Rehovot, Israel

Introduction

Both B and T lymphocytes are equipped with receptors that recognize antigenic determinants by virtue of their three dimensional complementarity to the determinant. However, whether or not a potential antigenic determinant on an immunogen will, in fact, be recognized may be influenced by immune response (Ir) genes linked to the major histocompatibility complex (MHC). The Ir genotype of an individual seems to regulate the magnitude of the T cell immune response to such determinants. The phenotype may be expressed as a relatively high response, a low response, or no detectible immune response to the determinant.

Since it was discovered that the immune response to insulin was under genetic control (1), and that MHC linked Ir genes regulated responses of T lymphocytes to various determinants on insulin (2), the insulin molecule has been an attractive immunogen for study. The amino acid sequence and conformation of the species variants of the molecule have been characterized (3). Thus, the immune response to insulins can provide information about which antigenic determinants T lymphocytes are permitted by Ir genes to see on the molecule.

Two classes of molecular structure could serve as the raw material from which the immune system might operationally define antigenic determinants

---

* Supported by a grant from the National Institute of Arthritis, Metabolism and Digestive Disease no. AM26766.

for T lymphocytes: the amino acid sequence of the immunogen, or the conformation of portions of the native, intact molecule.

Table 1A shows how T lymphocytes of mice might view antigenic determinants of ungulate insulins related to amino acid sequence.

TABLE 1

AMINO ACID SUBSTITUTIONS BETWEEN MOUSE, PORK, BEEF AND SHEEP INSULINS

A. Sequential Determinants:

	A Chain Loop			Non-Loop		
Insulin	A8	A9	A10	A4	B3	B30
Mouse	Thr	Ser	Ile	Asp	Lys	Ser
Pork	Thr	Ser	Ile	Glu	Asn	Ala
Beef	Ala	Ser	Val	Glu	Asn	Ala
Sheep	Ala	Gly	Val	Glu	Asn	Ala

B. Conformational Determinants:

	Non-Loop		Loop			Non-Loop
Insulin	B30	A4	A8	A9	A10	B3
Mouse	Ser	Asp	Thr	Ser	Ile	Lys
Pork	Ala	Glu	Thr	Ser	Ile	Asn
Beef	Ala	Glu	Ala	Ser	Val	Asn
Sheep	Ala	Glu	Ala	Gly	Val	Asn

The amino acid substitutions (4) that could contribute to foreign antigenic determinants are at positions 8-10 of the A chain loop, and at A4, B3 or B30 outside of the loop. The three ungulate insulins, pork, beef and sheep, share the non-loop substitutions at A4, B3 and B30. Beef and sheep, but not pork insulin differ from mouse insulin at A8-A10 of the A chain loop. Hence, an immune response to beef or sheep insulins that did not cross-react with pork insulin would map the response to the A chain loop substitutions. A response that cross-reacted equally well to all three insulins would be mapped to non-loop determinant(s) (5,6).

However, if we examine the conformation of the whole insulin molecule revealed by X-ray crystalography, we cannot very easily distinguish between loop and non-loop determinants. Analysis of the three dimensional structure of insulin (3,7) shows that the loop and non-loop substitutions are contiguous on the surface of the molecule and form a single patch of 6 amino acids: B30-A4-A8-A9-A10-B3. The sequence A8-A10 does not appear on the surface as part of a loop, but rather is sandwiched between non-loop substitutions (Table 1B). This substituted patch is about 24Å long and could be envisioned as a single determinant.

How do T lymphocytes view insulin? Do they see a conformational entity or do they see distinct sequential loop and non-loop determinants created during processing of the insulin molecule (8) ? In this paper we shall present the results of experiments designed to answer this question. One approach was to test whether Ir genes controlled responses to synthetic tripeptides A8-A10 of beef and sheep insulin and whether such responses cross-reacted with those elicited by immunization against the whole insulin molecule.

Another approach was to use anti-receptor antibodies that inhibited recognition by specific T lymphocytes of defined antigenic determinants. By analyzing the effects of anti-receptor antibodies on responses to various insulins we hoped to learn whether seemingly cross-reactive determinants were recognized by the same or diverse clones of T lymphocytes, and whether loop and non-loop determinants were recognized independantly.

The results presented here indicate that Ir genes influence responses to insulin determinants at the level of tripeptides. However, we also found evidence that the "loop" and "non-loop" substituted residues of insulin can be seen as a single conformational antigenic determinant by competing clones of T lymphocytes. Thus, some T lymphocytes under Ir gene control may recognize conformational determinants while other T lymphocytes recognize sequential determinants of insulin.

Material and Methods

Mice. The animal Breeding Center of this Institute supplied mice of strains

BALB/c (H-2^b) and H-2 congenic C3H.SW (H-2^b) and C3H.DiSn (H-2^k). Mice were used between two and three months of age.

Immunization against insulins. Mice were inoculated in each hind foot pad with 15 μg of pork insulin or 10 μg of beef or sheep insulins or tripeptides emulsified in complete Freund's adjuvant. Fourteen days later lymphocytes from the draining popliteal lymph nodes were assayed in a T lymphocyte proliferative assay as described (9).

Preparation of tripeptides. Ala-Ser-Val and Ala-Gly--Val tripeptides of beef and sheep insulin were synthesized under the supervision of Dr. M. Fridkin of the Department of Organic Chemistry, using a conventional procedue for peptide synthesis in solution employing N,N'-dicyclohexylcarbodiimide as a coupling agent (10). The tripeptides were found to be pure electrophoretically, chromatographically and by amino acid analysis.

Immunization against T lymphocyte receptors. BALB/c mice were immunized against beef insulin and T lymphocytes were generated by incubating suspensions of lymphocytes with beef insulin (100 μg/ml) for 3 days in RPMI 1640 medium supplemented with 1% normal syngeneic mouse serum. The lymphoblasts were washed and 2 x 10^7 emulsified in complete Freund's adjuvant were inoculated into multiple subcutaneous sites of syngeneic BALB/c mice. The mice were boosted every two weeks x5 with anti-beef insulin lymphoblasts emulsified in incomplete Freund's adjuvant and bled 2 weeks later. The antiserum was tested *in vitro* by using it in place of 1% normal mouse serum in proliferative assays against beef or pork insulins.

Results

H-2 Genetic Control of Response to A8-A10 Tripeptides

To learn whether H-2 linked Ir gene products regulated the responses of T lymphocytes to isolated peptide sequences of insulin, we prepared the A8-A10 tripeptides of sheep (Ala-Gly-Val) and beef (Ala-Ser-Val) insulins and immunized H-2 congenic mice of strains H-2^k and H-2^b. Table 2 shows the secondary proliferative responses *in vitro*. We found that H-2^b mice responded to the Ala-Ser-Val, but not to the Ala-Gly-Val tripeptide. In contrast, the H-2^k mice responded to the Ala-Gly-Val tripeptide. When

TABLE 2

H-2 REGULATION OF RESPONSE TO LOOP SEQUENCE TRIPEPTIDES OF SHEEP (Ala-Gly-Val) AND BEEF (Ala-Ser-Val) INSULINS

Strain	H-2	Immunization *in vivo*	Secondary proliferative response *in vitro* (cpm x 10^{-3})		
			Background	Sheep tripeptide Ala-Gly-Val	Beef tripeptide Ala-Ser-Val
C3H.DiSn	k	Ala-Gly-Val	30	83	43
		Ala-Ser-Val	9	38	14
C3H.SW	b	Ala-Ser-Val	8	8	19
		Ala-Gly-Val	4	4	4

Mice were immunized with tripeptides and the proliferative responses of T lymphocytes from the draining lymph nodes were measured.

these H-2^k mice were immunized with the Ala-Ser-Val beef tripeptide, they demonstrated no secondary response to the homologous Ala-Ser-Val tripeptide, but did show a response to the Ala-Gly-Val tripeptide with which they had not been injected. This phenomenon of cross-priming was also noted in immunization against whole beef or sheep insulins. We found that the H-2 "forbidden" variant activated little or no memory to itself. However, immunized H-2^k or H-2^b mice showed a secondary response to the H-2 "permitted" variant insulin (9). Thus, the responses to the loop tripeptides were influenced by the same H-2 haplotypes that were associated with responses to the intact insulin molecules, H-2^b responded to beef and H-2^k to sheep determinants (9). Furthermore, the phenomenon of cross-priming was also observed to some degree. Hence, many of the features of Ir gene control of the T lymphocyte proliferative response to whole insulin were seen at the level of isolated small peptides. These results would seem to be compatible with the notion that T lymphocytes see processed antigens.

Sheep Insulin Tripeptide Cross-Reacts with Intact Sheep Insulin, But Not *vice versa*

The above results indicated that H-2 genes can control the response to tripeptides possessing the sequences found in the A chain loops of sheep and beef insulins. However, the question remained whether these same tripeptide sequences were recognized in the course of immunization of mice against intact insulin.

TABLE 3

Ala-Gly-Val LOOP SEQUENCE TRIPEPTIDE OF SHEEP INSULIN PRIMES FOR A ONE-WAY SECONDARY RESPONSE TO ITSELF AND TO WHOLE SHEEP INSULIN

Strain	H-2	Immunization *in vivo*	Secondary proliferative response *in vitro* (cpm x 10^{-3})		
			Background	Sheep Insulin	Ala-Gly-Val
C3H.DiSn	k	Sheep	19	39	21
		Ala-Gly-Val	19	38	47

Mice were immunized with either whole sheep insulin or the sheep loop tripeptide and T lymphocyte proliferative responses were measured.

Table 3 shows the results of an experiment testing cross-reactivity between whole sheep insulin and the Ala-Gly-Val tripeptide. H-2^k responder mice were immunized against either molecule and the T lymphocyte secondary proliferative responses were measured. We found that immunization against the sheep A chain loop tripeptide activated a secondary response that could recognize either the tripeptide or the whole molecule. However, their cross-reactivity was not evident in the opposite directions. Mice immunized against whole sheep insulin failed to respond to the tripeptide.

It seems that the response of H-2^k mice to sheep insulin is directed primarily against an antigenic determinant associated with the A chain loop, since there was no cross-reaction to pork insulin and very little to beef insulin that both differ from sheep only in the loop region (9; Table 1). The lack of response to the tripeptide following immunization against the whole molecule suggests that the amino acid sequence of the loop is not the only element recognized by T lymphocytes responding to the intact molecule. It is probable that the conformation assumed by the amino acid chain contributes significantly to their specificity as an antigenic determinant. Hence, the Ala-Gly-Val tripeptide may not have the same conformation *in vitro* as it does when it is part of the A chain loop on whole insulin.

Anti-Receptor Antibodies Uncover a Functional Relationships between Loop and Non-Loop Determinants

In the experiments quoted above we investigated the reactivities and cross-reactivities of synthetic peptides as a means of analyzing the nature of antigenic determinants recognized on insulin by T lymphocytes. Another way of studying the selection of antigenic determinants by the immune system was to manipulate clones of insulin-recognizing lymphocytes by anti-receptor antibodies. We immunized $H\text{-}2^d$ mice against syngeneic lymphoblasts that had been raised *in vitro* against beef insulin to obtain antisera directed against receptors that recognize beef insulin. These antibodies to (anti-beef) receptors were added to secondary proliferative cultures responding *in vitro* to either beef or pork insulins to see if the responses to the sequential loop and non-loop determinants were distinct or related.

We had found earlier that immunizing $H\text{-}2^d$ mice against pork insulin produced lymphocytes that responded equally well to either pork or beef insulin (9). This total cross-reactivity suggested a response to the non-loop determinants shared by pork and beef insulin (Table 1A). In contrast, $H\text{-}2^d$ mice immunized against beef insulin showed a high secondary response to beef insulin and a much lower response to pork insulin (9). This lack of cross-reactivity indicated a response to the beef A chain loop determinant (Table 1A). Thus, it appeared that the A chain loop determinant was immunodominant.

Table 4 shows that in the absense of anti-receptor antibodies, these results were indeed obtained. Immunization against pork insulin led to cross-reactive secondary responses to pork (20,000Δ CPM) and to beef insulins (18,000Δ CPM). Immunization against beef insulin produced a strong secondary response to beef insulin (48,000Δ CPM) and a relatively weak response to pork insulin (9,000Δ CPM).

TABLE 4

ANTIBODIES TO THE ANTI-BEEF RECEPTOR AUGMENT, THE RESPONSE TO T LYMPHOCYTES TO PORK INSULIN

Immunizing Insulin	Secondary Proliferative Response			
	Secondary Insulin	Antiserum to (anti-beef) receptors	Δ CPM $\times 10^{-3}$	Percent change
Pork	Pork	-	20	
		+	30	+50
	Beef	-	18	
		+	7	-61
Beef	Beef	-	48	
		+	6	-88
	Pork	-	9	
		+	18	+100

Proliferative responses were measured in the presence or absence of 1% antiserum to the (anti-beef) receptor.
ΔCPM = (test CPM - control CPM without antigen).

However, the presence of antiserum to (anti-beef) receptors had striking effects on these reactivities (Table 4). The apparent cross-reactivity between pork and beef insulins that defined a response to non-loop determinant(s) was abolished. The response to pork insulin was increased by 50% in the presence of this anti-beef receptor antiserum while the response to beef insulin was decreased by about 60%. This indicates that distinct clones of lymphocytes recognized pork and beef insulins. Apparent cross-reactivity between the two insulins was, therefore, due to a mixture of clones each recognizing the putative sequentially identical non-loop segments of pork or beef isulin. These results cast doubt on the independent existence of the same sequential non-loop determinant(s) in both molecules.

This idea was strengthened by the effect of the anti-beef receptor antiserum on the responses induced by priming with beef insulin (Table 4). The response to beef insulin was inhibited by 88%, while the weak response to pork insulin was increased by 100%. This result argues against the independent existence of the beef A chain loop determinant as distinct from the pork non-loop determinant. Hence, the results obtained using anti-receptor antibodies are compatible with the conformational view of the insulin molecule that proposes an antigenic patch including both sequential loop and non-loop amino acid substitutions (Table 1B).

Discussion

The findings presented here raise a number of paradoxes. The observation that the tripeptides were immunogenic was unexpected. We supposed tripeptides to be too small to be immunogenic and, in fact, synthesized them to be used in inhibition studies. Contrary to expectation, the tripeptides were immunogenic and the response they elicited was found to be under control of H-2 genes. Their immunogenicity may have resulted from aggregation into larger immunogenic complexes, since the tripeptides were not easily soluble. B. Singh and E. Fraga report elsewhere in this volume that the beef tripeptide Ala-Ser-Val was not immunogenic in their hands. It is possible that their peptide preparation differed from ours; certainly our assay systems differ and such factors can cause discrepancies in results.

In addition to differences in the responses of $H\text{-}2^k$ and $H\text{-}2^b$ mice to the sheep and beef tripeptides, we also found a hint of cross-priming of H-2 "forbidden" and "permitted" tripeptides (Table 2). This indicates that some of the complex phenomena of H-2 gene control may be expressed at the level of very small sequences of the immunogen, and supports the idea that the H-2 gene products are involved in processing antigenic determinants (8).

However, cross-reactivity between the sheep tripeptide and the intact sheep determinant was only partial and this suggests that native conformation is also seen by T lymphocytes.

Our studies with anti-receptor antiserum also provided evidence for a role for conformation destinct from primary sequence in creating antigenic determinants seen by T lymphocytes. We found (Table 4) that different clones of lymphocytes recognized the seemingly identical sequential non-loop determinant(s) defined by a response to pork insulin. These conclusions were based on the findings that antiserum to the anti-beef receptor influenced the responses to both beef and pork insulins. Conformational analysis of the insulin molecule shows that the loop and non-loop substitutions are contiguous and can be seen to form a single patch on the insulin molecule (3,7; Table 1). Thus, it is conceivable that T lymphocytes recognized the substituted residues in their conformational contiguity as well as possibly in their sequence. In this way we can understand how loop and non-loop antigenic determinants on beef and pork insulins were seen at each others expense.

An element of competition seemed to characterize the relationship between clones of lymphocytes responding to beef versus pork insulins. Grossman and Cohen have developed a quantitative model to explain how competition between different, but related clones of lymphocytes could determine the phenotype of an immune response (11). Ir genes could regulate the Ir phenotype by influencing the outcome of clonal competition through small, quantitative differences in the way antigenic determinants are recognized. This model does away with the need to postulate discrete cellular defects as a cause for H-2 genetical low responsiveness. It also explains the variability of the phenotype of the response to insulin influenced by variation in the mode of presentation of the molecule (12). Whether or not the clonal competition model is accurate, it seems that some T lymphocytes recognize conformational entities on the surface of the intact insulin molecule. Other T lymphocytes seem to see small sequential fragments of the molecule. Both kinds of recognition are subject to influence by the products of H-2 linked Ir genes.

References

1. Arquilla, E.R., Finn, J.: Science 142, 400-401 (1963).
2. Keck, K.: Nature 254, 78-79 (1975).
3. Blundell, T.L., Dodson, G.G., Hodgkin, D.C., Mercola, D.A.: Adv. Protein Chem. 26, 279-402 (1972).
4. Dayhoff, M.O. ed. Atlas of Protein Sequence and Structure, Natl. Biomed. Res. Found., Washington, D.C. Vol. 5, 1972.

5. Rosenthal, A.S., Barcinski, M.A., Blake, J.T.: Nature 267, 156-158 (1977).

6. Barcinski, M.A., Rosenthal, A.S.: J. Exp. Med. 145, 726-742 (1977).

7. Ranghino, G., Talmon, J., Yonath, A., Cohen, I.R.: in Structural Aspects of Recognition and Assembly in Biological Macromolecules, Ed. M. Balaban, in press.

8. Benacerraf, B.: J. Immunol. 120, 1809-1812 (1978).

9. Cohen, I.R., Talmon, J.: Eur. J. Immunol. 10, 284-289 (1980).

10. Sheehan, J.C., Hess, G.P.: J. Amer. Chem. Soc. 77, 1065 (1955).

11. Grossman, Z., Cohen, I.R.: Eur. J. Immunol. 10, 633-640 (1980).

Ir GENE CONTROL OF THE INSULIN-SPECIFIC IMMUNE RESPONSE IN MICE.

J.A. Kapp and R.P. Bucy

Department of Pathology, The Jewish Hospital of St. Louis,
216 S. Kingshighway, St. Louis, Missouri, USA, 63110

Introduction

Antigens of limited heterogeneity, especially those antigens that differ only slightly from host proteins, have been very useful for the analysis of cellular interactions involved in the development and regulation of immunity. Study of responses to these antigens has led to the identification of autosomal, dominant genes linked to the major histocompatibility complex (MHC) that are intimately involved in the development of immunity. These MHC-linked immune response (Ir) genes are: 1) readily demonstrated in response to antigens that display a limited number of immunogenic determinants; 2) expressed in virtually all phases of T cell-dependent immune responses; and 3) able to discriminate between small structural differences between antigens (1). We believe that these Ir genes are involved in development of immunity to all T cell-dependent antigens and that the identification of a cell type(s) in which Ir gene defects are expressed will reveal the role that these genes play in the development of physiological immune responses.

The basis for our choice of insulin as a model antigen was the observations of Klaus Keck demonstrating that antibody responses to heterologous insulins were all-or-none responses and that antibody responses to beef, sheep, and pork insulin were distinct for inbred strains of mice bearing the $H\text{-}2^{b,d,k}$ haplotypes (2-4).

Basic and Clinical Aspects of Immunity to Insulin

We have previously shown that mice that were nonresponders to pork insulin could produce antibodies that bind to pork insulin if immunized with an immunogenic form of the antigen (5,6). For example, $H-2^b$ mice produce antibodies that bind to pork insulin if immunized with pork proinsulin or beef insulin. Therefore, it seems unlikely that the Ir gene defect in the immune response to pork insulin in $H-2^b$ mice lies at the level of the B cells. The studies reported here were initiated to determine the insulin-specific T cell functions in responder and nonresponder mice.

Results

Pattern of Ir gene control to insulin

A major feature in the rationale of using insulin responses as a probe of Ir gene control mechanisms is the diversity of the Ir gene control pattern to this series of proteins whose structures are defined. A summary of the Ir gene control of responses to fluorescein conjugated to four different insulin molecules is shown in Table I. The development of an immune response was assessed by measuring the primary plaque forming cell (PFC) response in lymph nodes of mice injected with 50 μg of fluorescein-insulin (FL-insulin) in CFA in the footpads. Fluorescein-specific PFC responses were measured using fluorescein conjugated to sheep erythrocytes and the insulin-specific PFC responses were measured using insulin conjugated to sheep erythrocytes (7). IgM PFC responses specific for fluorescein or insulin were infrequent and showed no differences between mice bearing different haplotypes (not shown). However, development of both fluorescein and insulin-specific IgG PFC are controlled concordantly by H-2-linked Ir genes.

Table I. Genetic Control of Responses to Fluorescein-Insulin

		Specific IgG PFC/Lymph Node[a]			
		B10.D2	C57BL/10	B10.BR	B10.S
Antigen	Indicator	$H\text{-}2^d$	$H\text{-}2^b$	$H\text{-}2^k$	$H\text{-}2^s$
FL-Pork	FL-SRBC	20,550	900	400	100
	INS-SRBC	37,300	200	400	200
FL-Beef	FL-SRBC	51,300	46,600	200	200
	INS-SRBC	35,700	28,300	<100	<100
FL-Sheep	FL-SRBC	27,100	11,000	7,800	<100
	INS-SRBC	7,500	6,300	4,300	<100
FL-Horse	FL-SRBC	20,900	20,400	3,400	<100
	INS-SRBC	57,900	18,800	6,400	<100

[a]Mice received 50 μg FL-Insulin in CFA in hind foot pads and PFC responses were measured 13 days later. Each value is the arithmetic mean of 3 mice/group.

Insulin-specific T cell activity in C57BL/10 mice

In order to explore the possibility that unresponsiveness in the insulin system might be associated with the induction of suppressor T cells, we examined the effect of preinjection of pork insulin on the subsequent response to beef insulin in C57BL/10 mice. The results demonstrated that pork insulin did not inhibit subsequent responses to beef insulin but actually primed $H\text{-}2^b$ mice for enhanced insulin-specific responses to the immunogenic forms of insulin (not shown). To pursue the characterization of the cells primed by pork insulin, we have developed an adoptive transfer protocol in which primed cells are isolated from different sources and recombined to generate a specific PFC response in normal, irradiated (700 rads) syngeneic mice. Spleen cells from normal mice and mice primed with beef insulin i.p. were separated into T cell and B cell enriched fractions by differential adherence to rabbit anti-mouse Ig coated plastic dishes (8). These cells were then injected alone or in mixtures into irradiated syngeneic recipients that were challenged with beef insulin i.p. and assayed for PFC responses nine days after challenge (Table II). Unfractionated normal spleen cells developed no PFC responses, while unfractionated spleen cells from beef insulin primed mice generated approximately 130,000 insulin-specific PFC per spleen. Recipients of normal T cells mixed with either normal or primed B cells failed to develop any insulin-specific responses. Primed T cells plus normal B cells gave no better response than primed T cells alone. Recipients of mixtures of primed T and B cells developed approximately 80,000 PFC per spleen. Therefore this adoptive transfer system requires the addition of both primed T cells and primed B cells for the development of insulin-specific PFC responses.

Table II. Transfer of Insulin-Specific PFC Responses

Whole Spleen 40×10^6 Cells[b]	T Cells 20×10^6	B Cells 20×10^6	Insulin Specific IgG PFC/Spleen[a]
Normal	--	--	≤ 200[c]
Primed	--	--	130,000
--	Normal	--	≤ 200
--	Primed	--	25,000
--	--	Normal	≤ 200
--	--	Primed	≤ 200
--	Normal	Normal	≤ 200
--	Normal	Primed	≤ 200
--	Primed	Normal	20,000
--	Primed	Primed	80,000

[a]C57BL/10 mice received 700 R, were reconstituted and injected with 50 μg beef insulin in CFA i.p. Splenic responses were assayed nine days later.

[b]Spleen cells from normal or beef insulin primed C57BL/10 mice.
[c]Arithmetic mean of responses of 3 recipients.

Since pork insulin did not suppress responses to beef insulin in H-2^b mice we asked whether pork insulin could prime cells for the generation of insulin-specific PFC responses in adoptive recipients (Table III). Mixtures of purified lymph node T cells from mice primed with beef or pork insulin and splenic B cells from mice primed with beef insulin generated strong PFC responses when challenged with beef but not pork insulin. Lymph node T cells from mice primed with the unrelated protein, Ovalbumin (OVA), failed to reconstitute the response to beef insulin, indicating that insulin-specific T cells are essential to the development of this PFC response. Furthermore, pork insulin appears to be as effective as beef insulin in priming a population of cells in H-2^b mice that can generate helper cell functions upon challenge with the immunogenic form of insulin, beef insulin. The ability of beef and pork primed lymph node T cells to provide helper T cell activity is abolished by treatment with anti-Thy 1.2 serum plus complement (data not shown).

Table III. Antigenic Specificity of Transferred Responses

Primed Lymph Node T Cells[b] (10×10^6)	Beef Insulin Primed[c] (20×10^6)	Insulin Specific IgG PFC/Spleen[a] by Recipients Challenged with: Pork Insulin	Beef Insulin
--	Whole Spleen	800 ± 100	56,400 ± 7,500
--	B Cells	500 ± 200	700 ± 300
OVA	B Cells	600 ± 100	1,000 ± 400
Beef	B Cells	700 ± 200	138,400 ± 20,000
Pork	B Cells	900 ± 100	109,000 ± 36,400

[a]C57BL/10 recipients treated as described in Table I and challenged with 50 μg beef or pork insulin in CFA i.p.

[b]Lymph node T cells from C57BL/10 mice primed with 50 μg antigen in CFA 11 days earlier.

[c]Spleen cells or anti-Thyl + C treated splenic B cells from C57BL/10 mice primed with beef insulin in CFA 6 weeks earlier.

There is a potential problem inherent in our experimental design that needed to be addressed before we could confidently interpret these results. The problem is that development of PFC responses in adoptive recipients requires primed B cells from syngeneic mice. In the previous experiments, these B cells were derived from mice that had been primed with beef insulin. It would not be inconceivable that a population of beef insulin primed spleen cells in the anti-Thyl treated, beef insulin primed cell pool could actually be responsible for the generation of specific helper cell function by beef and pork insulin primed lymph node T cells. Since the fluorescein-specific IgG PFC response to fluorescein-insulin conjugates is controlled by the same Ir genes that control the response to insulin (Table I) we could obtain primed B cells from mice injected with fluorescein conjugated to the unrelated carrier, fowl gamma globulin (FGG). Lymph node T cells from mice primed with OVA, beef or pork insulin were adoptively transferred with FL-FGG primed B cells and challenged with fluorescein-beef insulin (Table IV).

Table IV. Helper T Cell Activity for Haptenated Insulin

Primed T Cells[a] (15 X 10^6)	FL-FGG Primed Cells[b] (15 X 10^6)	Challenge Antigen	FL-Specific IgG PFC/Spleen[c]
--	Spleen	FL-FGG	232,000 ± 18,300
--	B Cells	FL-FGG	7,600 ± 1,500
OVA	B Cells	FL-Beef	13,700 ± 7,600
Beef	B Cells	FL-Beef	159,700 ± 10,700
Pork	B Cells	FL-Beef	121,000 ± 5,000

[a]Lymph node T cells from C57BL/10 mice primed with 50 μg antigen in CFA in the footpads 11 days earlier.

[b]Spleen cells or splenic B cells from C57BL/10 mice primed with 50 μg FL-FGG in CFA i.p. 8 weeks earlier.

[c]C57BL/10 irradiated recipients were challenged with 50 μg FL-FGG or FL-insulin in CFA i.p. and assayed 9 days later.

Quite clearly pork and beef insulin, but not OVA, primed lymph node T cells for the generation of fluorescein-specific PFC responses in these adoptive recipients. Insulin-specific PFC were also assayed in these recipients but none were detected, presumably because there was no source of insulin-primed B cells in these mice. These data rule out the possibility that the helper cell activity of pork insulin-primed T cells observed in the previous experiments was dependent upon beef insulin-primed cells in the B cell pools.

Discussion

We have demonstrated that although pork insulin fails to stimulate antibody formation in $H\text{-}2^b$ mice,this molecule can stimulate a specific T cell which can develop functional helper activity in irradiated recipients if these recipients are challenged with beef insulin. Thus, we must explain the dichotomy that pork insulin can prime helper T cells and that pork insulin binds to anti-beef insulin antibodies, and presumably insulin specific B cells, but that pork insulin cannot stimulate a significant plaque forming cell response in $H\text{-}2^b$ mice. To account for this observation, one could propose that a single insulin-specific helper T cell population could be initially stimulated by pork insulin, but somehow these T cells were unable to deliver a signal to B cells without the participation of a responder form of insulin (beef insulin). However, this model would require a change in the antigenic specificity of a particular clone of T cells resulting from antigenic exposure. Such a change in fine specificity would require a somatic modification of the antigen receptor structure such that a receptor which could originally recognize pork and beef insulin becomes able to discriminate the structural differences between beef and pork insulin. We find this notion unappealing since it is incompatible with all the evidence that clones of lymphocytes each bear a receptor whose precise antigenic specificity is not modified by antigenic exposure or the state of lymphocyte differentiation. Therefore, we have postulated that two independent T cells are required for the development of antibody responses to insulin. Our results then can be explained by proposing that $H\text{-}2^b$ mice have an antigen-specific T cell subpopulation which can be stimulated by both beef and pork insulin, but this T cell subset cannot interact directly with B cells. We have designated this type of cell as an amplifier T cell since the stimulation of this cell alone is not sufficient to generate helper T cells, but stimulation of this cell is required for the efficient generation of helper T cell function. The amplifier T cell is probably specific for some determinant that is shared between beef and pork insulin since both of these molecules can stimulate this activity. However, we suggest that the T cell which actually delivers the helper signal to the B cells is specific for the A chain loop structure of beef insulin, since this is the only structural difference between the two molecules and therefore must be involved in the Ir gene specificity. We suggest that beef insulin can mediate a functional interaction between the amplifier and helper T cells through an antigen bridge, since it presents these two determinants in a covalently linked arrangement. Pork insulin cannot mediate this interaction since this molecule does not contain the A chain structure required by the helper T cell. In pork insulin immunized lymph node T cells, the helper cell is presumably present as an unstimulated cell, but after stimulation with beef insulin in the presence of the amplifier T cell, the helper cell can deliver a functional signal to the B cell. Definitive demonstration that there are two distinct T cell subpopulations will require physical isolation and characterization of each of these cell types and the restoration of functional activity by their admixture. Such experiments are currently in progress.

There are numerous experimental systems in which two T cell subpopulations are required for the generation of optimal helper cell activity. Our suggestion that two T cells are required for the generation of responses to insulin is thus compatible with the observations of other investigators. Our interpretation that Ir gene control can operate at the level of T cell - T cell interaction has also been suggested by the data from Strassman et al. (9,10) and von Boehmer and Haas (11).

Ir genes have now been shown to operate at the level of T cell-macrophage interactions (12,13,14), T cell-B cell interactions (15,16,17) and more recently T cell-T cell interactions. These observations suggest that the mechanisms of nonresponsiveness are heterogeneous and consequently Ir genes must regulate cell-cell interactions at multiple sites in the pathway leading to an immune response.

Acknowledgements

The work reported in this manuscript was supported by US Public Health Service Research Grant AI-13987 and US Public Health Service Research Career Development Award AI00361 from the National Institute of Allergy and Infectious Diseases. We thank John Hauenstein for expert technical assistance and Paula Ryan for expert secretarial assistance.

References

1. Benacerraf, B. and Katz, D.H.: Adv. Cancer Res. 21, 121 (1975).
2. Keck, K.: Nature 254, 78 (1975).
3. Keck, K.: Eur. J. Immunol. 5, 801 (1975).
4. Keck, K.: J. Immunol. 7, 811 (1977).

5. Kapp, J.A., Strayer, D.S.: J. Immunol. 121, 978 (1978).

6. Kapp, J.A., Strayer, D.S., Robbins, P.F., Perlmutter, R. M.: J. Immunol. 123, 109 (1979).

7. Schroer, J.A., Inman, J.K., Thomas, J.W., Rosenthal, A.S.: J. Immunol. 123, 670 (1979).

8. Mage, M., McHugh, L.L., Rothstein, T.: J. Immunol. Meth. 15, 47 (1977).

9. Strassman, G., Eshhar, Z., Mozes, E.: J. Exp. Med. 151, 265 (1980).

10. Strassman, G., Eshhar, Z., Mozes, E.: J. Exp. Med. 151, 628 (1980).

11. von Boehmer, H., Haas, W.: J. Exp. Med. 150, 1134 (1979).

12. Rosenthal, A.S., Shevach, E.M.: The Role of Products of the Histocompatibility Gene Complex in Immune Responses. D.H. Katz and B. Benacerraf, editors. Academic Press, N.Y. 1976.

13. Yano, A., Schwartz, R.H., Paul, W.E.: Eur. J. Immunol. 8, 344 (1978).

14. Miller, J.F.A.P., Vadas, M.A., Whitelaw, A., Gamble, J.: Proc. Nat. Acad. Sci. USA 72, 5095 (1975).

15. Katz, D.H., Hamaoka, T., Dorf, M.E., Maurer, P.H., Benacerraf, B.: Proc. Nat. Acad. Sci. USA 70, 2624 (1973).

16. Marrack, P., Kappler, J.W.: J. Exp. Med. 149, 780 (1979).

17. Taussig, M.J., Mozes, E., Isac, R.: J. Exp. Med. 140, 30 (1974).

18. Taussig, M.J., Munro, A.J., Campbell, R., David, C.S., Stains, N.A.: J. Exp. Med. 142, 694 (1975).

INFLUENCE OF INSULIN MODIFICATION UPON THE IMMUNE RESPONSE TO INSULIN

J. W. Thomas, J.A. Kapp

Jewish Hospital of St. Louis. Department of Pathology and Laboratory Medicine. 216 S. Kingshighway, St. Louis, Missouri, USA, 63110

J. A. Schroer

Laboratory of Clinical Investigation, NIAID, NIH, Bethesda, Maryland, USA

A. S. Rosenthal

Department of Immunology, Merck Institute for Therapeutic Research, Rahway, N.J. USA

Introduction

The immunological responsiveness to numerous protein antigens has been shown to be closely associated with genes (Ir) linked to the major histocompatibility complex (MHC) in several species of laboratory animals. In humans similar association has been made between diseases involving immunological phenomenon and HLA antigens. In the case of insulin dependent juvenile diabetes certain HLA antigens appear to be closely associated with genes that are responsible for or are permissive of the autoreactivity leading to islet cell destruction. Identifying the particular antigen(s) or stimulus(i) involved in such a complex disease state is a major task, more so in view of the gap in the basic knowledge of Ir gene function. Understanding the basic mechanism of immune response gene function is key to the eventual understanding of such disease states.

Fortunately, the highly defined insulin molecule can be used as an antigen which is under the control of immune response genes (1,2). Through the use of species variants of mammalian insulins immune response genes can be deduced to have a unique relationship to specific amino acid residues. For example, mice of $H\text{-}2^b$ haplotype are able to respond when immunized with beef but not pork insulin; the two amino acid differences in the A chain loop are apparently responsible for this responsiveness (1,3). Mice of the $H\text{-}2^d$ haplotype on the other hand respond to both beef and pork insulin, suggesting that at least part of the response is directed at shared determinants (3). The specificities of such reactivity however appear to reside within the T cell since antibodies are highly cross-reactive and bind species variants equally well (4). In order to study the influences of such limited T cell responses upon an equally specific B cell population, we have modified the insulin molecule with a single trinitrophenol (TNP) group and analyzed the immune reactivity of such modified insulins in terms of antibody production and T cell reactivity. These data indicate that the response to modified insulin is similar in some but not all aspects of the response seen with the unmodified molecule. These differences include increased influence of non-H-2 genes on the anti-hapten response, increased ability of modified insulin to stimulate insulin immune T cells, and the ability of modified insulin to reset regulatory mechanism resulting in a decreased anti-insulin response.

Materials and Methods

Animals and immunization.

All animals indicated in the accompanying tables were adult mice of 8-20 weeks of age. Mice of the same sex were used for individual experiments. The animals were immunized in the hind foot pads with 25-50 μg of antigen emulsified in 0.1 ml of complete Freund's adjuvant (CFA).

Antigens and preparation.

The TNBS modified beef and pork insulin were prepared from single component insulins obtained from Dr. Ron Chance of The Eli Lilly Company. The reaction was allowed to proceed overnight in borate buffer pH 9.5 to obtain a molar ratio of 0.98 for TNP-pork and 1.06 for TNP-beef insulin. Insulin ester was prepared as reported previously (5) briefly methyl-4-mercaptobutyrimidate hydrochloride is allowed to react with the single lysine residue on the insulin B chain. The modified insulin is separated by precipitation in citrate phosphate buffer pH 5.3 and washed extensively.

Assays of antibody production and T cell proliferation.

To assay antibody production a slide modification of the Jerne plaque assay was employed. Draining lymph node cells were removed and cultured in soft agar with sheep red blood cells coated with TNP or insulin. Plaque forming cells were enumerated after addition of rabbit anti-mouse serum facilitating and complement or complement alone for determination of indirect (IgG) or direct (IgM) plaques.

The ability of T lymphocytes to incorporated ^{3}H-Thymidine in the presence of antigen was used to access T cell functions. Oil induced exudate cells were passed over nylon wool as previously described to yield a population of highly reactive T lymphocytes (6). These cells were cultured at 1 X 10^{5} cells/cc in microtiter plates for four days prior to determination of DNA synthetic activity.

Results

Both H-2 and non H-2 genes influence the anti-hapten plaque forming cell (PFC) response to TNP-insulin.

The secondary splenic PFC response of several inbred strains of mice immunized with TNP-insulin and boosted with TNP-insulin is shown in Table I. This pattern of responsiveness seen with anti-carrier PFC (5) and circulating antibody (1,4) is in general retained. Mice of $H\text{-}2^d$ haplotype respond to both pork and beef insulin. The antihapten response of TNP-beef is always greater than that seen with TNP-pork and probably indicates that additional clones of T helper cells are generated by beef insulin in $H\text{-}2^d$ mice. Other strains such as $H\text{-}2^{a,k,q}$ are nonresponders to either insulin. Mice of $H\text{-}2^b$ haplotype are able to respond well to TNP-beef insulin but poorly to TNP-pork insulin. Mice of the C3H background demonstrate a different pattern of response, that is influenced by the H-2 type. C3H/SW ($H\text{-}2^b$) mice are able to respond to both beef and pork TNP-modified insulins; however, beef generate a greater response than pork indicating a differential recognition process. C3H/HEJ ($H\text{-}2^k$) mice are able to generate anti-TNP responses only to TNP-beef insulin. Presumably, non H-2 genes on the C3H background are responsible for shifting the heirarchy of response. The mechanism responsible for this remains to be determined.

Table I. Anti-TNP Response of Secondary Spleen PFC to TNP-Insulin[a]

Strain	H-2	TNP-Beef αTNP Ind.PFC/10^6	TNP-Pork αTNP Ind.PFC/10^6
BALB/c	d	1,216.0 (1.1)	246.6 (1.3)
C57BL/6	b	274.6 (1.2)	17.9 (1.1)
B10.D2	d	777.8 (1.2)	231.7 (1.5)
DBA/1	q	1.4 (1.3)	<1.0
CBA	k	<1.0	<1.0
C3H/SW	b	838.9 (1.3)	316.7 (1.3)
C3H/HEJ	k	647.1 (1.3)	13.0 (1.6)

[a]Mice were immunized in the footpads $\bar{c}$ CFA, boosted i.p. for secondary PFC.
[b]Geometric mean and standard errors (x/÷).

In Table II the anti-hapten secondary response to TNP-beef insulin is mapped within the H-2 of B10 congenic mice. "Leakiness" of the anti-TNP response is seen in B10.BR and B10.A mice however as with anti-carrier PFC responses the high responsiveness requires the presence of H-2^b determinants to the left of I-B.

Table II. Mapping Within H-2 of the Ir Gene Control of PFC to Beef Insulin[a]

	H-2 KABJECSD	IgG PFC/10^6 (Anti-TNP)
B10.BR	kkkkkkkk	+
B10.A	kkkkkddd	+
B10.A(4R)	kkdddddd	0
B10.A(5R)	bbbkkddd	++++
B10	bbbbbbbb	++++

+ = 10-50 PFC/10^6

++++ = >200 PFC/10^6

[a]Protocol same as Table I.

Antihapten responses predominate over anti-carrier responses in mice immunized with modified insulins.

The recent development of a technique by which anti-insulin PFC could be detected has provided us with the unique ability to detect anti-hapten and anti-carrier responses simultaneously. Table III demonstrates the primary lymph node response of B10, B10.D2, and B10.BR mice immunized with TNP-pork or TNP-beef insulin. These peak responses occur eleven to fifteen days after immunization with antigen in Freund's complete adjuvant. The high responder strain B10.D2 (H-2^d) make very large anti-TNP responses (>500/10^6) to both TNP-beef and TNP-pork insulin. However, the anti-carrier responses are an order of magnitude lower. This difference does not appear to be explainable on the basis of denatration during the modification procedure since TNP-insulin can inhibit 95% of anti-insulin PFC responses (unpublished observations). Again "leakiness" of the anti-hapten response is demonstrated in that low levels of easily detectable anti-TNP PFC are present in the nodes of "nonresponder" $H\text{-}2^k$ mice immunized with beef and pork and $H\text{-}2^b$ with TNP pork insulin immunization. Further studies are in progress to determine if such responsiveness is due to a lower threshold for activation of anti-hapten B cells by low levels of help. Alternately such response may be due to determinants created in the modified molecule.

Table III. Primary Lymph Node PFC Response to TNP-Insulin[a]

Strain	Antigen	TNP(IgG) PFC/10^6	Insulin (IgG) PFC/10^6
B10.D2	TNP-PSC	1429.0 (1.5)[b]	45.0 (3.3)
B10.BR	"	58.0 (1.6)	5.6 (2.4)
B10	"	157.5 (1.4)	3.0 (2.2)
B10.D2	TNP-BSC	689.5 (1.6)	42.6 (1.4)
B10.BR	"	83.2 (1.7)	1.4 (1.4)
B10	"	369.1 (1.3)	17.3 (1.5)

[a]4-6 animals per group were immunized in the footpads with 50 μg of TNP-insulin; two weeks later the PFC were determined in the draining lymph nodes.

[b]Geometric mean and standard errors (x/÷).

Modified insulin is a more potent stimulator of T cell activation than the unmodified molecule.

To determine the nature of T cell reactivity to modified insulins peritoneal exudate T lymphocytes from B10 mice immune to beef insulin or TNP-OVA were tested for their reactivity to modified or unmodified insulin. As shown in Table IV, T cells immune to the control antigen do not respond when stimulated with either form of beef insulin. When immune to beef insulin a good response is obtained with both modified and unmodified insulin. The response to modified insulin is always greater than that of the unmodified molecule. This increased ability of modified insulins to activate T cells is seen in all strains tested. In addition, it does not appear to be specific for TNP-modification since other haptens produce the same result.

Table IV. Proliferative Response of Peritoneal Exudate T Lymphocytes[a]

Antigen in Culture	TNP-OVA Immune $\Delta CPM \times 10^{-3}$	Beef Insulin Immune $\Delta CPM \times 10^{-3}$
TNP-OVA	58.8 ± 2.2[b]	0.2 ± 1.4
Beef Insulin	.055 ± 1.1	52.3 ± 7.5
TNP Beef Insulin	.06 ± 2.2	83.7 ± 9.3
PPD	51.7 ± 0.35	45.3 ± 0.8

[a]Oil induced PETELES as described in Methods.

[b]Mean ± SEM ($\times 10^{-3}$) of three experiments.

When the reciprocal experiments were performed in which mice were immunized with TNP-modified insulin, the modified insulin was again more stimulatory. However, the degree of difference was no more than that seen when animals were immunized with unmodified insulin. Thus, T cell proliferation does not appear capable of detecting neoantigenic determinants on the haptenated insulin molecule. Other mechanisms must be proposed in order to explain the augmented T cell reactivity to modified insulins.

Modified insulins may effect important regulatory mechanisms of the insulin immune response.

Since perturbation of the molecule alone could not account for the poor anti-insulin response, we have studied the influence of pretreatment of various insulin preparations on the subsequent anti-insulin response. Table V shows the results in mice pretreated with soluble insulin, insulin ester, TNP-insulin, or saline alone which were subsequently immunized with insulin in CFA. Unmodified insulin was injected intraperitoneally in 0.5 cc of saline in order to avoid hypoglycemia. The beef insulin ester used was prepared by the same procedure used for coupling insulin to SRBC (5), and was given intravenously.

Table V. Modified Insulins Induce Non-Responsiveness in Responder (H-2^d) Mice[a]

Pretreatment	Day 0 Immunization	D7 α Insulin PFC/10^6 LNL	D14 α Insulin PFC/10^6 LNL
Beef Insulin	CFA Beef Insulin	231.6 (1.67)[b]	30.3 (1.47)
TNP-Beef Insulin	"	19.2 (1.34)	41.6 (1.41)
Ester of Beef Insulin	"	3.7 (1.9)	16.9 (1.84)
Saline Control	"	<1	301.6 (1.10)

[a] 4 mice in each group were pre-injected with the appropriate modified insulin, 7 days later they were immunized with unmodified insulin in CFA and PFC determined one and two weeks later.

[b] Geometric mean and standard errors (x/÷).

Pretreatment of mice with saline does not alter the subsequent response to insulin in CFA which peaks 14 days after immunization. However, pretreatment with unmodified insulin in saline is shown to prime these animals for an augmented response on day 7 (column one). This is in contrast to the data of Tada et al. who were able to induce suppression by carrier priming (7). More interesting still is the ability of both ester and TNP modified forms of insulin to prevent a subsequent response to insulin in CFA. A kinetic analysis has failed to show a normal peak response over a 3-4 week period. One should note however that some degree of priming does take place with the modified insulin, for under normal circumstances no detectable PFC are detected at the early points in time. Nonetheless modified insulins do tend to tip the balance of the anti-insulin response downward. Currently, studies are underway using adoptive transfer techniques to identify the cell(s) responsible for this unresponsiveness.

Discussion

In order to attain a more basic understanding of the genetic and cellular mechanisms controlling immune responsiveness we have evaluated the influence of antigen modification upon the immune response to insulin. The genetics of anti-TNP responses of TNP-beef or TNP-pork insulin are similar in some but not all aspects of the responses previously reported with unmodified insulin. The high responder status of $H\text{-}2^d$ mice to beef and pork insulin, and $H\text{-}2^b$ mice to beef insulin is preserved. However, there is a difference in the absoluteness of the response since low but easily detectable levels of anti-hapten PFC are demonstrable in strains which do not produce anti-insulin PFC. This difference is most striking when the animals bear C3H background genes. Recently, strains which are pretreated with "nonresponder insulin" have been found to be primed for an augmented response to insulin to which they respond (8,9). These observations would imply that some degree of helper differentiation is present even though an antibody response is not detected. In the case of anti-TNP responses such low level helper cells are potentially able to activate the anti-TNP precursor B cells. C3H mice could be even more easily activated because of the intrinsic nature of their B cell pool. Another explanation could be the creation of neoantigenic determinants via the modification procedure.

The creation of hapten specific T cell determinants has been described when the antigen modified is closely analogous to the animals own protein (10). In attempts to identify such determinants we studied the proliferative reactivity of immune T cells. Modification was found to augment the proliferative response _in vitro_ even if the immunizing antigen was not modified. This augmentation has prevented identification of a neoantigenic determinant via T cell proliferation.

In studying the PFC response of high responder mice immunized with TNP-insulin it was observed that the anti-insulin response was greatly reduced. In order to study the influence of modified insulins on the insulin specific response various pretreatment regimens were employed. Preinjection of carrier alone was found to prime for an accelerated anti-insulin PFC response. However, animals pretreated with soluble hydrosuccinimide-insulin ester or TNP-insulin were subsequently found to be hyporesponsive when immunized with insulin in CFA. On-going studies indicate that suppressor cells may be at least in part responsible for this reduced responsiveness. Modified insulins may reset the balance between helper events leading to antibody production and suppressor events which down regulate these responses. This could take place through the creation of suppressor determinants or perhaps from alteration of the normal helper determinants. These possibilities and others will require elucidation before the complexities of Ir gene function controlling the response to insulin can be fully understood.

References

1. Keck, K.: Nature 254, 78 (1975).
2. Barcinski, M.A., Rosenthal, A.S.: J. Exp. Med. 145, 726 (1977).
3. Rosenwasser, L.J., Barcinski, M.A., Schwartz, R.H., and

Rosenthal, A.S.: J. Immunol. 123, 471 (1979).

4. Kapp, J.A., Strayer, D.S., Robbins, P.F., and Perlmutter, R.M.: J. Immunol. 123, 109 (1979).

5. Schroer, J.A., Inman, J.K., Thomas, J.W., and Rosenthal, A.S.: J. Immunol. 123, 670 (1979).

6. Schwartz, R.H., Jackson, L., and Paul, W.E.: J. Immunol. 115, 1330 (1975).

7. Tada, T., Takemori, T.: J. Exp. Med. 140, 239 (1974).

8. Cohen, I.R., Talmon, J.: Eur. J. Immunol. 10, 284 (1980).

9. Bucy, R.P., Kapp, J.A.: Submitted for publication (1980).

10. Yamamoto, H., Hamoka, T., Yoshizwa, M., Kuroki, M., and Kitagawa, M.: J. Exp. Med. 146, 74 (1977).

FUNCTION AND COMPLEMENTATION OF Ir GENES CONTROLLING THE RESPONSIVENESS OF MICE TO INSULIN

E. Spaeth*), H. Stötter, A. Reske-Kunz, F. Zimmermann, E. Rüde
Institut für Immunologie der Joh. Gutenberg Universität,
D-6500 Mainz, FRG

H.J. Hedrich
Zentralinstitut für Versuchstiere
D-3000 Hannover, FRG

Introduction

The function of Ir genes is of remarkable specificity for the respective antigen. It has, therefore, been explained by an influence of Ir genes on the specificity of the antigen receptors of T cells. Recently, indirect mechanisms have been proposed for such a function of the Ir gene products which are assumed to be identical with the Ia antigens. It was suggested that in the thymic environment MHC antigens act by selecting somatic variants of T cell receptors, resulting in a limited range of specificities of the differentiated T cells for external antigens combined with a restriction specificity for the respective MHC haplotype (1). Alternatively, it has been proposed that Ir gene products or Ia antigens expressed in macrophages select the determinants of an antigen molecule which are presented to T cells (2, 3). These models in their simplest form would suggest that either functional T cells with receptors for a non-permissive antigen do not exist or effective presentation of the antigen is not possible. If,

*) This work was carried out in partial fulfillment of the requirement for a doctoral thesis at the University of Mainz D77

however, T cell functions for a normally non-permissive antigen could be detected in non-responder mice, more complicated mechanisms for Ir gene function have to be considered.

Results and Discussion

1) Detection of pig insulin specific helper T cells in low responder mice of $H-2^b$ haplotype. Although direct immunization of low or non-responder mice does not lead to a detectable activation of T helper cells or T cells mediating delayed type hypersensitivity, there are some indications that T cells capable of interacting with a non-permissive antigen might exist in certain low responder strains (4 - 7). In order to test whether functional T cells potentially reactive with a non-permissive antigen can be detected in non-responder mice, it was tried to activate such cells indirectly via immunization with a cross-reactive but permissive antigen.

For such studies bovine and pig insulins were used in an in vitro helper assay: nylon wool enriched T cells from mice primed with one of the insulins were co-cultivated with DNP-KLH primed spleen cells (DNP-primed "B" cells) and restimulated in vitro with the DNP-conjugate of bovine or pig insulin. DNP-specific IgG plaques were determined. With T cells from (C3H x B10)F_1 hybrids, which are capable of responding to both antigens, the insulins were found to cross-react completely (Fig. 1). Using B10 mice, which are responders to bovine insulin but non-responders to pig insulin, no response was observed upon priming with pig insulin, as expected. However, upon priming with bovine insulin a significant restimulation of T helper cells was not only seen with the homologous conjugate but also with the DNP-conjugate of the non-permissive pig insulin (Fig. 1). Thus, T helper cells capable of recognizing at least certain determinants of pig insulin must be present in non-responder H-2^b mice. Furthermore, the detection of functional T helper cells implies that low responder macrophages must be capable of presenting pig insulin for the restimulation of the primed T cells, since there is ample evidence that the secondary in vitro response of T cells is macrophage-dependent.

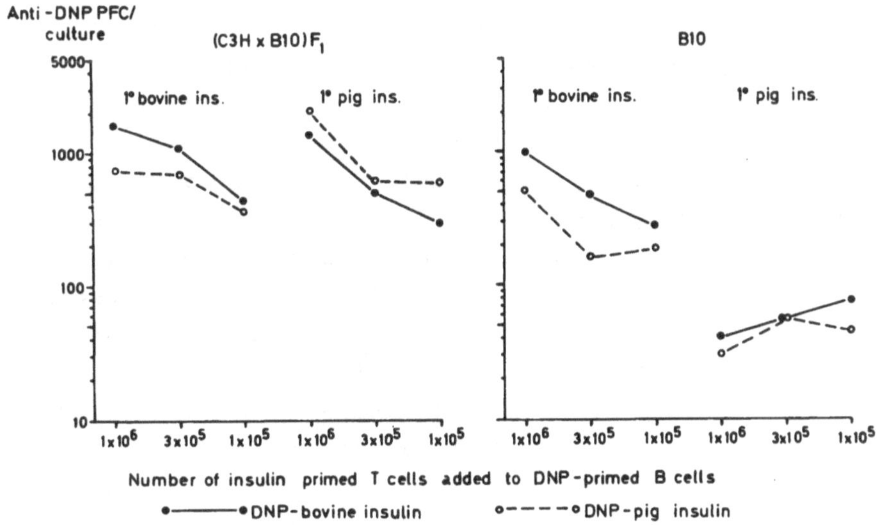

Fig. 1: Reciprocal cross-stimulation of primed T helper cells by bovine and pig insulin.
Nylon wool purified lymph node T cells primed in vivo with bovine or pig insulin were co-cultivated with spleen cells (3 x 10^6/culture) from mice primed and re-immunized 7 days before culture with DNP-KLH (DNP-primed "B" cells). The cells were restimulated with 1 µg/ml of either DNP-bovine or pig insulin. IgG anti-DNP plaque forming cells were determined on day 4.

This result is in agreement with and explains previous findings of Keck (8). In these experiments an anti-hapten response could be induced in H-2^b mice with a hapten-conjugate of the non-permissive pig insulin if this conjugate was injected together with the permissive bovine insulin.

Furthermore, functional T helper cells could be detected in low responder mice to synthetic polypeptide antigens using the same experimental approach as described here (9).

On the other hand, analogous experiments in which the cross-stimulation of closely related permissive and non-permissive antigens was assayed by T cell proliferation led to the conclusion that for a cross-reaction to occur, it was necessary that the mouse strain was of responder type not only for the priming antigen but also for the antigen used for the secondary stimulation (10). The same observation was made with T cells of B10 ($H-2^b$) mice primed with bovine insulin. In proliferation assays these cells could not be significantly cross-stimulated by pig insulin (data not shown). An obvious explanation for this apparent discrepancy between T helper and proliferation tests would be that the former, especially in the form used in this study, is more sensitive than the latter. Another interesting possibility to explain this discrepancy is based on the observation that two subsets of T cells may be required to provide help at different stages of B cell activation, i.e. induction of proliferation and B cell differentiation to Ig secretion (11). Since in the experiments described here primed B cells restimulated in vivo 7 days before culture (12) were employed, mainly the second subset of T helper cells may be effective in the co-operation with "pre-induced" B cells. Possibly T cells of this subset can be restimulated to a sufficient extent also by a non-permissive antigen, whereas priming of these cells occurs via the cross-reacting but permissive antigen.

According to the experimental data obtained it appears not very likely that low responsiveness to pig insulin in $H-2^b$ mice is due to the absence of T helper cells, at least of one subset, capable of recognizing this non-permissive antigen. The question rather arises why such T helper cells are not activated during primary immunization. One possibility is that helper cell induction requires an interaction of T cell subpopulations as, for instance, the activation of T inducer cells which, by production of Interleukin 2, cooperate in the induction of T helper cells from their precursors (13). The regulatory function of Ir genes would then mainly influence the stimulation of the inducer cell or the interaction of the T cells, whereas if these steps can be bypassed by cross-priming with a permissive antigen, functional T helper cells can be detected.

Evidence for T-T interactions has recently been described for the delayed-type hypersensitivity response to the polypeptide (T,G)-A--L (14). In the case of insulin the recognition of at least two different "carrier" determinants by T cells has been postulated to be of importance for the induction of an antibody response (8). Alternatively, the results described here could be explained by the preferential induction of suppression during primary immunization with the non-permissive pig insulin. Again, such suppressive effects could be bypassed if priming is carried out with a permissive antigen carrying cross-reactive determinants. No evidence has yet been obtained supporting this possibility, although with certain antigens and mice of certain H-2 haplotypes low responsiveness could be associated with suppression (5, 6, 15).

2) <u>Complementation of Ir genes controlling the immune response of mice to pig insulin</u>. The ability of F_1 hybrids of the mouse strains C57BL/10 (B10) and C3H to mount an antibody response to pig insulin was found by K. Keck (8) to depend on the complementation of Ir genes associated with the parental $H\text{-}2^b$ and $H\text{-}2^k$ haplotypes. In addition, genetic factors of the C3H background seem to be involved, since (B10 x B10.BR)F_1 hybrids did not produce significant amounts of antibody (8). This system of complementing Ir genes was chosen for further studies on the expression of Ir genes in

T cells and/or macrophages and for studying cross-reactivities.

The test system used was the antigen induced secondary proliferation of T cells in vitro as measured by the incorporation of tritiated thymidine. Mice were primed with insulin in complete Freund's adjuvant subcutaneously and after seven days T cells from the draining lymph nodes were purified by passage through nylon wool for the stimulation experiments.

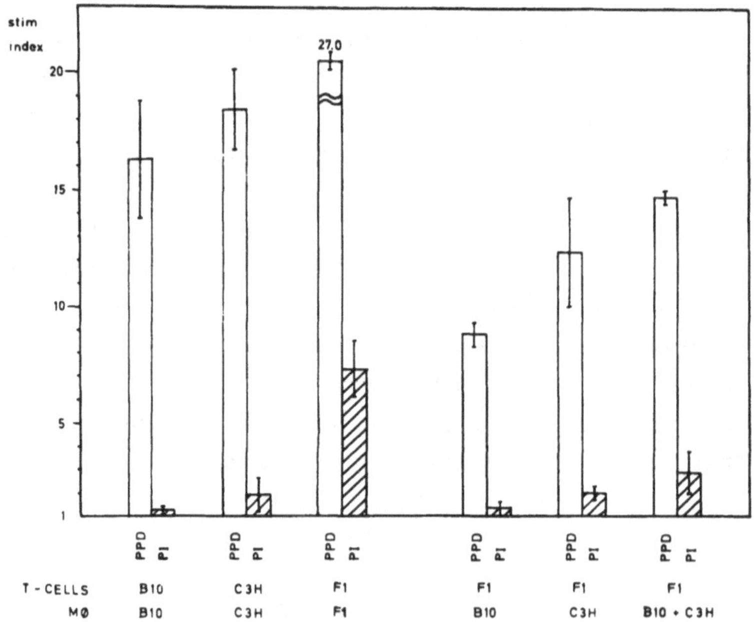

Fig. 2: Ir gene complementation in responsiveness of mice to pig insulin:
Nylon wool purified lymph node T cells (2 x 10^5/culture) from mice primed with pig insulin (PI) in complete Freund's adjuvant were added to irradiated spleen cells (4 x 10^5/culture) as a source of macrophages and were restimulated by 100 µg/ml of pig insulin or by PPD as a control. T cell proliferation was measured by incorporation of ^{3}H-thymidine. Arithmetic means of quadruplicate cultures were calculated and expressed as stimulation ratio.

The results of such experiments confirmed that mice of H-2^b and H-2^k haplotypes are non-responders to pig insulin while H-$2^{b/k}$ heterozygotes responded to this antigen (Fig. 2). No influence of the C3H background was observed since (B10 x C3H) and (B10 x B10.BR)F_1 hybrids responded to a comparable extent (Fig. 3). Furthermore, in helper assays of the type described above, no significant difference between pig insulin primed T cells from (B10 x C3H) and (B10 x B10.BR)F_1 hybrids was found in their capacity to provide help for the induction of anti-DNP responses (data not shown). The apparent discrepancy between these results and those obtained by testing for antibody production in vivo (8) could be due

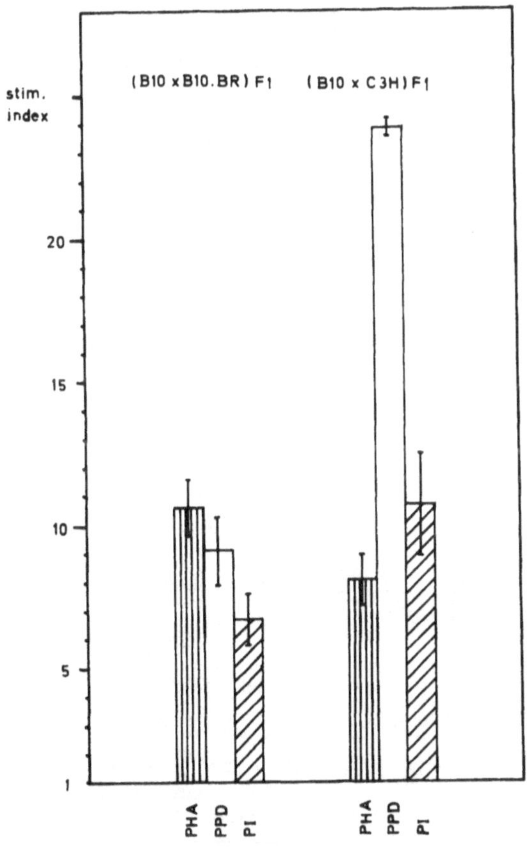

Fig. 3: Localization of the complementating Ir genes in the H-2 complex; independence of the C3H genetic backbround. Restimulation of pig insulin (PI) primed T cells as measured by ^{3}H-thymidine incorporation was carried out as described in Fig. 2.

to the influence of C3H background genes, for instance of immunoglobulin genes, on the ability of B cells to respond to pig insulin.

Mapping of the complementing Ir genes was carried out by testing F_1 hybrids derived from several H-2 recombinant strains as shown in Fig. 4. It can be concluded from the data obtained that these genes map to the left of the $I\text{-}B^b$ and $I\text{-}B^k$ subregions, most probably in the A subregions of the two haplotypes. In more recent experiments, using (B10.A(5R) x A.TL) and (B10.A(5R) x A.TH)F_1 hybrids, the K^k region could also be excluded, because the former showed positive and the latter negative reactions. This confirms the mapping of one of the genes in the A^k subregion. Very few examples of A/A-subregion complementation, so-called β-β complementation (15), have been described based on antibody production in vivo. Only very recently it was pos-

	MHC - REGIONS										
	K	A	B	J	E	C	S	G	D	response	complementing subregions
4R x	k	k	b	b	b	b	b	b	b	–	not $I\text{-}B^b$ to D^b
C3H	k	k	k	k	k	k	k	k	k		⇒ K^b and/or $I\text{-}A^b$
4R x	k	k	b	b	b	b	b	b	b	+	K^k and/or $I\text{-}A^k$
CSW	b	b	b	b	b	b	b	b	b		
3R x	b	b	b	b	k	d	d	d	d	+	K^b to $I\text{-}J^b$
C3H	k	k	k	k	k	k	k	k	k		
3R x	b	b	b	b	k	d	d	d	d	–	not $I\text{-}E^k$
CSW	b	b	b	b	b	b	b	b	b		

Fig. 4: Mapping of the complementing Ir genes within the H-2 complex by assaying for T cell proliferation in vitro (see Fig. 2). H-2 haplotypes of F_1 hybrids immunized with pig insulin are listed; + indicates stimulation rates $\geq$ 3, - indicates stimulation ratios $\leq$ 2.

sible to demonstrate this phenomenon also at the T cell level using the polypeptide antigen G-A--L in the proliferation assay (16).

It was of particular interest to test in this system whether pig insulin could be presented to primed F_1 T cells only by F_1 or also by parental macrophages. The results of such experiments (Fig.2) demonstrate that only weak stimulations, which cannot be considered as significant, were observed with each of the parental macrophages or a mixture of the parental macrophages. On the other hand, highly significant stimulation was seen with F_1 macrophages. Thus, both parental Ir genes must be expressed in the antigen-presenting macrophages for the induction of T cell proliferation. This could be explained by the assumption that only F_1 macrophages can present pig insulin in a correct way because of the presence of Ia structures resulting from an interaction of products coded for by the complementing Ir genes. Alternatively, all clones of F_1 T cells which are specific for pig insulin are at the same time restricted for a complementing Ia-structure which is expressed only on F_1 macrophages, although the parental macrophages can possibly also present pig insulin as indicated by the experiments reported above.

The requirements for an F_1 restriction specificity of T cells and its relation to the role of the thymus in the ability to respond to pig insulin was studied in thymusless (C57BL/6 x C3H)F_1 hybrid mice. These mice were reconstituted with either parental or F_1 thymus.

Each nude mouse at the age of 6 - 8 weeks received two neonotal thymi of either one parental type, of both parental types, or of F_1 type. The thymi were implanted subcutaneously in the shoulder region. After 60 - 70 days the animals were immunized with pig insulin in complete Freund's adjuvant into the foot pads and the T cell proliferation assay was carried out as usual .

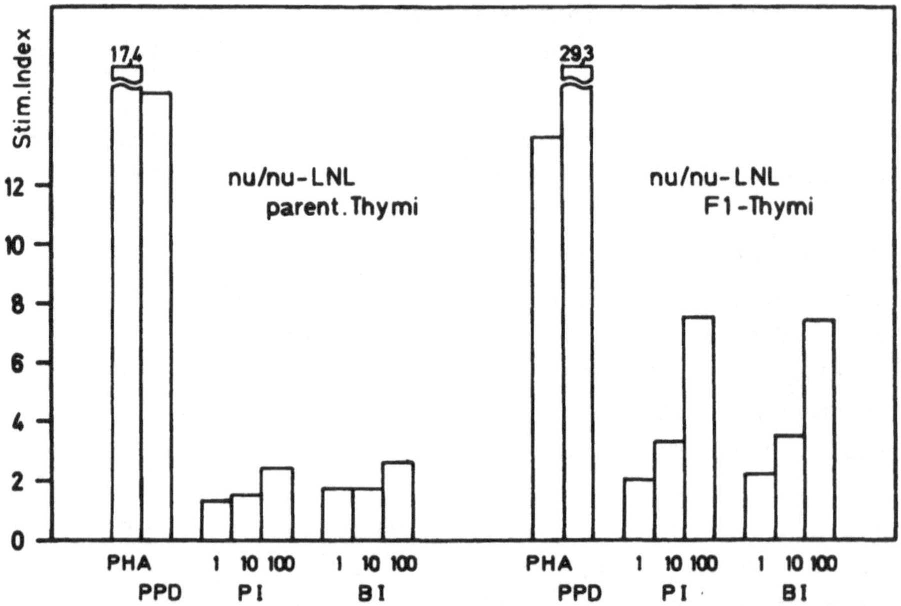

Fig. 5: Responses of (C57BL/6 x C3H)F_1 nude mice reconstituted with either both parental thymi or two F_1-thymi to pig insulin. Primed T cells were restimulated in vitro with three doses (1, 10 and 100 µg/ml) of the homologous pig insulin (PI) or bovine insulin (BI) and with PPD and PHA as controls. T cell proliferation was measured by incorporation of ^{3}H-thymidine and results expressed as stimulation ratios.

The results of a typical experiment are presented in Fig.5. The cells of F_1 nude mice reconstituted simultaneously with both parental thymi (C57BL/6, H-2^b and C3H, H-2^k) and immunized with pig insulin showed only a weak response of borderline significance when rechallenged in vitro with either pig or bovine insulin. Upon reconstitution with F_1 thymi a response comparable to that of normal mice was obtained. Both types of reconstituted nude mice showed strong responses with PPD or PHA, indicating that reconstitution was successful in both cases.

This result shows that T cell precursors of the complementing F_1 genotype which differentiated in both parental thymi respond very poorly to pig insulin, although F_1-type macrophages, which in the previous experiments (Fig.2) were found to be important for the presentation of pig insulin, were present in these animals. This indicates that the presentation of pig insulin on F_1 macrophages alone is not sufficient for the induction of a significant response, even though the F_1 T cells are presumably restricted for the two parental I region haplotypes expressed on the F_1 macrophages. It rather appears to be important that the T cells of the F_1 genotype also differentiate in an F_1 thymus. One can expect that this leads to the selection of T cell clones which are restricted for an F_1-specific Ia determinant resulting from trans-complementation between $I\text{-}A^k$ and $I\text{-}A^b$ subregions in form of hybrid molecules. The existence of such F_1-specific determinants has also been inferred from the specificity of certain alloreactive T cell clones and some biochemical evidence supporting the existence of hybrid molecules has been obtained (17).

As shown recently in studies with nude mice, the function of the thymus is not required for the differentiation of T cells which can develop into TNP-specific cytotoxic T cells restricted for their own K and D subregion antigens (18,19). One could assume that such self-restricted T cells, in our case for a hybrid Ia determinant, are potentially also present in the (C57BL/6 x C3H)F_1 nudes. If reconstitution with a thymus would only have a hormonal influence on the differentiation and/or expansion of these self-restricted T cells one could expect to find reactivity to pig insulin not only in those nude mice reconstituted with the F_1 thymus but also in those reconstituted with one or both parental thymi. Therefore, the F_1 thymus appears to have at least a selective function in the development of F_1 hybrid restricted T cells and concomitantly responsiveness to pig insulin.

Acknowledgements

This work was supported by a grant of the Deutsche Forschungsgemeinschaft SFB 107 (Mainz).

References

1. von Boehmer, H., Haas, W., and Jerne, N.K.: Proc. Nat. Acad. Sci. USA 75, 2439 (1978).
2. Rosenthal, A.S.: Immunol. Rev. 40, 136 (1978).
3. Schwartz, R.H., Yano, A., and Paul, W.E.: Immunol. Rev. 40, 153 (1978).
4. Howie, S., Feldmann, M., Mozes, E., and Maurer, B.H.: Immunology 32, 291 (1977).
5. Araneo, B.A., Jowell, R.L., and Sercarz, E.E.: J. Immunol. 123, 961 (1979).
6. Kapp, J.A., Pierce, C.W., and Benacerraf, B.: J. exp. Med. 142, 50 (1975).
7. Cohen, I.R., and Talmon, J.: Eur. J. Immunol. 10, 284 (1980).
8. Keck, K.: Eur. J. Immunol. 7, 811 (1977).
9. Stötter, H., and Rüde, E.: Immunobiology 156, 221 (1979).
10. Schwartz, R.H., Horton, C.L., and Paul, W.E.: J. exp. Med. 145, 327 (1977)
11. Keller, D.M., Swierkosz, J.E., Marrack, P., and Kappler J.W.: J. Immunol. 124, 1350 (1980).
12. North, J.R., and Maizels,R.M.: Immunology 32, 771 (1977).
13. Stötter, H., Rüde, E., and Wagner, H.: Eur. J. Immunol. 10, 719 (1980).
14. Strassmann, G., Eshhar, Z., and Mozes, E.: J. exp. Med. 151, 628 (1980).
15. Benacerraf, B., and Dorf, M.E.: Cold Spring Harbor Symposia on Quant. Biol. XLI, Part 2, 465 (1976).
16. Solinger, A.M., and Schwartz, R.H.: J. Immunol. 124, 2485 (1980).
17. Fathman, C.G.: Transplantation 30, 1 - 4 (1980).
18. Hünig, T., and Bevan, M.J.: J. exp. Med. 152, 688 (1980).
19. Wagner, H., Hardt, C., Bartlett, R., Pfizenmaier, K., Röllinghoff, M., and Heeg, K.: Behring Institute Mitteilungen (1980), in press

THE XID GENE CONTROLS Ia.W39 ASSOCIATED IMMUNE RESPONSE GENE FUNCTION FOR INSULIN INDUCED T CELL ACTIVATION

L.J. Rosenwasser and B.T. Huber

Allergy Division, Department of Medicine, CRC, Department of Pathology, Tufts University School of Medicine, Boston, Massachusetts 02111, U.S.A.

Introduction

The control of the expression of major histocompatibility complex (MHC) linked immune response (Ir) gene function and its mechanism remain an area of intense research and speculation in the understanding of antigen mediated immune response (1). Over the years, an attractive hypothesis has emerged which suggests that the antigenic determinants involved in stimulating specific primed helper, delayed type hypersensitivity, or proliferating T cell clones are a complex of antigen fragment in association with the glycoprotein alloantigens, the immune response associated (Ia) molecules. This functional complex of antigen fragment and Ia is suitably displayed to T cells by antigen presenting cells of variable origin including some that are of mononuclear phagocyte (MØ) lineage. Previous work with insulin has contributed much to our present understanding of the nature and mechanism of Ir gene function in antigen recognition (2-5). For example, MHC linked Ir genes control the murine T cell proliferative response of $H\text{-}2^b$ mice to beef insulin (6). This control is dependent on a determinant selection process expressed by the Ia positive antigen presenting MØ and maps to the K^b and/or $1\text{-}A^b$ subregion(s) of the H-2 gene complex.

Mutant CBA/N mice possess on X-linked recessive defect, which has been recently mapped (xid) (7). This xid gene regulates the expression of the late appearing B cell differentiation antigens Lyb3, Lyb5, Lyb7, and the newly defined Ia.W39. Recently, Ia.W39, a new private specificity of $I\text{-}A^b$, has been described (8). It is selectively expressed on a functional subset of B cells in mice of the $H\text{-}2^b$ haplotype, which is absent in newborn normal and adult mutant mice carrying the xid gene. Furthermore,

Basic and Clinical Aspects of Immunity to Insulin

this Ia molecule is synthesized in the cytoplasm of B cell in xid defective and neonatal normal mice, although it is not expressed on the B cell membrane (9). Biochemical studies have revealed that Ia.W39 has a similar 2-chain structure as the conventional Ia molecule, but data from several experiments suggest that Ia.W39 is expressed independently from the classical Ia specificities encoded by the I-A^b subregion of the MHC (9). This Ia molecule with its unique specificity and selective expression represents a potentially powerful probe in the dissection of the specific mechanism of Ir gene function for beef insulin in the H-2^b mouse.

The experiments described in this report have unequivocally shown, using different approaches, that the responsiveness to beef insulin in the H-2^b haplotype is dependent on the expression of Ia.W39 on antigen presenting MØ. Moreover, we have demonstrated for the first time a specific non-MHC gene (xid) linked regulation of an H-2 linked Ir gene function.

Materials and Methods

Animals: C57 Bl 6/J (B6) mice were purchased from Jackson Laboratories, Bar Harbor, ME. (CBA/N x C57 Bl 6)F_1 (N x B6)F_1, and (C57 Bl 6 x CBA/N)F_1 (B6 x N)F_1 mice were bred in the animal facilities at Tufts University School of Medicine from breeding stock originally obtained from the National Institutes of Health.

Antigens: Beef and pork insulin were obtained from Eli Lilly and Co., Indianapolis, IN. and were the kind gifts of Dr. Alan S. Rosenthal of Merck, Sharp and Dohme, Rahway, New Jersey. Both beef and pork insulin contained less than 0.05% of proinsulin contamination.

Alloantisera: Anti I-A^b alloantisera, (A x B10.A)F_1 anti B10.A (5R) was obtained from the Research Resource Branch, National Institute of Allergy and Infectious Disease, and its anti-K^b activity was absorbed with E1-4 tumor cells. Anti-Ia.W39 was prepared by immunizing (N x B6)F_1 male mice with B6 spleen cells, as previously described (8). Normal mouse sera (NMS) from non immune (N x B6)F_1 mice was used as a control.

Immunization, Cell culture techniques, antigen pulsing techniques: These methods are well described and are previously published (6,10-13).

Results

Effect of anti-Ia sera on the insulin specific T cell proliferative response. The ability of anti Ia.W39 serum to block insulin specific T cell proliferation in B6 mice was tested. As can be seen in Table I, experiment 1, 1% anti-Ia.W39 serum markedly inhibited beef insulin induced proliferation (89%) and to a lesser extent PPD induced cell division (62%). Anti I-A^b serum also significantly blocked both beef insulin (89%) and PPD (100%) induced activation.

TABLE I

Effect of Anti-Ia Sera on Proliferative Responses of B6 T Cells[a]

	HTdR incorp.[b] Δcpm	
Exp: 1	Beef Insulin - 100ug/ml	PPD - 10ug/ml
1% NMS	11,901	10,055
1% α Ia.W39	1,287	3,786
Exp: 2	Beef Insulin - 100ug/ml	PPD - 10ug/ml
1% NMS	19,463	12,727
1% α I-A^b	3,190	0

a - 2 x 10^5 LNL T cells 5 x 10^4 AAC (MØ) per well cultured for 4 days in round bottom microtiter plates

b - Δcpm= Experimental (Ag) - Control (No Ag)

Immune proliferative response of normal and xid defective F_1 mice to beef insulin. A series of experiments is summarized in Table II which depicts the comparative ability of beef insulin primed T cells from normal

(N x B6)F_1 female and (B6 x N)F_1 male mice and from defective (N x B6)F_1 male mice to respond to beef and pork insulin and other immunogens[b]. Both normal (N x B6)F_1 ♀ and (B6 x N)F_1♂ mice mounted a good T cell response to beef insulin with very little cross reaction to pork insulin stimulation (indicative of H-2^b type recognition of the A chain loop determinant within beef insulin). The xid defective (N x B6)F_1♂ mice, however, could not develop a significant primed T cell proliferative response to beef insulin. All three groups of mice made comparable responses to TNP-OVA and PPD. Since the defective F_1♂ mice express all conventional Ia^b specificities but lack Ia.W39, the striking conclusion offered by these data is that beef insulin responsiveness in the H-2^b mouse is associated with the expression of Ia.W39.

TABLE II

Proliferative Response of Immune F_1 T Cells[a]

^{3}HTdR Incorp.[b]
(Δcpm $\pm$ SEM) x 10^3[c]

	(N x B6)F_1 ♀	(N x B6)F_1 ♂	(B6 x N)F_1 ♂
Beef Insulin 100ug/ml	12.28 ± 2.74	2.30 ± 0.69	12.31 ± 4.86
Pork Insulin 100ug/ml	2.51 ± 0.91	1.33 ± 0.47	2.64 ± 1.32
TNP-OVA 200ug/ml	49.68 ± 3.73	42.08 ± 5.69	N.D.[d]
PPD 10ug/ml	6.98 ± 1.10	4.91 ± 1.29	7.58 ± 2.72

a - Usual proliferative technique as in Table I

b - Mean (Δcpm ± SEM) x 10^{-3} for 4 experiments

c - Control Baselines: (N x B6)F_1 ♀: 3.45 ± 1.16
(N x B6)F_1♂: 3.37 ± 1.66
(B6 x N)F_1♂: 2.12 ± 1.19

d - Not done

Response of immune F_1 female T cells to antigen pulsed presenting cells. Potential cellular defects in the beef insulin response of (N x B6)F_1 male mice were probed by comparing the ability of antigen (beef insulin) pulsed MØ from xid defective F_1 male and normal F_1 female mice to activate syngeneic F_1 female T cells, immune to beef insulin and CFA. As is shown in Table III, the F_1 female MØ presented beef insulin to the immune T cells, while the F_1 male MØ, pulsed with beef insulin, were unable to induce proliferation in the same group of T cells. Although a T cell defect cannot be ruled out, these data infer that the <u>xid</u> associated unresponsiveness to beef insulin is at the level of the antigen presenting cell which lacks Ia.W39 determinants. In controls not shown, both male and female F_1 MØ, pulsed with PPD and TNP-OVA, activated the primed T cells significantly.

TABLE III

Response of Immune (N x B6)F_1 Female T Cells to Antigen Pulsed Adherent Presenting Cells[a]

Ag Pulsed MØ[c] (AAC)	^{3}HTdR incorp.[b] (Δcpm ± SEM) x 10^{-3}
F_1 ♀ Beef Insulin	11.09 ± 0.58
F_1 ♂ Beef Insulin	1.77 ± 0.62

a) - 5 x 10^4 MØ (AAC) ± antigen pulse mixed with 2 x 10^5 LNL T cells per well cultured for 4 days in round bottom microtiter plates.

b) - Δcpm = Ag pulsed MØ activation of LNL T cells - Media pulsed MØ activation of LNL T cells.

<u>Ontogeny of presenting cell competence for beef insulin is Ia.W39 related.</u> Expression of Ia.W39 on the B cell membrane is not evident until 21 days after birth, while conventional Ia is present on B cells from neonatal mice. With this in mind, we compared the ability of MØ from neonatal (8 days old) and adult (N x B6)F_1 female mice to present beef insulin to adult primed syngeneic T cells. As can be seen in Table IV, the neonatal MØ were specifically deficient in presenting beef insulin, while presenting TNP-OVA efficiently. The adult MØ were able to present both

antigens. These results highlight once again the association of Ia.W39 with beef insulin responsiveness at the level of the antigen presenting MØ.

TABLE IV

Response of Immune Adult (N x B6)F_1 Female T Cells to Antigen Pulsed Adherent Presenting Cells[a]

Ag Pulsed MØ (AAC)	^{3}HTdR incorp.[b] Δcpm
Adult F_1 ♀ Beef Insulin	9,064
Adult F_1 ♀ TNP-OVA	20,339
Neonatal F_1 ♀ Beef Insulin	0
Neonatal F_1 ♀ TNP-OVA	21,753

a) - Usual proliferative technique as described in Table III

b) - Δcpm = Ag pulsed MØ activation of LNL T Cells - Media pulsed MØ activation of LNL T cells
Baseline: spontaneous incorp. of ^{3}HTdR in cultures of MØ (AAC) and LNL T cells without Ag Pulse (cpm)
Control Baseline: Adult F_1 ♀ MØ (AAC): 1,157 ± 398
Neonatal F_1 ♀ MØ (AAC): 883 ± 243.

Discussion

With the preceding experiments we have shown that monospecific anti-Ia.W39 serum could block beef insulin induced T cell proliferation in H-2^b mice. Conventional anti-I-A^b serum also blocked beef insulin T cell proliferation; however, it should be noted that the anti-I-A^b antisera may contain anti-Ia.W39 antibodies. This is a likely possiblity, since it was found in immunoprecipitation experiments that anti-I-A^b serum could preclear Ia.W39, but not vice versa (9). Over the years, on the basis of multiple studies in both mice and guinea pigs, it has been implied that alloantisera blockade is at the level of the antigen presenting MØ (14,15). It therefore follows from these blocking experiments that Ia.W39, a B cell differentiation marker expressed an a subpopulation of B cells, is also functionally expressed by antigen presenting MØ.

With a different approach, we have shown that beef insulin responsiveness is associated with the expression of Ia.W39, by demonstrating that normal (N x B6)F_1 female and (B6 x N)F_1 male mice as opposed to defective (N x B6)F_1 male mice could mount a T cell proliferative response to beef insulin. The same pattern was seen in the secondary IgG plaque forming cell (PFC) response to beef insulin, measured in these groups of mice (Huber and Rosenwasser, manuscript in preparation). Furthermore, we have shown that defective F_1 male MØ cannot present beef insulin to responder F_1 female beef insulin primed T cells.

Finally, we have shown that neonatal antigen presenting MØ, which presumably do not acquire Ia.W39 until 21 days after birth but have conventional Ia antigens analogous to neonatal B cells, are deficient in presenting beef insulin to primed adult T cells, again suggesting the association on Ia.W39 with beef insulin responsiveness at the level of the MØ. It is reasonable to infer from our stuides that neonatal MØ acquire the ability to present insulin as they acquire Ia.W39; therefore, it may be likely that functional maturation and acquisition of Ia.W39 and perhaps all other Ia molecules by antigen presenting MØ may be under the influence of X-linked regulatory gene(s).

In sum, we have found in (N x B6)F_1 male mice a defect in insulin related Ir gene function and expression of Ia.W39 on antigen presenting MØ. In the xid defective (N x B6)F_1 male B cells, it is felt that lack of Ia.W39 represents a maturation arrest in the differentiation pathway, where certain subsets of B cells do not develop. By analogy, the mechanism of xid regulated defective Ir gene function may be due to deletion or faulty maturation of a subpopulation of antigen presenting MØ or alternatively, a selective defect in Ia.W39 expression on the MØ membrane may be evident on all Ia bearing MØ. The molecular mechanism of this xid regulated Ir gene deficit is unknown and investigation in this area may provide a key to the precise workings of Ir genes. Another potential point of interest that is immediately apparent is whether this xid regulatory gene is operative in other haplotypes as a general regulatory phenomenon.

Two further points should be made concerning the results reported here. First, the data in this paper highlight the strong association of the Ia.W39 specificity with Ir gene function for beef insulin in $H-2^b$ mice. Other examples of the association of Ia antigens with Ir gene functions have been documented in previous studies in both guinea pigs and mice (16, 17). Second, these findings document for the first time a potential MØ defect associated with the mutant CBA/N mouse. Thus we have shown that beef insulin responsiveness in the $H-2^b$ mouse is dependent on the expression of Ia.W39 by antigen presenting MØ. The defect in beef insulin reactivity in mutant (N x B6)F_1 male mice is due to lack of expression of Ia.W39, regulated by the xid gene. The discovery of an X-linked regulatory gene for Ir gene function is a new and provocative finding and should provide the basis for future studies on the regulation and mechanisms of insulin responsiveness.

Acknowledgement

Supported by the Ziskind and Posner funds of Tufts New England Medical Center and by National Institute of Health Grant AI-14910 and AC-24530. The authors wish to thank Dr. Sheldon M. Wolff for his continuing support of this project. The enthusiastic and expert technical assistance of Tom Brown and Tom Parrish is greatly appreciated. The authors also gratefully thank Mrs. Joanne Quigley for her secretarial assistance.

1. Benacerraf, B., and H.O. McDevitt: Science, 175:273, (1972).
2. Barcinski, M.A., and A.S. Rosenthal: J. Exp. Med. 145:726, (1977).
3. Rosenthal, A.S., M.A. Barcinski, and J.T. Blake: Nature 267:156, (1977).
4. Keck, K.: Nature 254:78, (1975).
5. Keck, K.: Eur. J. Immunol. 5:801, (1975).
6. Rosenwasser, L.J., M.A. Barcinski, R.H. Schwartz, and A.S. Rosenthal: J. Immunol. 123:471, (1979).
7. Berning, A., E. Eicher, W.E. Paul, and I. Scher: J. Immunol. 124: 1985 (1980).
8. Huber, B.T.: Proc. Nat'l Acad. Sci. (USA), 76:3460, (1979).
9. Huber, B.T., P.P. Jones, and D.A. Thorley-Lawson: Manuscript submitted for publication, (1981).
10. Rosenwasser, L.J., and A.S. Rosenthal: J. Immunol. 121:2497, (1978).
11. Rosenwasser, L.J., and A.S. Rosenthal: J. Immunol. 123:1141, (1979).
12. Rosenwasser, L.J., R.S. Bhatnagar, and J.D. Stobo: J. Immunol. 124: 2854, (1980).
13. Rosenwasser, L.J., and B.T. Huber: J. Expt. Med. 153:, in press (1981).
14. Schwartz, R.H., C.S. David, D.H. Sachs, and W.E. Paul: J. Immunol. 117:531, (1976).
15. Thomas, D.W., U. Yamashita, and E.M. Shevach: J. Immunol. 119:223, (1977).
16. Shevach, E.M.: Springer Seminars in Immunopathology 1:207, (1978).
17. Schwartz, R.H., C.S. David, M.E. Dorf, B. Benacerraf, and W.E. Paul: Proc. Nat'l. Acad. Sci. USA 75:2387, (1978).

INDUCTION OF IMMUNITY AND SUPPRESSION BY PIG INSULIN IN MICE

M. Momayezi and K. Keck
University of Konstanz, Faculty of Biology, D-7750 Konstanz, Germany

Introduction

Our earlier studies (1,2) and the experiments of others (3,4) have demonstrated that in mice the immune response to insulin is controlled by H-2 linked Ir-genes. The A-chain loops of sheep- and horse insulin act as immunogenic determinants in $H\text{-}2^k$ mice, whereas $H\text{-}2^b$ mice recognize in addition the A-chain loop of bovine insulin as an immunogenic determinant. Pig insulin, which lacks this determinant, is not immunogenic in all mouse strains and reactivities to insulin is presented in the paper by K. Keck (this Symposium).

We have studied the induction of immunity and suppression by pig insulin in mice. Previous studies have shown that pre-immunization with nonimmunogenic pig insulin suppresses the IgG response to an immunogenic insulin for example to sheep insulin or pig proinsulin in $H\text{-}2^k$ mice (6,7). In other words, the less immunogenic pig insulin induces tolerance to one of the more immunogenic insulins.

This work was supported by the Deutsche Forschungsgemeinschaft, Sonderforschungsbereich 138, "Biologische Grenzflächen und Spezifität".

Basic and Clinical Aspects of Immunity to Insulin

Suppression of IgM response

For the investigation of the IgM response, we used FTC-coupled insulin (FTC-B_1-insulin) as antigen (2), because IgM antibodies to the FTC-group can be determined easily and reproducibly by an hemolysis test (8).

C3H.He mice were immunized with pig insulin 3 to 21 days before challenge with FTC-B_1-sheep insulin. Fig. 1 shows that, similar to the IgG response the IgM response is also suppressed, if the animals are preimmunized with pig insulin. Suppression can be induced as long as 3 weeks before challenge with the immunogenic sheep insulin. However, simultaneous immunization with both insulins does not suppress the immune response to sheep insulin.

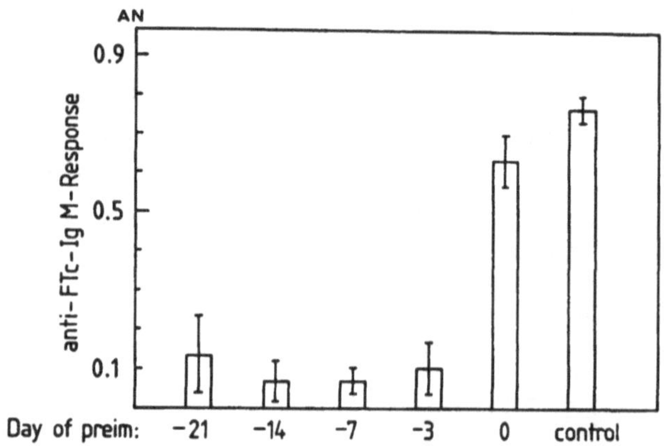

Fig. 1 Effect of time between Preimmunisation with nonimmunogenic pig-insulin and immunization with immunogenic FTC_1-sheep-insulin

Demonstration of suppressor cells

We have asked whether in vivo suppression of antibody production is due to specific suppressor cells. As shown in Fig. 2, one group of Balb.K mice ($H-2^k$) was injected with sheep insulin, which induces T-helper cells. A second group was treated with pig insulin, for the induction of tolerance. Seven days later spleen cells were transferred into X-irradiated syngenic mice. All mice were then immunized with 30 µg FTC-B1-sheep insulin in CFA. Ten days later the animals were bled and anti-FTC IgM antibodies were measured by a hemolysis test.

Control group A did not receive any cells and can produce specific antibodies to FTC-B1-sheep insulin. Sheep insulin primed spleen cells, including insulin specific T-helper cells, were transferred together with naive cells into group C mice. These animals show a normal IgM response to the FTC-haptene. Pig insulin primed spleen cells, which certainly include no helper cells, were given to mice of group D, again together with naive cells. No IgM production is observed in this group, as expected. The mice of group B received both sheep insulin primed spleen cells (including helper cells) and pig insulin primed cells (including putative suppressor cells). The presence of suppressor cells is demonstrated by the dramatically decreased response in these animals.

Genetic control of tolerance induction

We have investigated, whether other mouse strains, which are also nonresponders to pig insulin, can by means of pretreatment with pig insulin be made nonresponsive to sheep insulin.

DEMONSTRATION OF SUPPRESSOR CELLS INDUCED BY PIG INSULIN IN BALB.K MICE

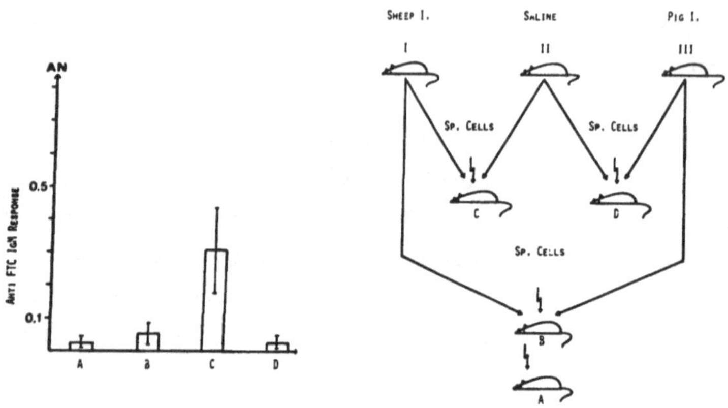

Fig. 2 Balb.k mice were injected:
I with 30 µg sheep insulin in CFA
II with 100 µg salin in CFA
III with 20 µg pig insulin in CFA
seven days later, spleen cells were transfered into three groups x-iradiated (700R) syngenic mice.

a) The animals of group A did not receive any cells (control group).
b) Group B received 5 x 10^7 sheep insulin and 5 x 10^7 pig insulin primed cells.
c) 5 x 10^7 sheep insulin primed cells were transfered together with 5 x 10^7 naive cells into the mice of group C.
d) 5 x 10^7 pig insulin primed cells were given to mice of group D again together with 5 x 10^7 naive cells. All mice were immunized with 30 µg FTC_1-sheep insulin. Anti FTC-IgM antibodies were measured 10 days later by a hemolysis test.

a) H-2 influence

Three groups of H-2^k mice were immunized with sheep insulin, pig insulin or with pig insulin followed 5 days later by sheep insulin. The results are shown in Fig. 3. The IgG production to sheep insulin is suppressed in H-2^k mice by pretreatment with pig insulin as previously shown. However, if H-2^b mice which are likewise nonresponders to pig insulin were treated similarily, the response to a successive immunization does not differ from control values. In other words, these mice can not be tolerized by pig insulin. Since Balb.B and Balb.K mice as well as C3H.SW and C3H.He differ only in their H-2 haplotypes,genes associated with the H-2-complex must be responsible for this difference in their susceptibility to tolerance induction.

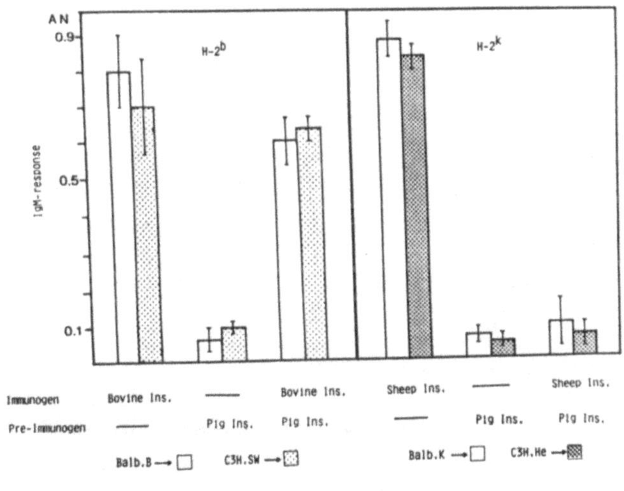

Fig. 3 Successive immunisation experiment and H-2-effect on suppressor induction

b) Allotype influence

The following experiments demonstrate, that genes outside of the H-2 complex also controle the susceptibility of mice to tolerance induction by pig insulin. We have examined four $H-2^k$ mouse strains, which respond with IgG antibody production to sheep - but not to pig insulin. As shown in Fig. 4, only mice having the allotype $Ig-1^a$ are tolerized by a preimmunization with pig insulin. Thus immunoglobulin heavy-chain genes influence tolerance induction. We have also demonstrated previously (9, 10) that in those mouse strains which are unable to produce IgG antibodies to pig insulin (IgG nonresponder strains) the IgM response is linked to Ig-1 allotype. $H-2^k$ mice carrying the allotype $Ig-1^b$, but not those carrying the allotype $Ig-1^a$, produce IgM-antibody to pig insulin.

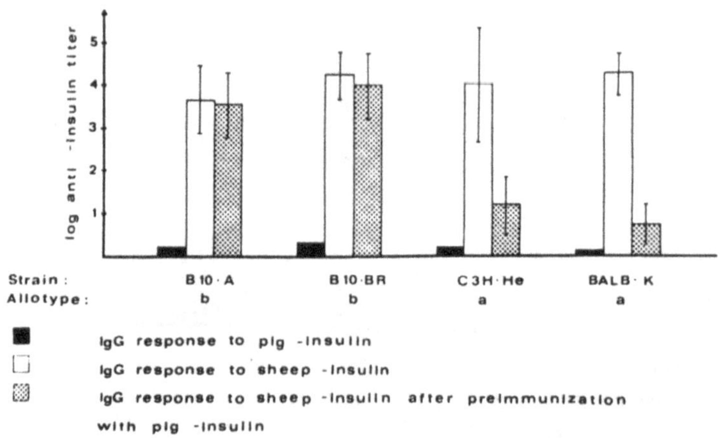

Fig. 4 Anti insulin IgG-response to pig- and sheep-insulin and tolerance induction in $H-2^k$ mouse strains, carrying different allotype

It seems that an inverse relationship exists between the intensity of the immune response (IgM response) and the induction of tolerance. The genes mentioned above are involved in the regulation of the antibody response to insulin. As shown in Table 1, the IgG-nonresponder mouse strains, which are able to produce IgM antibody to pig insulin, can not be tolerized by this insulin (B10.BR, B10.S, B10.A). In contrast, pig insulin induces tolerance in those mice, which do not produce insulin specific IgM antibody (C3H.He, Balb.K). Experiments with hybrid strains show a dominant inheritance of IgM-production and hence the susceptibility to tolerance induction is inherited recessively.

Table 1: Correlation between allotype related IgM-response and immune-suppression

Mousestrain	H-2 Haplotype	Allotype	IgG-Resp.	IgM-Resp.	Suppr.
C3H.He	k	a	-	-	+
BALB-K	k	a	-	-	+
B10.BR	k	b	-	+	-
B10.S	s	b	-	+	-
B10.A	a	b	-	+	-
C3H.He x B10.BR	k	a/b	-	+	-
C3H.He x B10.S	k/s	a/b	-	+	-
BALB-K x B10.BR	k	a/b	-	+	-

In summarizing we have shown that the induction of tolerance is influenced by at least three parameters: As far as the antigen is concerned, carrier determinants induce helper cells and thus prevent the induction of tolerance. In what concerns the animals,H-2 as well as allotype linked genes decide whether antibody production is turned on or tolerance induction is allowed.

Usually we expect tolerance induction to take place at antigen doses much lower than the dose needed for antibody production. However in the experiments described here, we use the same standard dose of antigen (20 µg/mouse) for both tolerance induction and antibody production. Nevertheless, we claim that we are dealing with a typical low zone tolerance for the following reasons: A low zone dose of antigen does not mean just a low amount of antigen expressed as mg antigen per mouse, but it means an antigen dose which can not induce antibodies of either class under the same experimental conditions (carrier determinants, H-2, allotype, adjuvants). Thus, starting from an immunogenic antigen dose, an effective low zone dose for tolerance induction can be reached by either lowering the dose of antigen (9), or by using the same standard dose of antigen and at the same time changing the experimental parameters, (11,12,13) so that the dose response curve is shifted to higher anigen doses. Under these conditions the standard dose as compared to the "present" immunogenic dose is an effective low zone dose.

This is illustrated by Fig 5 to 7. Sheep insulin is immunogenic in C3H/He mice at the standard dose of 20 µg, as shown by the DRC in Fig 5. The same dose of pig insulin does not lead to antibody production but to induction of tolerance. The dose response curve of pig insulin probably starts in this strain at much higher doses. Up to 60 µg of antibody do not induce significant amounts of IgM or IgG antibody. Thus 20 µg of pig

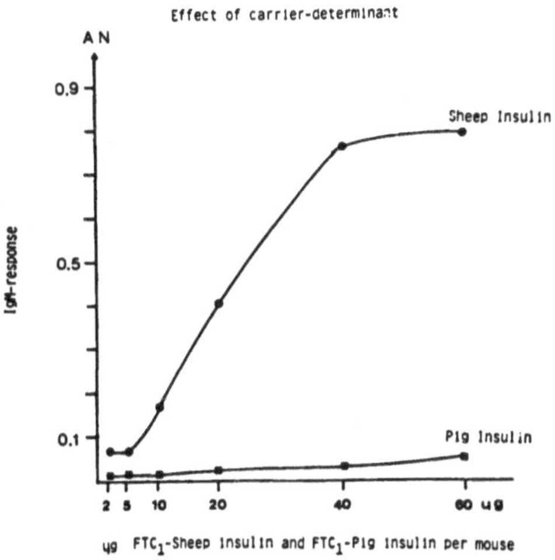

Fig. 5
Effect of carrier-determinant
Anti FTC IgM-response of C3H.He (H-2^{k}, Ig-1^{a}) mice to FTC_1-pig insulin and FTC_1-sheep insulin

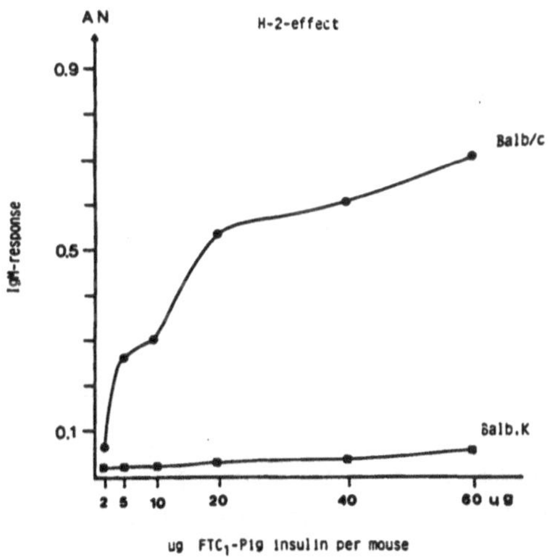

Fig. 6
H-2-effect
Anti FTC IgM-response of Balb/c (H-2^{d} Ig-1^{a}) and Balb.k (H-2^{k}, Ig-1^{a}) mice to FTC_1-pig insulin

insulin is a low zone dose in this strain, which induces tolerance.

In Fig 6 DRC of Balb/c and Balb.k mice to pig insulin are given. The standard dose of pig insulin is immunogenic in Balb/c but tolerogenic in congenic Balb.k mice, demonstrating the influence of H-2 linked genes at the dose response curve.

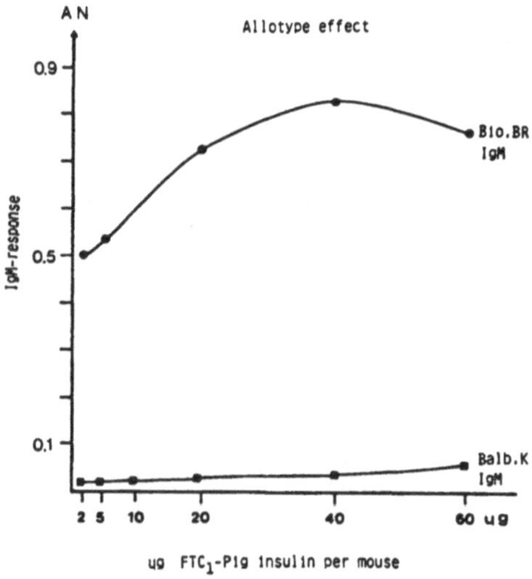

Fig 7
Allotype effect
Anti FTC IgM-response of Balb.k ($H-2^k$ $Ig-1^a$) and B10.BR ($H-2^k$, $Ig-1^b$) mice to FTC_1- pig insulin

In Fig 7 the shift of the dose response curve is caused by allotype linked genes. Pig insulin induces IgM antibody in B10.BR mice at all antigen doses tested. However, Balb.k mice, which have the same H-2 haplotype by a different allotype, do not produce antibody of any class (IgM or IgG) but, as demonstrated above, can be tolerized by the standard dose of pig insulin.

A similar shift of the dose response curve can be achieved even in responder animals by changing the adjuvant, as shown by others (14). This type of approach can be used to answer the question, why tolerance can not be induced with the standard dose of pig insulin in the H-2^b mice. The mouse strains bearing H-2^k and H-2^b haplotypes are defined as non-responders at standard dose of antigen. However, when H-2^b mice are tested at higher doses, they are able to respond to pig insulin (Fig 8). At this lower dose, therefore, there has been no induction of tolerance or T-suppressor cells, indeed perhaps T-helper cells have been triggered in insufficient numbers for antibody production.

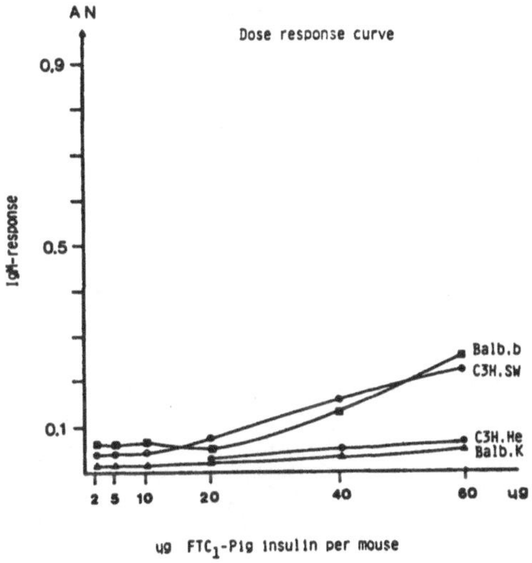

Fig. 8
Dose response curve in H-2^b and H-2^k mice. The animals were immunized with FTC_1-pig insulin. IgM-antibodies to FTC-group were determined

Acknowledgment
The expert technical assistance of Mrs. B.Bergmann is gratefully acknowledged.

Literatur

1) Keck, K. (1975) Natur 254, 78
2) Keck, K. (1975) Eur. J. Immunol. 5, 801
3) Rosenthal, A.S. (1978) Immunological Reviews 40, 136
4) Cohen, I.R. and Talmon, J. (1980) Eur. J. Immunol. 10, 284
5) Keck, K. and Momayezi, M. (1979) D. Brandenburg (Ed) Insulin Chemistry and Related Hormones, W. de Gruyter co. Berlin - New York 1980
6) Keck, K. and Momayezi, M. (1978), J. Immunol. 121 1612
7) Keck, K. 1977, Diahetologia 13: 407
8) Kolb, H., Keck, K., Momayezi, M., Schicker, C. and Trissel, D. (1977), J. Immunol. 118: 427
9) Momayezi, M., Dissertation 1980, University Konstanz (FRG)
10) Momayezi, M., Keck, K. and Kolb, H. (1978), Z. Immun.-Forsch. (Immunbiology), 155 44
11) Parish, C.R. (1974), Progress in Immunology II, Biological Aspects I, Vol. 2, 39, North-Holland Publishing Company
12) Adonini, L., Harvey, M.A., Miller, A. and Sercarz, E.E. 1980, J. Exp. Med. 150, 293
13) Araneo, B.A., Yowell, R.L. and Sercarz, E.E. 1979, J. of Immunol. 123, 961
14) Baskin, B.L. and Rosenthal, A.S. (1980), J. of. Immunol. 124: 184

GENETIC CONTROL OF ANTI-INSULIN RESPONSES IS ASSOCIATED WITH ACTIVATION OF DIFFERENT T-CELL SETS

By Sara Abromson-Leeman,[o] Bonnie J. Rapp, and Harvey Cantor[oo]

Harvard Medical School
Department of Pathology
Farber Cancer Center
Boston, Massachusetts 02115

Introduction

Immune responses to many protein antigens are controlled by genes linked to MHC (major histocompatibility complex) (1). "Non-responder" phenotypes are conventionally difined by failure to develop significant levels of specific antibody after immunization with a particular antigen. The cellular and molecular mechanisms that underlie MHC-linked unresponsiveness are not precisely understood. Two general explanations have been discussed: (1) antigen in association with I-region gene products fails to activate T-cells, including T-helper cells (TH) (2,3) or (2) antigen, (possibly in association with I-region gene products) selectively stimulates T-cell sets that generate suppression which preempts delivery of the helper signal to the appropriate B-cell (4,5).

We have approached this problem by analyzing the types of T-cell sets activated in mice after immunization with purified insulin molecules from two different species, sheep and cow. These two insulins differ in their primary amino acid sequences at a single position in the A chain, A9. $H-2^a$ mice

---

This work was supported by USPHS Grant AI-13600
o Supported by NSF fellowship
oo Scholar of the Leukemia Society of America

Basic and Clinical Aspects of Immunity to Insulin

generate substantial antibody responses after immunization with sheep but not cow insulin; genes controlling antibody responses to these insulins have been mapped to the I-region of the MHC (6,7). Utilizing a modification of the lymphocyte proliferation assay described originally by Corradin et al. (8), we show that: (1) immunization with both insulins is followed by substantial and specific T-cell activation, as judged by incorporation of ^{3}H-thymidine after re-stimulation of T-cells in vitro, (2) both responses depend upon adherent "accessory" cells, and (3) cow ("non-responder") and sheep ("responder") insulins activate different types of cells.

Materials and Methods

Animals. A/J and B10.A mice were obtained from the Jackson Laboratory, Bar Harbor,ME. 6-10 wk old female mice were used in these experiments.

Antigens. Crystalline bovine, sheep, and rat insulins were generous gifts of Dr. Ronald Chance of the Lilly Research Laboratories, Division of Eli Lilly and Co., Indianapolis, IN. The proinsulin content of the bovine insulin lot was 0.06%.

Immunizations. Mice were immunized with .05 ml. of an emulsion containing equal volumes of CFA (complete Freund's adjuvant, Difco Labs) and 20 µgs insulin in PBS (phosphate buffered saline), either in the hind footpads or at the tail-base as described by Corradin et al. (8).

Measurement of in vitro lymphocyte proliferation. Proliferation was assessed using a modification of the technique of Corradin et al. (8). Briefly, draining lymph nodes (inguinal and periaortic after tailbase immunization and popliteal and inguinal after footpad immunization) were removed two to three weeks after immunization (unless otherwise stated).

Single cell suspensions were made in SBSS (special balanced salt solution) supplemented with antibiotics by gently teasing with 26-gauge needles. Cells were cultured in complete Click's medium as modified by Maizels et al. (8,9). Cultures were supplemented with 0.5% heat-inactivated ($56^{o}C$ x 30 min) homologous pooled normal mouse serum (NMS) obtained on the day of culture initiation. Unless otherwise stated, 4 x 10^{5} viable cells were dispensed into each well of a microtiter plate (Falcon 3040) along with either medium alone or medium containing the appropriate concentration of insulin, to give a final volume of 200 µl. Each culture group was set up in triplicate and incubated for 5 days in an atmosphere of 5% CO_2 95% air. 18-24 hours before harvest, 1 µCi (^{3}H-methylthymidine, sp act 20 Ci/mH, New England Nuclear, Boston, MA) in a ^{3}H-T volume of 10 µl was added to each well. All values represent the means of triplicate cultures.

Preparation and use of antisera. NMS was obtained from C3H/HeJ mice, absorbed with spleen, lymph node, and thymus cells of A/J, C57BL/6, and Balb/c mice (1:1 volume), and used at a final dilution of 1:40. Ly1.2 and Ly2.2 antisera were prepared, tested for specificity and used as described (10). Monoclonal antiy-Thy 1.2, a gift from Dr. M. Gefter (MIT) was used at a final dilution of 10^{-4}. Preparation and use of anti-Qa1 serum, (B6xA-T1a^{b}) anti-A strain leukemia ASL-I, is described elsewhere (11,12). Specificity of this serum for products of the Qa1 locus was confirmed by absence of cytotoxic effects on cells from the T1a^{b} congenic strain. Specificity was also tested functionally by differential effects of antiserum + C treatment on the proliferation responses after absorption with cells from either the B6 or B6-TL^{+} congenic mouse strains.

As described previously, 20 x 10^6 cells/ml were incubated 1/2 hour at $4^{o}C$ with antisera at the final concentrations indicated, washed, and incubated with selected rabbit sera as a source of C (complement) for 40 min at $37^{o}C$ (10). After treatment, all cell populations were readjusted to 4 x 10^6/ml in complete medium and 0.1 ml (4 x 10^5 cells) dispensed into each well of a microtiter plate.

Preparation of purified T cells. Highly enriched populations of T cells were obtained by incubating lymphocyte suspensions on rabbit anti-mouse $F(ab')_2$ - coated culture dishes according to Wysocki and Sato (14). Approximately 35-40% of the starting population was recovered; Ig^+ cells accounted for 3% of this population.

Immunization and assay of anti-insulin antibodies. Mice were immunized with 20 µg insulin in CFA i.p.; 3 weeks later they were boosted with the same amount of insulin i.p. Sera were collected 8-10 days later. Serum antibody determinations were performed using a modification of the solid phase radioimmunoassay technique, as previously described (15).

Depletion of adherent cells. Lymph node populations were depleted of adherent cells by sequential passages over plastic plates, according to the method of Mosier et al. (16).

Preparation of adherent spleen cells. Spleen cells (5 x 10^6/ml) from normal mice were incubated in SBSS with 0.5% NMS ($37^{o}C$ x 2 hrs) in plastic tissue culture dishes (Falcon 3003), washed vigorously to remove non-adherent cells. After three such incubations, the cells were incubated overnight, washed vigorously and chilled at $4^{o}C$ for 20 minutes. Adherent cells were then recovered by scraping with a teflon policeperson. Recovery of cells after this procedure was 1% of the starting population.

Plaque forming cell assay. Assay for antibody producing cells was performed by the Cunningham modification of the Jerne plaque assay as previously described (11). Conjugation of insulin to sheep erythrocytes was performed according to Schroer et al. (17). Only indirect plaques were detectable.

Cell phenotyping. Phenotypes of in vitro cultured cells were determined using a micro-^{51}Cr release assay as previously described (11).

Results

A/J mice were immunized with either sheep or cow insulin, and cell populations from lymph nodes draining the immunization site were tested for antigen-induced proliferative activity. Substantial proliferative responses to both sheep and cow insulins are obtained from lymph node cells of these mice after stimulation in vitro with the homologous insulin (Figure 1, Panel A).

The responses were maximal two to four weeks after in vivo priming. The magnitude and tempo of proliferative responses of lymph node cells draining the tailbase or footpad were indistinguishable (data not shown).

The finding that lymphocytes of A/J mice primed to cow insulin proliferate in vitro to cow insulin was somewhat surprising because cow insulin does not elicit antibody production in mice of this haplotype (6,7). We confirmed this point by measuring both the plaque-forming cell response in these lymphocytes as well as serum antibody titers to the two insulins. Panel B of Figure 1 shows that although plaque-forming cells with specificity for sheep insulin are easily detected in lymph nodes of A/J mice immunized 2-3 weeks earlier with sheep insulin, virtually none arise after immunization

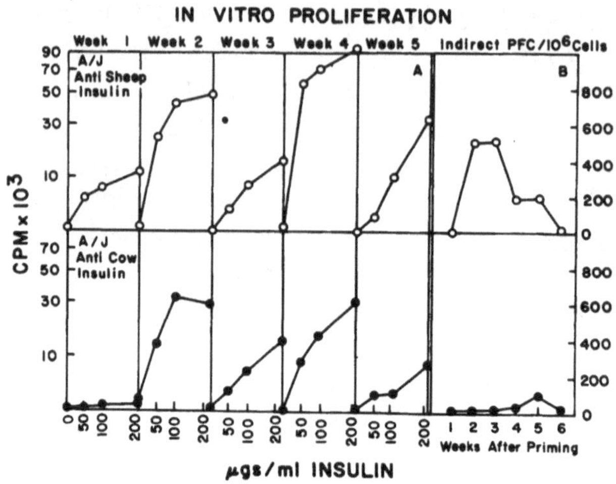

Figure 1. A/J mice were immunized in the hind footpads with 20 ugs insulin in CFA. From one to five weeks later, popliteal and inguinal nodes were removed, an aliquot plaqued with insulin-conjugated sheep erythrocytes, and the remainder set up in vitro for 5 days with the indicated concentrations of the homologous insulin to assay for proliferative activity.

Table 1

SECONDARY IN VIVO ANTIBODY RESPONSES TO INSULIN

Serum Titer: ugs/ml			
A/J Anti-Sheep Insulin		A/J Anti-Cow Insulin	
Mouse #1	233.0	Mouse #1	13.8
#2	527.0	#2	15.6
#3	307.8	#3	17.5
#4	118.8	#4	3.5
		#5	22.5
		#6	4.6
$\bar{x}$ =	296.5	$\bar{x}$ =	12.9

Table 1: The figures represent serum titers of specific antibody as assayed in a solid phase radioimmunoassay using the homologous insulin. Sera were obtained 8 days after boosting with insulin in saline i.p.

of A/J mice with cow insulin. An analysis of serum antibody titers also confirms this point. Significant titers of specific antibody are elicted in A/J mice after priming and boosting with sheep but not cow insulin (Table I). Since previous studies have shown that T-cells from "non-responder" mice do not proliferate when re-stimulated in vitro (3,9,20), it was essential to establish whether or not this proliferative reaction represented an antigen specific T-cell response.

Proliferative responses to insulin are not a result of its hormonal activity. To rule out the possibility that CFA-activated lymph node cells are stimulated to divide by insulin, the proliferative response of lymph node cells in cultures supplemented with rat insulin (structurally identical to mouse insulin) was assessed. After stimulation with CFA, draining lymph node cells do not proliferate in the presence of rat insulin in vitro. (CPM incorporated by medium control = 1060 $\pm$ 28; cpm in the presence of 100 μgs/ml rat insulin = 1482 $\pm$ 142).

Secondary proliferative responses are mediated mainly by T cells. Depletion of lymphocytes bearing surface Thy1.2 before stimulation eliminated 80-95% of the proliferative reaction to either insulin (Figure 4) and approximately 80% of cells stimulated with either insulin for 5 days were lysed by anti-Thy1.2+C (Table 2). Furthermore, depletion of sIg^+ cells from lymph node cell populations resulted in populations enriched in proliferative activity to both insulins (Figure 2). Taken together, these data show that although immunization of A/J mice with sheep insulin elicits strong antibody response while cow insulin does not, both specifically activate T-cells to the same degree. We therefore asked whether the responses to the two insulins reflected different cellular reactions.

Table 2

PHENOTYPES OF CELLS HARVESTED FROM SECONDARY CULTURES ON DAY 5

% Cells Killed With:	Sheep Insulin Primed	Cow Insulin Primed
NMS+C	0	0
ANTI-THY 1.2+C	80	79

Table 2: After stimulation with antigen for 5 days in culture, cells were harvested, dead cells removed using Ficoll-Hypaque, and phenotype of the remaining cells determined using a micro^{51}Cr release assay.

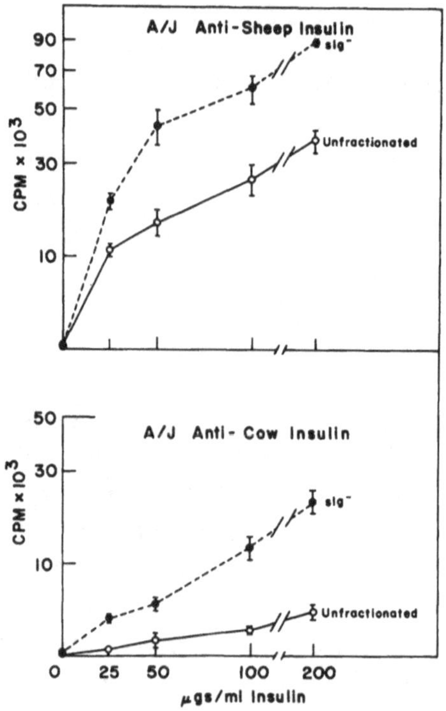

Figure 2: Two weeks after tailbase priming, inguinal and periaortic nodes were removed from A/J mice and assayed either as unfractionated populations or after depletion of B-cells as described

Different activation of T cell sets by sheep (responder) and cow (non-responder) insulins. Cow and sheep insulins differ from one another at a single amino acid at position 9 in the A chain (Figure 3). Although both insulins stimulate T-cells equally well, we asked whether this difference was sufficient to initiate different types of responses. Cells responsible for the proliferative reactions were analyzed by treating lymph node populations primed to the different insulins with various antisera and complement before in vitro restimulation of equal numbers of the remaining cells with the homologous insulin. The results (Figures 4 and 5) can be summarized as follows: (a) proliferative responses to both insulins are virtually eliminated by treatment with either anti-Thy1.2 and C or anti-Ly1.2 and C, (b) proliferative responses to sheep insulin are not decreased by treatment with anti-Ly2.2 or anti-Qa1 + C, or anti-Ly2.2 + antiQa1 + C, and (c) in contrast, although $Ly1^{+}2^{-}$ cells also account for the major proliferative response to cow insulin, treatment of these cells with anti-Qa1 and C reduces this response to less than 1/3 that of NMS + C treated lymphocytes. Analysis of the effects of depleting $Qa1^{+}$ cells was also done using B10.A mice (Figure 5). Similar results were obtained; the response to sheep insulin was not affected by elimination of cells bearing the $Qa1^{+}$ phenotype whereas the response of B10.A mice to cow insulin is abrogated after elimination of $Qa1^{+}$ cells. Thus, the T-cell response to cow insulin depends mainly on the presence of $Qa1^{+}$ cells, either for the actual proliferation, or for induction of proliferation of $Ly1{:}Qa1^{-}$ cells. Proliferative responses to sheep insulin, on the other hand, do not require $Qa1^{+}$ cells.

Responses to both sheep and cow insulin are adherent cell dependent. We next asked whether both types of responses require the presence of macrophages. Adherent cells were depleted from immune lymph node populations by sequential passages over plastic dishes. These adherent cell-depleted

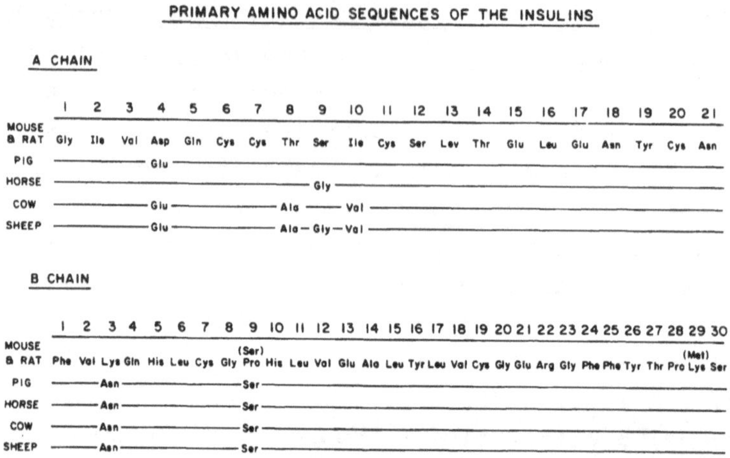

Figure 3: Primary amino acid sequences of insulins (from ref. 18). Identity with mouse insulin is indicated by a solid line.

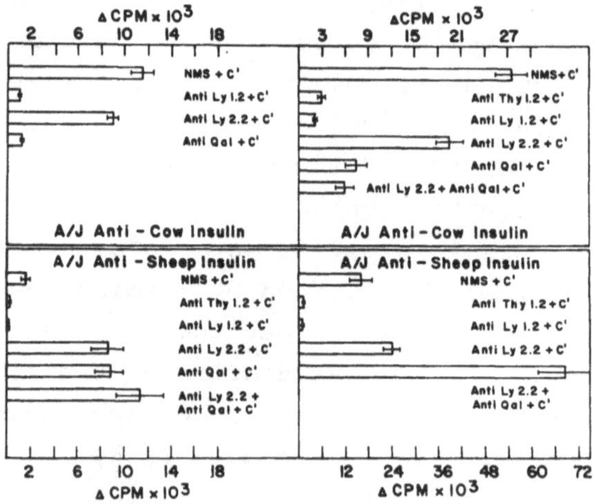

Figure 4: Three weeks after tailbase priming, cells from draining lymph nodes were treated with the indicated antisera before stimulation of 4 x 10^5 viable cells with 100 ugs/ml of the homologous insulin.

populations were assayed for their ability to proliferate to the insulins, either alone, or when reconstituted with 5×10^4 adherent spleen cells. Figure 6 shows that both the response to sheep insulin as well as that to cow insulin are reduced by depletion of adherent cells. Both responses are reconstituted upon addition of adherent cells derived from syngenic non-immune spleen cell populations.

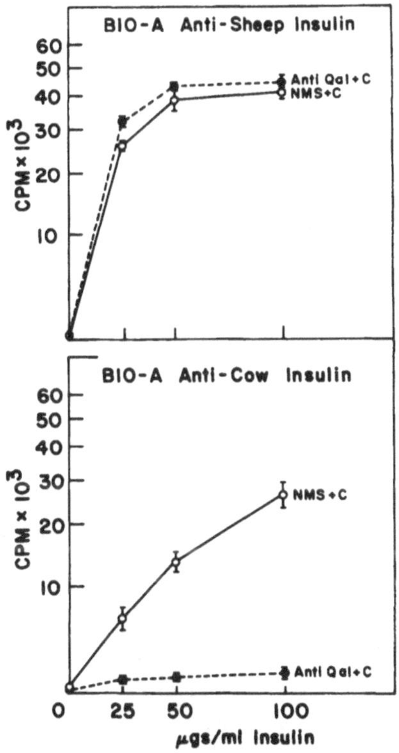

Figure 5: Lymph node cells from B10.A mice taken 3 weeks after tailbase priming. After antiserum + C treatments, 4×10^5 viable cells were dispensed into each well, with either medium or homologous insulin at concentrations indicated.

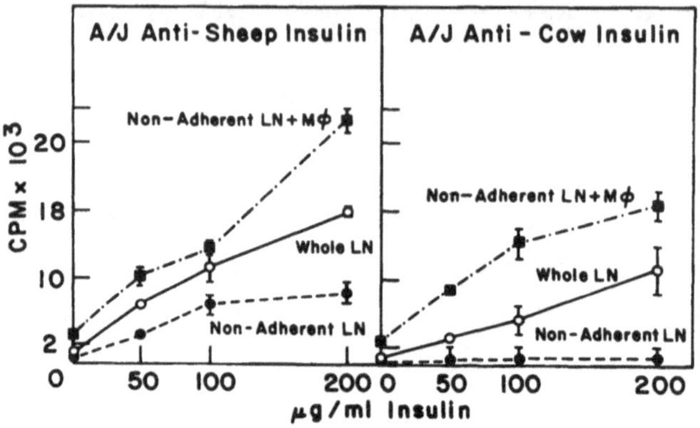

Figure 6: 4×10^5 non-adherent cells, obtained by passage over plastic dishes, were tested alone or in combination with 5×10^4 non-immune splenic adherent cells.

Discussion

The T-cell proliferation assay is a useful in vitro measure of antigen-induced activation of the immune system (8,24). We used this assay to determine whether lack of an Ir-gene controlled immune response to cow insulin reflected failure to specifically active T-cells. These data show that the inability of $H\text{-}2^a$ mice to produce antibody to cow insulin cannot be ascribed to an absence of antigen-specific T-cell activation.

Cow and sheep insulin molecules differ from one another by a single amino acid, and from mouse insulin by five and six amino acids, respectively (18). Confirming results obtained by Keck (7), we found that H-2^a mice produce significant titers of specific antibody and develop plaque forming cells in draining lymph nodes after immunization with sheep but not cow insulin. However, both insulins specifically activate T-cells, as judged by ^{3}H-T incorporation after restimulation in vitro. This response is immunologic because (a) rat insulin, identical to mouse insulin, did not stimulate populations of CFA-activated lymph node cells to incorporate ^{3}H-T, (b) the response is T-cell dependent, as judged by abrogation of the response after removal of Thy-1^+ cells, and (c) the response requires the presence of macrophages.

A more detailed analysis of the surface phenotype of cells required in the response to sheep ("responder") and cow ("non-responder") insulins revealed striking differences. The proliferative reaction to cow insulin is dependent upon a $Qa1^+$ subpopulation of cells; in contrast, the reaction to sheep insulin is mediated by a $Qa1^-$ subset(s) of cells. Some antisera to I-J subregion products (13) provided an additional distinguishing phenotype: the reaction to cow but not sheep insulin depends upon I-J^+ cells. (Unpublished results, Leeman, Murphy, Gershon, Cantor.) Taken together, these findings demonstrate that molecules differing by a single amino acid presumably in combination with the appropriate gene product(s) on macrophages can activate different sets of cells, depending on the MHC haplotype of the host.

Our data do not indicate whether dependency on a particular subset of cells is due to actual proliferation of that set or to inducing functions of that subset upon other sets of cells. Reduction of responses to cow insulin after treatment with anti-Qa1 and C may indicate that: (1) $Qa1^+Ly1^+2^-$ cells are themselves proliferating, (2) $Qa1^+$ $Ly1^+2^-$ T-cells are inducing other T-cells to proliferate, or (3) a set of $Qa1^+$ antigen-presenting cells initiates this response (but not the response to sheep insulin). Support for the first explanation comes from analysis of long term cell lines from "non-responder" B10.A mice stimulated with cow insulin; about 80% of these cells express the $Ly1^{+}2^{-}:Qa1^{+}$ phenotype (Leeman and Cantor, manuscript in preparation). Previous studies have demonstrated that (a) $Ly1:Qa1^{+}$ cells but not $Ly1:Qa1^{-}$cells induce other T-cells (surface phenotype $Ly1^{+}2^{+}3^{+}:Qa1^{+}$) to generate 'feedback' suppressive activity and (b) both the $Qa1^{+}$ and the $Qa1^{-}$ subsets of Ly1 cells appear to be required for optimal activation of antigen-specific B-cells (11,21) (although $Ly1:Qa1^{-}$ cells alone help B-cells, albeit less efficiently). The studies reported here suggest that an Ir-gene controlled antibody response may depend on the relative level of activation of $Qa1^{+}$ as opposed to $Qa1^{-}$ subsets of Ly1 cells. Activation of Ly1 cells that are predominantly $Qa1^{+}$ (as opposed to $Qa1^{-}$Ly1 cells) may not lead to the generation of efficient T-helper acitvity. Alternatively, activation of the "$Qa1^{+}$" immunoregulatory circuit may preempt delivery of T_H signals to B-cells due to eihter excessive T_S activity or to an increased sensitivity of these inducer T-cells to inhibitory signals. Analysis of the influence of these cells sets upon anti-insulin antibody responses should distinguish between these possibilities.

Although there is good evidence that some instances of MHC-linked unresponsiveness reflect T-suppressor cell (T_S) activation (4,5), these same antigens have failed to stimulate T-cells to proliferate in vitro (9,22). Previous analysis of in vitro T-cell reactions to insulins have indicated that peritoneal exudate T cells from mice of the H-2^b haplotype proliferate after restimulation in vitro with cow insulin, which elicits antibody, but not with pig insulin, which does not (20,23). Several possibilities may account for these discrepant results. Possibly the mechanism of unresponsiveness of the H-2^b haplotype to pig insulin differs from that of the H-2^a haplotype to cow insulin. Alternatively, failure to detect proliferative reactions to "non-responder" antigens may reflect differences in the in vitro assay used to measure T-cell activation. For example, stimulation of lymph node cells as opposed to PETLES, and/or differences in culture medium and serum supplements that may selectively support reactivity of different cell sets may allow detection of "non-responder" proliferative reactions.

In sum, these data show that Ir-gene controlled unresponsiveness does not necessarily reflect a lack of T-cells that recognize antigen, but can result from antigen-specific activation of sets of T-cells that do not generate effective T-helper function. We are currently investigating the precise sequences of cellular interactions that occur in responder and non-responder immunologic circuits, as well as the molecular bases for these interactions.

Summary

Mice of the $H\text{-}2^a$ haplotype generate substantial antibody responses after immunization with sheep insulin but not with cow insulin. The amino acid sequences of these two insulins are identical at all but a single position. Control of antibody responses to these insulins has been mapped to the I-region of the MHC. Utilizing a lymphocyte proliferation assay to assess cellular activation, we show that: (1) immmunization with either sheep or cow insulin is followed by substantial and specific T-cell activation, as judged by incorporation of ^{3}H-thymidine after re-stimulation of T-cells in vitro, (2) the T-cell responses to both sheep and cow insulins require the presence of an adherent cell population, and (3) cow and sheep insulins activate different types of cells.

References

1. Benacerraf, B., and H.O. McDevitt: Science 175, 273 (1972).
2. Schwartz, R.H.: Scand. J. Immunol. 7, 3 (1978).
3. Barcinski, M.A. and A.S. Rosenthal: J. Exp. Med. 145, 726 (1977).
4. Kapp, J.A., C.W. Pierce, S. Schlossman, and B. Benacerraf: J. Exp. Med. 140, 648 (1974).
5. Adorini, L., Miller, A., and E.E. Sercarz: J. Immunol. 122, 871 (1979).
6. Keck, K.: Eur. J. Immunol. 5, 801 (1975).
7. Keck, K.: Eur. J. Immunol. 7, 811 (1975).
8. Corradin, G., H.M. Etlinger, and J.M. Chiller: J. Immunol. 119, 1048 (1977).
9. Maizels, R.M., Clarke, J.A., Harvey, M.A., Miller, A. and Sercarz, E.E.: Eur. J. Immunol. 10, 509 (1980).
10. Shen, F.W., E.A. Boyse, and H. Cantor: Immunogenetics 2, 591 (1975).
11. Cantor, H., J. Hugenberger, L. McVay-Boudreau, D.D. Eard ley, J. Kemp, F.W. Shen, and R.K. Gershon: J. Exp. Med. 148, 871 (1978).
12. Stanton, T.H. and E.A. Boyse: Immunogenetics 3, 525 (1976).
13. Murphy, D.B., L.A. Herzenberg, K. Okumura, L.A. Herzenberg, and H.O. McDevitt: J. Exp. Med. 144, 1099 (1976).
14. Wysocki, L. and V. Sato: Proc. Natl. Acad. Sci. USA 75, 2844 (1978).
15. Woodland, R. and H. Cantor: Eur. J. Immunol. 8, 600 (1978).
16. Mosier, D.: Science 158, 1575 (1967).
17. Schroer, J.A., J.K. Inman, J.W. Thomas and A.S. Rosenthal: J. Immunol. 123, 670 (1979).
18. Smith, L.F.: Diabetes 21 (Suppl 2), 457 (1972).
19. Schwartz, R.H. and W.E. Paul: J. Exp. Med. 143, 529 (1976).
20. Rosenthal, A.S.: Immunol. Rev. 40, 135 (1978).
21. Eardley, D.D., J. Hugenberger, L. McVay-Boudreau, F.W. Shen, R.K. Gershon, and H. Cantor: J. Exp. Med. 147, 1106 (1978).
22. Yano. A., R.H. Schwartz, and W.E. Paul: Eur. J. Immunol. 8, 344 (1978).
23. Rosenwasser, L.J., M.A. Barcinski, R.H. Schwartz, and A.S. Rosenthal: J. Immunol. 123, 471 (1979).
24. Schwartz, R.H., L. Jackson, and W.E.Paul: J.Immunol. 115, 1330 (1976).

SUPPRESSION OF INSULIN RESPONSES IN VITRO

Sirkka Kontiainen and Tom Scheinin
Department of Bacteriology and Immunology
University of Helsinki, Finland

Introduction

Immune response (Ir) genes associated with the major histocompatibility locus (MHC) are of major importance in the control of immune responsiveness (1,2). Immune responses are also regulated by multiple cell interactions either enhancing (helping) or decreasing (suppressing) the response (3,4). Thus only mice of the responder haplotype will make antibodies to antigens such as certain synthetic polypeptides ((T,G)-A--L or GAT), lysozyme or insulin analogues (5-8). Although unable to trigger antibody production these antigens may be able to induce suppressor pathways. This has been shown with (T,G)-A--L and GAT, where both responder and nonresponder strains make specific suppressor factors which abolish the response by responder helper cells (9,10). These findings suggest that immune suppression and immune responsiveness may have different genetic control (2). The leasons in nonresponder mice are not fully understood but one may be at the level of antigen presenting cells, macrophages (11,12).

The cellular pathways of T cell mediated suppression and help have been extensively studied in mice (13,14) and their analysis in humans has started (15,16). In mice helper effector cells have Ly1 surface antigens while suppressor effector cells have Ly2.3 (17,18). The human analogues on effector precursors may be the Fc receptors for μ and γ on peripheral T cells (19). Helper and suppressor cells may secrete their ef-

Basic and Clinical Aspects of Immunity to Insulin

fector molecules, termed factors, which replace the function of the parent cells (13,14,19a). Some of these factors are MHC restricted in their function (13), while some lack MHC and even species restriction (16,19a,20).

Responses to insulin have also been studied in detail. Keck and his co-workers demonstrated that only certain strains of mice make antibodies to e.g. pork or beef insulin and correlated this to the MHC type of the mice (21,22). Rosenthal and his co-workers showed MHC restricted T cell proliferation to insulin analogues (23-25). They were also able to locate the lesion in nonresponder mice or guinea-pigs to macrophages (24) and to show the same reactivity pattern in T cell help measured in adoptive antibody responses (25).

Although T cell proliferation (23-25), induction of T helper cell activity _in vivo_ (25) or _in vitro_ (26) and _in vivo_ antibody responses to insulins (21,22) have been studied in detail, it is not clear whether insulin specific suppression can be induced, and whether insulin specific suppression is important in the regulation of responsiveness to insulin. These studies were started to test whether insulin molecules are able to induce suppression, and to characterize the suppressive molecules.

Materials and Methods

Animals. BALB/c mice bred at the Department were 3-4 months old when used.

Tissue culture conditions. The induction of insulin specific helper and suppressor cells as well as the cooperative cultures were as previously described (27-29), as was the production of suppressor factors (30). The helper cells (HC) and factors (HF) were usually induced with 0.01 µg/well of pork (or beef) insulin as follows:

spleen cells 10^7/ml + pork insulin 0.01 µg/ml → HC_{pork}
4 d. in vitro

HC_{pork} $5x10^6$/ml + pork insulin 0.01 µg/ml → HF_{pork}
24 h. in vitro

To test whether suppressor cells (SC) and factors (SF) to insulins could be induced the first 4 d. culture was performed with 10, 30 or 100 µg/ml of insulin (instead of 0.1 or 0.01 µg/ml); the second, 24 h. culture, however, was with 0.01 µg/ml. The cooperative cultures were usually as follows:

$3x10^5HC_{pork}$/well+$3x10^6$ spl.cells/well+0.05µg/ml of TNP-pork insulin
4 d. in vitro

For the cultures the cells were suspended and placed in the inserts of Marbrook-Diener culture vessels in Hepes (10 mM) buffered Eagle's Minimum Essential Medium (MEM) supplemented with glutamine (2mM), penicillin (100IU/ml), streptomycin (100 µg/ml) and 5% of foetal calf serum (Gibco, batch 401201B). The outer medium in the culture vessels was bicarbonate buffered MEM supplemented as above but having 5% of donor horse serum (Flow, batch 2929070) instead of foetal calf serum and containing 2-mercaptoethanol ($5x10^{-5}$M).

The cultures were performed in a humidified atmosphere of 10% CO_2 in air. All the cooperative cultures were started in triplicates.

Human insulin factors were produced from peripheral blood lymphocytes derived from normal, healthy laboratory personnel with informed concent. SF were produced as with mouse cells after Ficoll-Isopaque separation (29) of the mononuclear cells.

Antigens. Pork or beef insulins and their DNP-derivatives kindly given by Dr. Alan Rosenthal were mainly used. In some experiments beef and pork insulins from NOVO (NOVO, batches

08581126 and S8381104.) were used without further purification.

Assay of help vs. suppression. The numbers of anti-DNP antibody forming cells (AFC), assayed as previously described (27) and shown as anti-DNP AFC/10^6 cultured cells ± SE express the activity of HC_{pork} induced *in vitro*. Suppression was measured as a decrease in the numbers of AFC after SF_{pork} or SF_{beef} was added to the mixture of HC_{pork}, normal spleen cells and DNP-pork in the beginning of the culture. The results are interpreted as follows:

HC_{pork}	spleen cells	SF	DNP-pork	
-	+	-	+	background
+	+	-	+	help (response)
+	+	+	+	suppression

The percentage of suppression (%S) is calculated

$$\%S = 100 \times \frac{\text{suppression - background}}{\text{help - background}}$$

Proliferative assays. To test whether proliferation could be induced in normal spleen cells or PBL, 3×10^5 cells in 0.1 ml of medium were added to flat bottomed 96 microtitre wells together with 1, 10, 30 or 100 µg of insulin or 5µg of concanavallin A in 0.1 ml of medium per well. After 72 h of culture, 1 mCu of 3H-thymidine was added. The cells were harvested 6 h later, and the radioactivity bound to the cells counted. The results are expressed as stimulation indexes (Sl)

$$Sl = \frac{\text{cpm in experimental}}{\text{cpm in background}}$$

Characterization of suppressor factors. The following immunoadsorbents, prepared and used as previously described (19a) were used: pork or beef insulins, rabbit anti-mouse immunoglobulin (RαMIg), keyhole limpet haemocyanin (KLH) and rabbit anti-SF antisera.

Results

1) <u>Induction of insulin specific suppressor cells.</u> BALB/c spleen cells cultured with 10, 30 or 100 µg/ml of either pork or beef insulin did not contain helper activity e.g. did not generate anti-DNP AFC when added to normal spleen cells and stimulated with DNP-insulins. This was in contrast to spleen cells cultured with 0.01 to 1 µg of insulin (helper cells) which yielded good helper activity. However, the cells cultured with a high dose of antigen (suppressor cells, SC) when added to the mixture of insulin helper cells (HC) and normal spleen cells suppressed the response by HC. Small numbers of suppressor cells (SC) were required for suppression e.g. as few as 10^4 SC caused a significant suppression of helper activity.

The suppressor cells however seem to lack analogue specificity e.g. SC induced with beef insulin suppressed pork insulin responses equally well and in similar numbers as pork insulin induced SC (Table 1). SC induced with other antigens e.g. keyhole limpet haemocyanin did not affect insulin help (data not shown).

Table 1. Suppression of insulin help

STIMULUS		SUPPRESSION		RESPONSE	
HC_{pork}	TNP-pork	SC		anti-DNP AFC/10^6	%S
-	+	-		27 ± 8	-
+	+	-		191 ± 2	-
+	+	$SC_{pork}10$	10^4	129 ± 10	38
+	+		10^5	138 ± 22	32
+	+	$SC_{pork}30$	10^4	133 ± 17	35
+	+		10^5	120 ± 8	43
+	+	$SC_{pork}100$	10^4	184 ± 9	4
+	+		10^5	131 ± 2	37
+	+	$SC_{beef}10$	10^4	147 ± 8	27
+	+		10^5	89 ± 10	62
+	+	$SC_{beef}30$	10^4	78 ± 2	69
+	+		10^5	133 ± 4	35
+	+	$SC_{beef}100$	10^4	107 ± 4	51
+	+		10^5	98 ± 12	55

$3x10^5$ HC_{pork} of BALB/c origin were added to $3x10^6$ normal spleen cells together with 1 µg of TNP-pork/well in the presence or absence of 10^4 or 10^5 suppressor cells induced with 10, 30 or 100 µg of either pork or beef insulin as indicated. Anti-DNP AFC assayed on day 4 of the cooperative culture. Results expressed as AFC/10^6 cultured cells.

This lack of analogue specificity is in contrast to the results with HC where poor stimulation of help was obtained when HC_{pork} were stimulated with DNP-beef instead of DNP-pork (Fig.1).

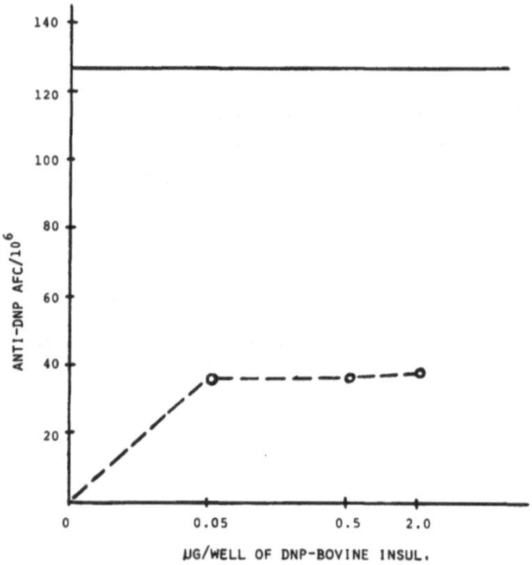

Fig.1. $3x10^5$ HC_{pork} of BALB/c origin where added to $3x10^6$ normal BALB/c spleen cells and stimulated with 0.05, 0.5 or 2.0 µg DNP-beef/well (o---o) instead of the optimum dose 0.05 µg/well of DNP-pork (solid horizontal line).

2) Insulin suppressor factors lack analogue specificity.
Suppressor factors (SF) released by pork insulin induced SC upon further *in vitro* culture with 0.1 µg/ml of pork insulin efficiently decreased the response by pork insulin specific helper cells. However, when SF derived from beef insulin induced SC further cultured with a small dose of beef insulin were tested for the suppression of pork insulin induced help they also suppressed pork insulin help to the same degree as SF_{pork} (Fig.2). Neither of these factors

suppressed KLH-specific help (Table 2), nor did KLH specific suppressor factors affect insulin help.

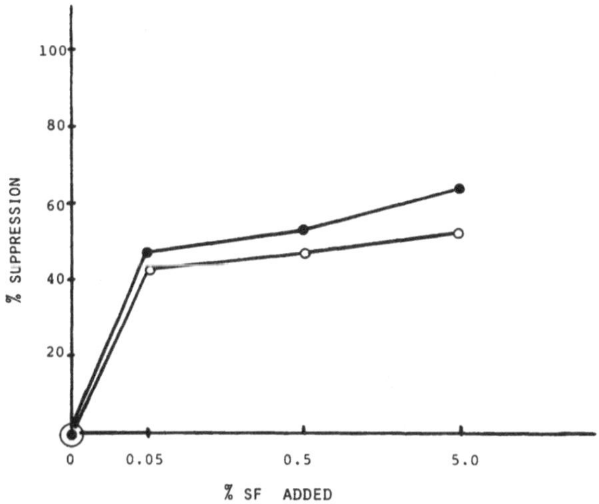

Fig.2. $3x10^5$ HC_{pork} of BALB/c origin were added to $3x10^6$ normal BALB/c spleen cells together with 1.0 µg/ml of TNP-pork in the presence or absence of SF_{pork} (●——●) or SF_{beef} (o——o) of B10.D2 origin.

Table 2. Specificity of insulin suppressor factors

STIMULUS TNP-KLH 1° spl.cells	TNP-KLH	SUPPRESSION SF	RESPONSE IgG anti-DNP AFC/10^6	%S
+	-	-	30 ± 30	-
+	+	-	4300 ± 270	-
+	+	SF_{KLH} 2.5%	1900 ± 150	58
+	+	0.25%	2600 ± 360	40
+	+	SF_{pork} 2.5%	4100 ± 560	6
+	+	0.25%	4200 ± 290	3

$3x10^6$ TNP-KLH primed CBA spleen cells were stimulated with TNP-KLH and cultured in the presence or absence of SF. Anti-DNP AFC were assayed on day 6 of the culture. Both SF_{KLH} and SF_{pork} were of human origin, and derived from the same donor.

3) <u>Comparison of insulin suppressor factors of human and mouse origin.</u> Pork or beef insulin induced suppressor factors from normal human peripheral blood monocytes suppress-

ed responses by HC_{pork} to the same degree as insulin suppressor factors of mouse origin (Fig.3). Human factors also lacked analogue specificity e.g. both pork and beef insulin induced SF decreased pork insulin specific help to the same degree (Fig.3), but did not affect KLH specific help (Table 2).

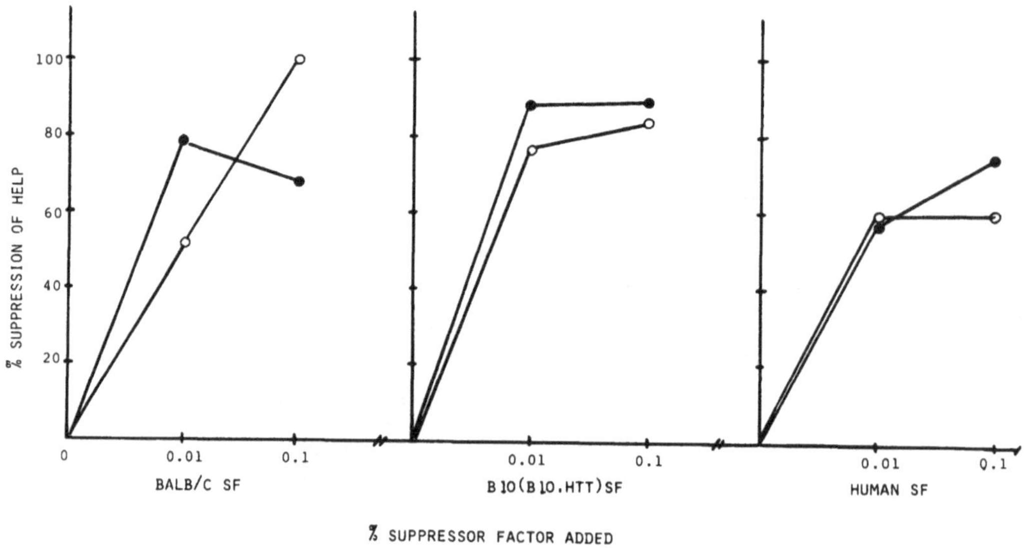

Fig. 3. $3x10^5$ BALB/c HC_{pork} were added to $3x10^6$ normal BALB/c spleen cells together with 0.05 µg/well of DNP-pork in the presence or absence of SF. Suppressor factors were induced with pork (•——•) or beef (o——o) insulins.

4) <u>Charasteristics of insulin suppressor factors.</u> The activity of suppressor factors induced with pork or beef insulin could be absorbed out with either beef or pork insulin immunoadsorbent but not with an unrelated antigen, keyhole limpet haemocyanin (KLH) neither with anti-mouse immunoglobulin. The lack of analogue specificity on functional tests was thus confirmed with the immunoadsorbance of results. In addition SF insulin activity was adsorbed out with the antisera reacting with the constant region of the antigen specific SF (Table 3).

Table 3. The effects of immunoadsorbent treatment on insulin SF.

STIMULUS HC_{pork}	DNP-pork	SUPPRESSION SF 5%	RESPONSE anti-DNP AFC/10^6	%S
-	+	-	7 ± 4	-
+	+	-	51 ± 4	-
+	+	SF_{pork}	22 ± 10	66
+	+	ads.pork	56 ± 4	0
+	+	" beef	52 ± 3	0
+	+	" KLH	21 ± 6	68
+	+	" RαSF	49 ± 21	5
-	+	-	33 ± 12	-
+	+	-	493 ± 17	-
+	+	SF_{beef}	271 ± 8	48
+	+	ads.αMIG	293 ± 32	43
+	+	" KLH	278 ± 19	47

$3x10^5$ BALB/c HC pork were added to $3x10^6$ normal BALB/c spleen cells together with 0.05 µg/well of DNP-pork in the presence or absence of SF_{pork} of human origin, unadsorbed or adsorbed as indicated.

5) Lack of proliferative responses to pork insulin by cells from normal BALB/c spleen or human peripheral blood.

Whether cells from normal donors would proliferate in the presence of insulin was tested by incubating normal spleen cells or PBL with various concentrations of insulin using concanavallin A as a control. Stimulation indexes (SI) in Table 4 indicate that no proliferative responses were obtained with any of the insulin concentrations used.

Table 4. Stimulation of normal cells by pork insulin.

STIMULUS		SI BALB/C SPLEEN CELLS	SI HUMAN PBL
Concanavallin A	5 µg/ml	3.5	28.0
Pork insulin	0.1 µg/ml	1.0	0.8
	1 "	0.9	0.8
	10 "	0.9	1.1
	30 "	1.0	1.0
	100 "	1.0	1.4

Discussion

Insulin specific suppressor cells and factors could be induced *in vitro* and effectively abolished the function of pork insulin specific helper cells. They resemble other antigen specific suppressor factors, and in addition to antigen combining site carry determinants coded for by the central (I) region of the MHC, but lack immunoglobulin (Fc) determinants (13,14). Serological analysis also revealed the presence of constant region determinants (Table 3), determinants shared (or cross reacting) with all antigen specific factors whether of mouse, monkey or human origin (31,14,20,29,31).

A puzzling feature of insulin suppressor factors is their apparent lack of analogue specificity e.g. although the factors are insulin specific and do not suppress for instance KLH responses they do not differentiate between pork and beef. Thus suppressor factors generated with either pork or beef insulin abolished the function of pork insulin specific helper cells. This is in contrast to insulin help or proliferation which is strictly analogue specific (23-26). If the lack of analogue specificity is not due to inpurities in the insulin preparations used (which is not excluded at present) it implies that suppression is directed against different (and possibly shared) determinants of the insulin molecule unlike help where difference in two or three amino acids of the B-chain are recognized. It may well be that insulin molecules are like lysozymes where different determinants are recognized by helper and suppressor cells (32,33).

An interesting feature of the insulin suppression is that also nonresponder mice e.g. mice in which T cell help or T cell proliferation cannot be generated (e.g. CBA) do produce insulin specific suppressor factors. This is like certain other antigens to which only part of the mice respond (9,10) and suggest a different control for immune "responsiveness" measured as help or T proliferation and "nonresponsiveness" measured as suppression.

Insulin analogues readily induced human insulin specific helper and suppressor factors. The suppressor factors reported here are like mouse factors in lacking insulin analogue specificity with the two analogues, pork and beef, tested. This suggests that one reason for the failures in the regulation of anti-insulin responses in some diabetics producing anti-insulin antibodies may be due to inefficient suppression. The possibility of testing insulin specific help and suppression in humans, however, offers one way of exploring the parameters of specific immune responses against a disease associated antigen in normal people as well as in diabetics.

Acknowledgements: We thank Ms. Pirkko Himberg and Pirjo Ranttila for excellent technical assistance and Liisa Suonio for her help in preparing the manuscript. These studies were supported by a grant from the Juvenile Diabetes Foundation.

References

1. Benacerraf, B., McDewitt, H.O.: Science 175, 273-279 (1972).
2. Benacerraf, B., Katz, D.H.: Immunogenetics and Immunodeficiency, B.Benacerraf (ed.), William Clowes and Sons, Ltd. London 1975.
3. Gershon, R.: Contemp. Top. Immunobiol. 3, 1-40 (1975).
4. Cantor, H., Gershon, R.: Fed. Proc. 38, 2058-2064 (1979).
5. McDewitt, H.O.: J. Immunol. 100, 485-492 (1968).
6. Munro, A.J., Taussig, M.J.: Nature 256, 103-106 (1975).
7. Hill, S.W., Sercarz, E.: Eur. J. Immunol. 5, 317-324 (1975).
8. Keck, K.: Eur. J. Immunol. 5, 801-807 (1975).
9. Kontiainen, S., Howie, S., Maurer, P.H., Feldmann, M.: J. Immunology 122, 253-259 (1979).
10. Kapp, J.A.: J. Exp. Med. 147, 997-1006 (1978).
11. Pierres, M., Germain, R.N.: J. Immunol. 121, 1306-1314(1978).
12. Erb, P., Meier, B, Feldmann, M.: J. Immunol. 122, 1916-1919 (1979).
13. Tada, T., Taniguchi, M., Okumura, K.: Progr. Immunol. 3, 369-377 (1977).
14. Feldmann, M., Baltz, M., Erb, P., Howie, S., Kontiainen, S., Woody, J., Zwaifler, N.: Progr. Immunol. 3, 331-337 (1977).
15. UytdeHaag, F., Heijnen, C.J., Ballieux, R.E.: Nature 271, 556-557 (1978).
16. Kantor, F., Feldmann, M.: Clin. Exp. Immunol. 36, 71-77 (1979).
17. Cantor, H., Shen, F.W, Boyse, E.A.: J. Exp. Med. 143, 1391-1403 (1976).
18. Feldmann, M., Beverley, P.C.L., Dunkley, M., Kontiainen,S.: Nature 258, 614-616 (1975).
19. Moretta, L., Webb, S.R., Grossi, C.E., Lydyard, P.M., Cooper, M.D.: J. Exp. Med. 146, 184-200 (1977).

19a. Kontiainen, S., Feldmann, M.: J. Exp. Med. 147, 110-122(1978).

20. Lamb, J.R., Kontiainen, S., Lehner, T.: Inf. Immun. 3, 903-907 (1979).
21. Keck, K.: Nature 254, 78-79 (1975).
22. Keck, K.: Eur. J. Immunol. 7, 811-816 (1977).
23. Barcinski, M.A., Rosenthal, A.S.: J. Exp. Med. 145, 726-742 (1977).

24. Rosenwasser, L.J., Barcinski, M.A., Schwartz, R.H., Rosenthal, A.S.: J. Immunol. 123, 471-476 (1979).

25. Rosenthal, A.S., Barcinski, M.A., Blake, J.T.: Nature 267, 156-158 (1977).

26. Erb, P.: Immunology, in press (1980).

27. Kontiainen, S., Feldmann, M.: Nature New Biol. 245, 285-286 (1973).

28. Kontiainen, S., Feldmann. M.: Eur. J. Immunol. 6, 296-301 (1976).

29. Kontiainen, S., Woody, J.N., Rees, A., Feldmann, M.: Clin. exp. Immunol., in press (1980).

30. Kontiainen, S., Feldmann, M.: Eur. J. Immunol. 7, 310-314 (1977).

31. Kontiainen, S., Feldmann, M.: Thymus 1, 59-79 (1979).

32. Adorini, L., Miller, A., Sercarz, E.E.: J. Immunol. 122, 871-877 (1979).

33. Yowell, R.L., Araneo, B.A., Miller, A., Sercarz, E.E.: Nature 279, 70-71 (1979).

IMMUNE RESPONSE PHENOTYPE OF INSULIN-PRESENTING CELLS MODIFIED BY INSERTION OF H-2 GENE PRODUCTS INTO CELL MEMBRANES

Aya Prujansky-Jakobovitz*, Ayala Frenkel†, Nathan Sharon* and Irun R. Cohen†
Departments of Biophysics* and Cell Biology†, The Weizmann Institute of Science, Rehovot, Israel

Introduction

T lymphocytes bearing specific receptors recognise and respond to their respective antigens through the agency of antigen-presenting cells. Soluble protein antigens will not stimulate helper or effector T lymphocytes unless the antigens have first been processed and served up to the T lymphocytes by appropriate antigen-presenting cells. Hence, the immunogenicity of an antigenic determinant may be seen as a function of communication between an antigen-presenting cell and a specific T lymphocyte.

The immune response to specific antigenic determinants appears to be controlled to a significant degree by products of genes in the major histocompatibility complex (MHC). This conclusion has emerged from genetical experiments which have shown that antigen-presenting cells will not communicate antigenic signals to T lymphocytes, unless both cell types share alleles within the MHC (1). Furthermore, the nature of these shared MHC alleles influences the choice of antigenic determinants recognized on the immunogenic molecule. For example, the response of T lymphocytes of guinea pigs to defined antigenic determinants on the porcine insulin molecule is regulated by the MHC genotype of the cells presenting insulin to responding T lymphocytes (2,3). A high or low response phenotype to a particular antigenic determinant is associated with particular alleles in the MHC of the immunized individual. Genetic loci that so influence the immune response phenotype are termed immune response (Ir) genes (4,5).

Supported in part by a Grant from the National Institute of Arthritis, Metabolism, and Digestive Diseases no. AM26766.

Much information has been gained about Ir genes by investigating the inheritance of Ir phenotypes and the influence of genotype on immunological behaviour. However, to learn more about molecular mechanisms underlaying Ir gene expression, it would be helpful to study the function of the products of Ir genes, in isolation from the genes themselves.

To achieve this end, we have developed an experimental model whereby it is possible to study immune effects of structural products of the MHC. Our strategy has been to insert membrane components from cells of one MHC genotype into recipient cells of a different MHC genotype, and to study the effect of this membrane engineering on the ability of antigen-presenting cells to communicate with T lymphocytes.

As vehicles for inserting membrane components, we use liposome vesicles compose of donor cell plasma membranes and Sendai virus envelopes (6). Specific glycoproteins of the Sendai virus envelope fuse the liposome to the recipient cell and the donor membrane components are integrated along with the vesicle into the plasma membrane of the recipient cell. By using MHC congenic mice as sources of donor and recipient cells, we can measure the contribution of products of MHC-linked Ir genes. This paper reports results showing that presentation of antigenic determinants of insulin to T lymphocytes can be achieved by membrane-engineered antigen-presenting cells. This indicates that structural products of MHC genes, expressed and active at the plasma membrane, are sufficient to mediate an Ir phenotype of the response to beef insulin.

Material and Methods

Mice. H-2 congenic C3H.DiSn ($H-2^k$) and C3H.SW ($H-2^b$) were used in the experiments described here. The mice were bred and supplied by the Animal Breeding Center of this Institute, matched for sex and used at 2-3 months of age.

Immunization. Mice were inoculated into the hind foot pads, with 10 µg of beef insulin, emulsified in complete Freund's adjuvant and 14 days later the draining popliteal lymph nodes were removed and suspensions of cells were tested for their proliferative response to antigen-presenting cells that had been pulsed with beef insulin.

Antigen-presenting cells (1). Spleen cells from naive mice were fused with membrane vesicles, irradiated with 1,500 R of gamma irradiation, and 10^7/ml viable cells were incubated for 1 h at 37°C with beef insulin, 100 µg/ml in RPM1 medium without added serum. The cells were washed extensively and 2 x 10^5 antigen-presenting cells were mixed with 4 x 10^5 lymph node lymphocytes in microtiter wells and cultured for 3 days. The proliferative response was measured in triplicate wells by incorporation of ^{3}H-tymidine as described (7).

Membrane vesicle fusion. The method of insertion of membrane vesicles was adapted (6) from that described by Volsky and his colleagues (8). The strategy was to exploit the fusigenic properties of Sendai virus envelope glycoproteins as transfer vehicles. Briefly, purified Sendai virus envelopes were solubilized in detergent (2% Triton X-100) and mixed with detergent solubilized plasma membrane components of donor spleen cells. Donor plasma membranes were purified and isolated on a sucrose density gradient. Plasma membrane enzyme markers were enriched up to 70 fold and no cytoplasmic enzymes, RNA or DNA were detectible. Vesicles containing plasma membrane components and Sendai virus fusigenic glycoproteins were formed by removing the detergent by dialysis. The reconstituted vesicles were isolated by centrifugation (100,000 G). The vesicles were fused with antigen-presenting cells by incubating 10^7 cells with 5-10 µg protein of vesicles in 1 ml fusion buffer at 4°C for 60 min. The bound vesicles were incorporated into recipient cells by further incubation at 37°C for 30 min. The cells were extensively washed, pulsed with insulin, and used as antigen-presenting cells. Control vesicles included those that contained Sendai virus envelopes without donor plasma membranes or plasma membranes without Sendai virus envelopes. Neither control preparation had any activity.

Results

Table 1 shows the results of inserting H-2^k or H-2^b plasma membranes into antigen presenting cells. Lymph node lymphocytes were taken from C3H.SW

($H-2^b$) responder mice that had been immunized against beef insulin. Antigen-presenting cells originated from C3H.SW responder or from C3H.DiSn ($H-2^k$) non-responder mice. C3H.SW spleen cells presented beef insulin to syngeneic responder C3H.SW lymph node T cells (net response of 26,000 cpm). The insertion of allogeneic C3H.DiSn ($H-2^k$) membranes into these C3H.SW antigenic presenting cells had two effects. There developed a proliferative response of 27,000 cpm in the absence of insulin that was caused most probably by a mixed-lymphocyte-reaction (MLR) of the $H-2^b$ responder lymph node cells against the stimulator spleen cells presenting inserted allogeneic $H-2^k$ antigens. Despite the MLR, these antigen presenting cells could activate a net response to insulin of 19,000 cpm above the background MLR.

The allogeneic C3H.DiSn ($H-2^k$) spleen cells produced an MLR of 43,000 cpm, but little or no net response to insulin (7,000 cpm). However, insertion of C3H.SW ($H-2^b$) membrane components into the allogeneic $H-2^k$ spleen cells, led to a net response to insulin of 62,000 cpm above the allogeneic MLR of 65,000 cpm measured in the absence of insulin.

TABLE 1

INSERTED H-2 GENE MEMBRANE PRODUCTS INFLUENCE PRESENTATION OF BEEF INSULIN TO T LYMPHOCYTES FROM PRIMED C3H.SW ($H-2^b$) MICE

Insulin presenting spleen cells	Origin of inserted membrane	Proliferative Response (cpm x 10^{-3})		
		Without Insulin	With Insulin	Net response to Insulin
C3H.SW ($H-2^b$)	None	2	28	26
	C3H.DiSn	27	46	19
C3H.DiSn ($H-2^k$)	None	43	50	7
	C3H.SW	65	127	62

Discussion

The results presented here indicate that insertion of syngeneic $H-2^b$ membrane components into allogeneic spleen cells from $H-2^k$ non-responder mice endows them with the capacity to present beef insulin to H-2^b responder T lymphocytes.

The response to insulin was measured as the increment in cpm above the background cpm that in effect comprised an allogeneic MLR in those cases where allogeneic H-2^k antigens were inserted or indigenous to the membranes of the antigen-presenting spleen cells. We hope that it may be possible to develop a model of presentation of insulin free of any possible allogeneic effects by using lines or clones of responder T lymphocytes that can recognize antigenic determinants of insulin, but no other antigens including allogeneic MHC products (A. Ben-Nun, H. Wekerle and I.R. Cohen, in preparation). However, despite the uncomfortably high MLR background, it is evident from the results that untreated allogeneic H-2^k spleen cells could not present insulin. Furthermore, the addition of H-2^k membrane components to H-2^b presenter spleen cells produced an MLR that not only did not enhance, but seemed to decrease the presentation of insulin by these cells to syngeneic H-2^b lymphocytes. Therefore, it seems reasonable to conclude that inserted H-2 membrane components activated the response to insulin by presentation of the antigen and not by non-specific allogeneic effects.

Control experiments (not shown) involving insertion of viral envelope components without H-2 antigens, or of non-specific H-2 antigens, showed no effect on presentation of insulin. Therefore, it appears that specific H-2 components were active in mediating presentation of insulin. The role of non-H-2 membrane components was excluded since we used H-2 congenic mice that shared identical non-H-2 genes.

In these experiments we have not identified the particular H-2 components responsible for presenting insulin. Mapping of H-2 subregions can be done by inserting membranes obtained from H-2 recombinant mice. Ultimately we hope to insert purified, isolated H-2 gene products and so characterize the functional molecules. Preliminary evidence suggest that the active components may not be serologically defined Ia antigens.

We do not yet know whether inserted H-2 membrane components allowed presentation of beef insulin because they merely allowed effective communication between the presenter and responder cells. It is also possible that in addition to a cell-cooperation function, the inserted membrane components facilitated the "processing" of a critical antigenic determinant on the insulin by the presenter cells (3,4). In any case, it seems that structural membrane components are sufficient to mediate an Ir phenotype. Hidden regulatory genes, or intracellular products were most probably not transferred in our experiments. Hopefully, our insertion procedure will enable us to identify the precise H-2 products needed for antigen presentation.

References

1. Yano, A., Schwartz, R.H., Paul, W.E.: J. Exp. Med. 146, 828-843 (1977).
2. Rosenthal, A.S., Barcinski, M.A., Blake, J.T.: Nature 267, 156-158 (1977).
3. Barcinski, M.A., Rosenthal, A.S.: J. Exp. Med. 145, 726-742 (1977).
4. Benacerraf, B.: J. Immunol. 120, 1809-1812 (1978).
5. McDevitt, H.O.: Ir Genes and Ia Antigens, Academic Press, New York 1978.
6. Prujansky-Jakobovits, A., Volsky, D.J., Loyter, A., Sharon, N.: Proc. Natl. Acad. Sci. (USA), in press.
7. Cohen, I.R., Talmon, J., Lev-Ram, V., Ben-Nun, A.: Proc. Natl. Acad. Sci. (USA) 76, 4066-4070 (1979).
8. Volsky, D.J., Cabantchik, Z.I., Beigel, M., Loyter, A.: Proc. Natl. Acad. Sci. (USA) 76, 5440-5444 (1979).

DIFFERENCES IN INSULIN ANTIBODIES INDUCED WITH VARYING ANTIGENIC FORMS

E. R. Arquilla, I. Valdes, R. Thompson, R. E. Michalski and K. Thomas

Department of Pathology, University of California, Irvine Medical Center

INTRODUCTION

Previous results from our laboratory suggested that the humoral response of guinea pigs to insulin resulted in different antibody populations when immunization was performed with different quarternary forms of insulin antigen (1). The antisera showed wide variations in antibody concentration, determinants on the insulin molecules to which antibodies were directed and avidity of the various antibodies. In view of these observations, experiments were designed firstly to examine the differences between the humoral response of guinea pigs immunized with various forms of insulin and secondly, to characterize the antigenic determinants to which these various antibodies react. As it was not clear whether or not these humoral immune response differences were due to the quarternary structure of the insulin antigen or to other factors such as immunization procedures and antigen preparation, these experiments were also designed to carefully control these parameters.

Outbred Hartley Mongrel guinea pigs were subjected to identical immunization regimens with four forms of insulin as the antigen: Zinc (Zn)-insulin crystals, Nickel (Ni)-insulin crystals, Fibrillar (Fib)-insulin and Zinc-free mono component (MC)-insulin. Because previous studies demon-

Basic and Clinical Aspects of Immunity to Insulin

strated that antibodies in the radioimmune titration assay (AB_R) and antibodies in the immune hemolysis titration assay (AB_H) are directed towards differing determinants on the insulin molecule (1, 2), the antiserum harvested from each guinea pig was individually titrated in each of the two systems. In view of the results found by these studies and the assumption that antibodies directed against the perturbed site on the molecule would react to a lesser degree than antibodies directed toward determinants distant from the perturbed site, further experiments were designed in order to characterize the antigenic determinants with which the various antibodies interact. Utilizing insulin derivatives containing known perturbations, inhibition studies were conducted in order to better define portions of the insulin molecule with which antibodies raised against MC-insulin and Ni-insulin crystals react. The results of these experiments not only help to establish the relationship between the structure of the antigen and antibody production, but also give insight into certain important intramolecular interactions that stabilize the conformation of insulin.

EXPERIMENTAL

Antigenic Preparation

MC-insulin was prepared from twice crystallized bovine insulin by chelation with EDTA and purification on a DEAE-Sephadex (A-25) column equilibrated with 0.01M Tris (hydroxymethyl aminomethane), 0.01M glycine, 0.8M NaCl and 7M urea buffer, pH 9 (3, 4). A single lot of MC-insulin was used as the starting material to prepare each of the other three antigens. MC-insulin as an antigen was suspended in buffered saline (0.01M Na_2PO_4, 0.85% NaCl, pH 7.4) to a concentration of 5 mg/ml. Zn-insulin crystals and Ni-insulin crystals were prepared from MC-insulin according to the method described by Schlichtkrull (5, 6). The pelleted crystals were suspended in buffered saline to a concentration of 5 mg/ml.

Fib-insulin was prepared according to Waugh (7). The resulting thixotropic gel was diluted to 5 mg/ml with buffered saline.

Each of the four forms of the insulin antigen was suspended in buffered saline. Alum (0.05%) Al $NH_4(SO_4)_2 \cdot 12H_2O$ was added bringing a final concentration of antigens to 4.76 mg/ml antigen. Each antigen suspension was divided into aliquots and stored at -80°F. For sensitization, 2.25 ml of antigen (0.5 ml) suspension was added to 15 ml of complete Freund's Adjuvant. For the booster injections, each of the antigen suspensions was diluted in buffered saline to 1 mg/ml immediately prior to the injection.

Immunization Procedure

The immunization procedure was a modification of the method described by Brugman and Arquilla (8). Outbred Hartley Mongrel guinea pigs were divided into four groups, each consisting of 13 to 14 animals. Each group was immunized with either MC-insulin, Zn-insulin crystals, Ni-insulin crystals or Fib-insulin, Figure 1.

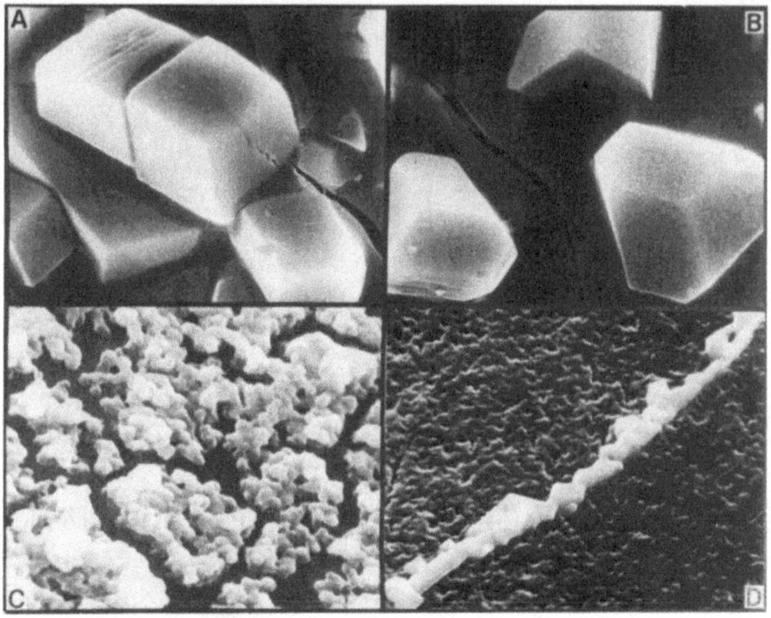

Figure 1: Scanning electron micrographs of four forms of insulin used as antigens: (a) Zn-insulin crystals (B) Ni-insulin crystals (C) Zn-free monocomponent (MC) insulin and (D) fibrillar (Fib) insulin were prepared from MC bovine insulin and processed for scanning electron microscopy.

The sensitization was accomplished with a total of 0.5 mg of each antigen per guinea pig administered in four divided injections of 0.2 ml containing 0.15 mg antigen into each paw pad. Following sensitization, glucose (15-20 g) was added to each 100 ml of drinking water, and sugar cubes were placed in cages to prevent hypoglycemic shock. When symptoms of hypoglycemia were noted, the guinea pigs were injected intraperitoneally with 5 ml of 50% glucose.

Two weeks following sensitization, the guinea pigs received their first of 9 booster injections. Three booster injections equally spaced over 9 days were given with a two-week interval between each set of 3 booster injections. Each antigen suspension (0.1 ml, 0.1 mg) was injected intradermally at the hip after the hair had been plucked. Following each booster injection, 15-20 g glucose was added to each 100 ml of drinking water, and sugar cubes were placed in cages to prevent hypoglycemic shock.

One week following the ninth booster (73 days after sensitization), all the guinea pigs were exsanguinated. The blood of each animal was allowed to clot at room temperature for 1 hour, and then at $4^{o}C$ for 2 hours. The serum was separated by centrifugation at 700 g for 10 minutes at $4^{o}C$. Each insulin antiserum was divided into appropriate aliquots and stored at $-80^{o}F$.

RESULTS

Differences in Humoral Immune Response of Guinea Pigs Immunized with Various Forms of Insulin

The titer of antibodies operative in the radioimmune system (AB_R) and antibodies operative in the immune hemolysis system (AB_H) of each antiserum was measured as previously described (2, 9). The AB_R titer was the reciprocal antiserum dilution of which 0.1 ml will bind 50% of 2×10^4 cpm of (^{125}I)monoiodoinsulin (approximately 200 mCi/mg, 0.059 ng) in a volume of 0.3 ml following incubation for 1 hour at $4^{o}C$. The free (^{125}I)monoiodoinsulin was adsorbed on 0.4 ml 1.5% charcoal/0.15% dextran (w/v) in buffer and separated from the antibody bound (^{125}I)monoiodoinsulin by centrifugation at 1500 g according to Herbert, et al. (10).

The AB_H titer is the reciprocal antiserum dilution of which 0.1 ml will, in the presence of excess complement, hemolyze 50% of 8.7×10^6 sheep red blood cells coated with Zn-insulin (11). Antiserum and the Zn-insulin-coated sheep red cells were incubated for 1 hour at $4^{o}C$. Excess complement in 0.1 ml was added, the mixture was incubated at $37^{o}C$ for

30 minutes, and the degree of specific immune hemolysis was determined as previously described (9, 11).

Elevated titers of antibodies operative in the immune hemolysis system were observed in antisera raised against Zn- and Ni-insulin crystals. The mean AB_H titer of the Zn-insulin antisera was significantly greater ($p<0.05$) than the mean AB_H titers of the MC- and the Fib-insulin antisera, but not significantly different from the mean AB_H titer of the Ni-insulin antisera. Likewise, the mean AB_H titer of the Ni-insulin antisera was also significantly greater ($p<0.05$) than the mean AB_H titers of the MC- and the Fib-insulin antiserum. The two individual antisera with the highest AB_H titers were raised against Ni-insulin crystals (Table 1, GP#N1, N2) while the two individual antisera with the lowest AB_H titers were raised against MC-insulin (Table 1, GP#M5, M9).

TABLE 1: Radioimmune and Immune Hemolysis Titers of Antisera Raised Against Four Different Forms of Insulin

GP#	MC-Insulin Antisera		Zn-Insulin Antisera		FIB-Insulin Antisera		Ni-Insulin Antisera	
	AB_r	AB_h	AB_r	AB_h	AB_r	AB_h	AB_r	AB_h
1	420	2500	55	1150	3900	300	6533	13417[d]
2	500	4300	1200	2900	2500	165[c]	5550	10240[d]
3	575	400	4700	3900	1300	300	4300	2080[d]
4	920	1600	760	4000[b]	2400	430[c]	1075	4000
5	190	125	900	5900[b]	2700	780	2087	507
6	2600	1350	330	850	95	880	1125	2067
7	1300	420	940	3000[b]	74	135	600	1287
8	330	710	155	5200	350	160	580	1576
9	,10	25	3200	4000	1800	750	1225	3180
10	1400	1700	2400	4100	4700	980[c]	590	2360
11	1650	1050	700	1000	620	3600	350	2437
12	24000	1025[a]	870	320	580	3125	11000	760
13	16500	1250[a]	160	180	4000	880	2700	2800
14			1900	870	3600	250		

+ - AB_R titer is the reciprocal antiserum dilution of which 0.1 ml will bind 50% of 20,000 cpm of ^{125}I-monoiodoinsulin.

* - AB_H titer is the reciprocal antiserum dilution of which 0.1 ml will hemolyze 50% of 8.7 x 10^6 sheep red cells coated with Zn-insulin.

a - Pooled to form the MC-insulin antiserum pool.

b - Pooled to form Zn-insulin antiserum pool.

c - Pooled to form Fib-insulin antiserum pool.

d - Pooled to form Ni-insulin antiserum pool.

No significant differences were demonstrable when the mean titers of antibodies operative in the radioimmune assay of the four groups of antisera were compared to one another.

The variance, however, of the AB_R titers amongst the guinea pigs immunized with MC-insulin was significantly greater (P,0.02) than the variance of the AB_R titers within each of the other 3 groups. Amongst the group of guinea pigs immunized with MC-insulin were the antisera with the lowest (M9, 10) and highest (M12, 24,000) AB_R titers, respectively, as shown in Table 1.

These results are submitted as evidence that the conformation of the insulin antigen modifies the humoral immune response of guinea pigs as measured by the respective AB_R and AB_H titers of the antisera raised. When either Zn- or Ni-insulin crystals are the antigen, significantly higher levels of antibodies operative in the immune hemolysis system (AB_H) are produced. When MC-insulin is the antigen, occasional very high levels of antibodies operative in the radioimmune system (AB_R) are produced.

Sensitivity of the Four Insulin Antisera Pools in the Radioimmune Assay

In previous experiments (1), it was observed that antibodies raised against Zn-insulin demonstrated decreased avidity when compared to antibodies raised against other forms of insulin. This suggests that the frequency of high-avidity antibodies raised against Zn-insulin is considerably lower than that of high-avidity antibodies raised against Ni-, Fib- and MC-insulin. In order to test this, radioimmunoassays using ^{125}I monoiodoinsulin as the indicator and MC-insulin as the inhibitor were performed with the four pools of antisera designated in Table 1. The titer of each of the antiserum pools (a dilution of antiserum capable of binding 50% of the indicator as described in the titration method) was used for each of the four respective pools. Plots (standard curve) of the pmoles of MC-insulin versus the percent inhibition of antibody binding to indicator by each of the four antiserum pools when incubated for 1 and 22 hours are presented in Figure 2.

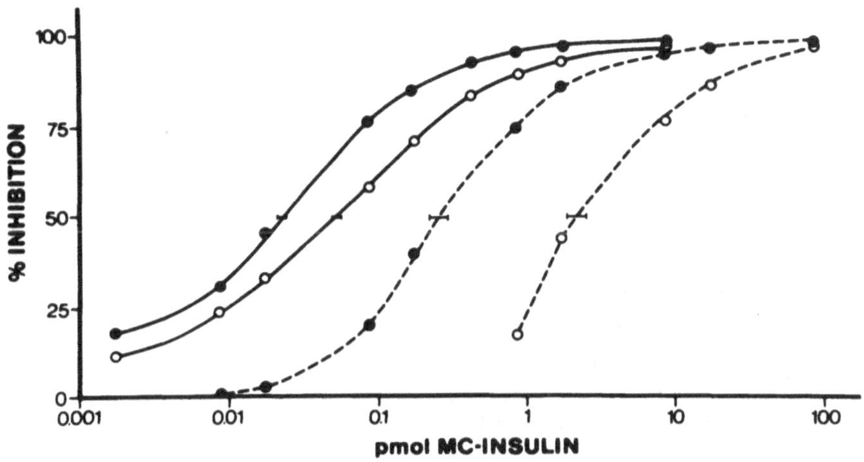

Figure 2: Relative Sensitivities of the four insulin antiserum pools in the radioimmunoassay after 1 hour and 22 hour incubations

Each insulin antiserum pool was diluted as described in the text and incubated with 2 x 10^4 cpm (^{125}I)monoiodoinsulin (approximately 200 mCi/mg, 0.059 ng), for either 1 hour or 22 hours at 4^oC, with the indicated amounts of MC-insulin in a final volume of 0.3 ml. Each point represents the mean of at least two assays. 0, Ni-insulin antiserum pool (AP), MC-insulin AP, and Fib-insulin AP were very similar and are represented by a single line, both after 1 hour (---) and after 22 hours (——) incubation; 0, Zn-insulin AP after 1 hour (---) and 22 hours (——) incubation.

The amount (pmoles of MC-insulin) required to inhibit 50% of the maximum binding was calculated from these plots and is presented in Table 2.

TABLE 2: Relative Sensitivities of the four insulin antiserum pools in the radioimmunoassay after 1 hour and 22 hour incubations

Antisera	1 Hour	22 Hour	Ratio*
Zn-insulin	2.35 ± 0.36	0.052 ± 0.002	45.2
Ni-insulin	0.30 ± 0.02	0.023 ± 0.002	13.0
Fib-insulin	0.26 ± 0.02	0.021 ± 0.000	12.4
MC-insulin	0.27 ± 0.02	0.021 ± 0.002	12.9

The radioimmunoassay was performed as described in the text. Values presented are means ± S.E.M.

* Pmoles for 50% inhibition at 1 hr over pmoles for 50% inhibition at 22 hrs. Pools of various antisera were derived from the individual antisera described in Table 1.

The one-hour standard curves for the Ni-insulin, MC and Fib-insulin antiserum pools were very similar. Approximately 0.28 pmoles of MC-insulin were needed for 50% inhibition of maximum binding. An order of magnitude less insulin was required for 50% inhibition when the reaction for these three antisera with inhibitor and indicator was permitted to continue for 22 hours. The standard curve for Zn-insulin antiserum however was significantly less sensitive. Approximately ten times more MC-insulin (2.35 pmoles) was needed for 50% inhibition after one hour incubation than the amount (0.2 pmoles) required for inhibition of the antibodies in the other three antiserum pools.

There was a 45-fold increase in sensitivity when the antiserum pool against insulin crystals was incubated 22 hours compared to 1 hour incubation (Table 2). This large increase in sensitivity as the incubation time was increased can best be attributed to equilibrium phenomena. The MC- and Fib-insulin antiserum pools were approximately ten times more sensitive than Zn-insulin antiserum pool after 1 hour incubation and 2½ times more sensitive after 22 hour incubation (Table 2).

These observations are consistent with the interpretation that the reactions between MC-insulin and the antibodies present in the antiserum pool from guinea pigs immunized with Zn-insulin crystals are slower to reach equilibrium than the antibodies raised against the other three forms of insulin. It is possible that this is due to a decreased rate of association or an increased rate of dissociation. In any case, it is clear that antibodies raised against Zn-insulin are less avid than the antibodies raised against the other three forms of insulin.

In these experiments, the decreased avidity of the Zn-insulin antibodies was measured against the heterologous MC-insulin standard. In previous studies where the homologous antigen Zn-insulin was used as the standard (1) a similar decreased avidity of antibodies raised against Zn-insulin was observed. It appears that when Zn-insulin is used as the antigen, it is likely that antibodies of low avidity and therefore, inferior sensitivity will be raised when employed in radioimmune assays.

Characterization of the Antigenic Determinants to Which Antibodies of Various Antiserum Pools React

In order to better characterize the portion of the insulin molecule with which antibodies raised against MC-insulin and Ni-insulin crystals interact, inhibition studies were performed with insulin derivatives containing known perturbations. In these studies, it was assumed that antibodies directed against the perturbed site on the molecule would react to a lesser degree than antibodies directed to determinants distant from the perturbed site. The selection of the monocomponent antisera pools and the nickel antisera pool was based upon previous studies (1). where it was observed that the Ni-insulin reacts poorly in the radioimmune assay in comparison to the MC-insulin which reacts poorly in the immune hemolysis assay.

The RIIA measures the interaction of a particular inhibitor with the antibodies operative in the radioimmune assay system (AB_R). Correspondingly, the IHIA measures the interaction of inhibitor with antibodies operative in immune hemolysis system (AB_H). The inhibition (%) of the antibody indicator reaction was plotted against the logarithm of the concentration (pmols) of each of the insulin derivatives used. The immunologic reactivity of each derivative is inversely related to the pmols required for 50% inhibition of antibody indicator reaction.

The respective antiserum pools were employed at a dilution where the insulin antibodies present were capable of binding 50% using, in both cases, the indicator (20,000 cpm) ^{125}I-monoiodoinsulin (approximately 0.04 ng). In the case of the radioimmune inhibition assay, the MC-insulin antiserum pool was diluted to 11,800 and Ni-insulin antiserum pool was diluted to 2,800-fold respectively. Therefore, an equivalent number of indicator molecules were bound in the RIIA by the Ni-insulin antiserum and the MC-insulin antiserum.

Three sets of insulin inhibitors were tested against both antiserum pools in each system. One group of inhibitors were prepared from the MC-insulin used for the preparation of the Ni-insulin crystals, Zn-insulin crystals, Fib-insulin and the MC-insulin used for immunization. The desasparagine desalanine insulin (DAA) was prepared in our laboratory (8) from the same MC-insulin.

A second group of derivatives was prepared from synthetic human insulin as described by Sieber and Marki (12, 13). The derivatives of interest that were tested against the two antisera pools contained perturbations of the A6 to A11 disulfide and the A7 to B7 disulfide. Finally, a third group of derivatives that were prepared also from the synthetic organic synthesized of human insulin contained perturbations in the α helix of the B-chain, specifically of B13 and B16. The data is presented in tabular form (Table 3).

TABLE 3. Characterization of Antibodies Against MC-insulin and Ni-insulin Crystals

INHIBITOR	RADIOIMMUNE INHIBITION ASSAY		IMMUNE HEMOLYSIS INHIBITION ASSAY	
	MC-INSULIN ANTISERA	NI-INSULIN ANTISERA	MC-INSULIN ANTISERA	NI-INSULIN ANTISERA
MC-insulin	0.27	0.30	16.27	204.74
DAA-insulin*	0.43	5.89	509.32	2415.99
Zn-insulin	0.24	0.25	2.28	2.77
Ni-insulin	0.81	0.94	1.65	1.19
human insulin	0.31	0.32	378.0	322.5
d-cys A6†	0.83	0.53	---	---
d-cys A6+11†	24.94	1.20	911.6	688.0
d-cys A7†	4.13	0.65	1599.6	(817.0)
d-cys A11†	21.50	2.06	756.8	576.2
d-cys B7†	4.21	0.64	842.8	636.4
Iso 1†	17.20	0.60	1076.0	705.2
Iso 2†	79.12	1.71	---	---
gln B13°	0.55	1.15	---	---
d-tyr B16°	0.49	1.03	---	---
des-tyr B16°	146.91	31.86	761.1	902.7
endo-tyr B16°	100.20	15.03	(584.5)	(734.8)

Values presented are mean pmoles ± S.E.M. of inhibitor required for 50% inhibition. Values in parentheses are pmoles of inhibitor required for 25% inhibition. The variation as calculated from standard error was approximately 10% for those which interacted well with antibodies and 30% for those which interacted poorly.

* DAA-insulin was prepared in our laboratory from the bovine MC-insulin used to prepare the Zn, Ni and Fib insulins used as antigens. This is the same MC-insulin used as antigen and also as an inhibitor in these studies (8).

† These are derivatives of synthetic human insulin with perturbations of the A6 to A11 and A7 to B7 disulfides.
Iso 1 is a synthetic human insulin with disulfide bonds, A7 to A11 and A6 to B7.
Iso 2 is a synthetic human insulin with disulfide bonds, A6 to A7 and A11 to B7 (12, 13).

° These are derivatives of synthetic human insulin with perturations of the B-chain, alpha-helix, B13 and B16.

The data presented in Table 3 suggests that the antibodies raised against MC-insulin interact with the extreme C-terminus of the B-chain, the N-terminus of the B-chain, the A-chain loop (A8, 9, 10) and the surface residues in proximity to disulfide A6 to B11 and A7 to B7 (Fig. 3 vertical lines). The evidence for this interpretation is based on the markedly attenuated interaction of MC-insulin antibodies with derivatives containing perturbations of the A6 to A11 disulfide and the A7 to B7 disulfide. A second interpretation which follows is that the majority of antibodies raised against Ni-insulin crystals interact with determinants on the insulin molecule which are distant from the surface residues in proximity to the A6 to A11 disulfide and the A7 to B7 disulfide.

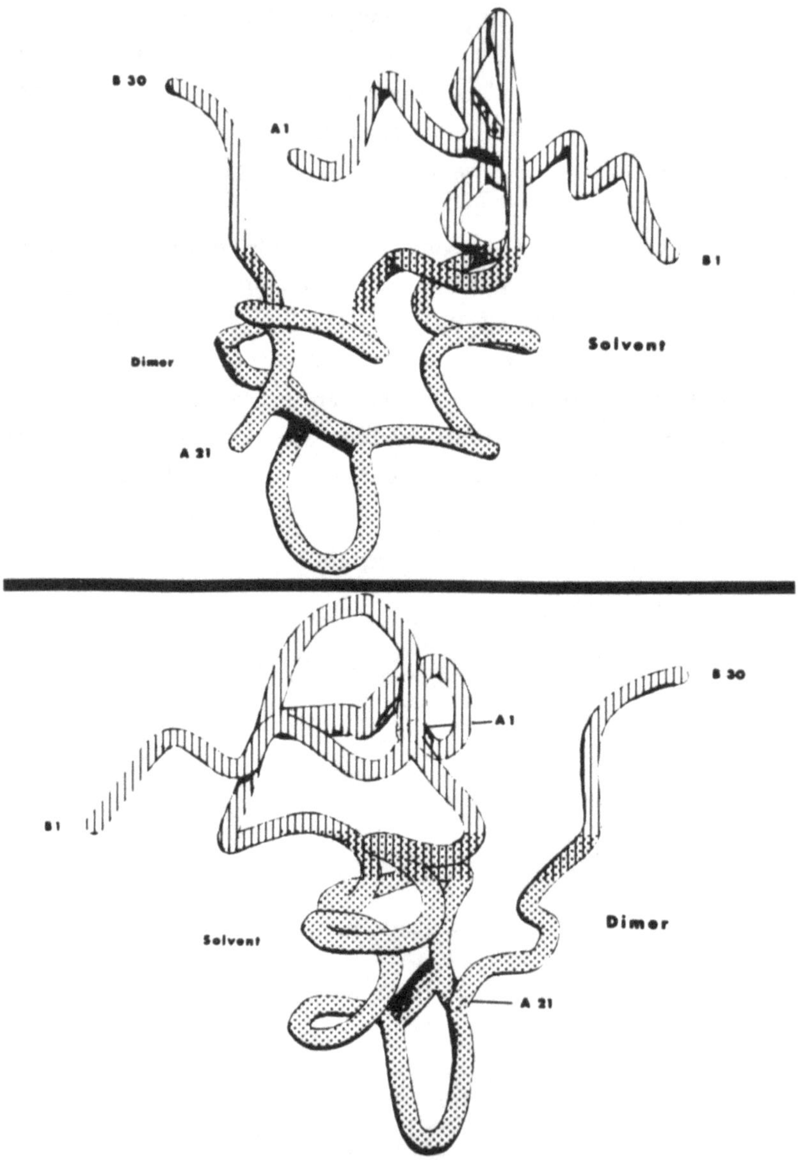

Figure 3: A view of a worm model of insulin constructed from the alpha carbon coordinates of the 51 amino acid residues in insulin (graciously supplied by Professor Dorothy Hodgkin and Guy Dodson).

The results obtained with derivatives that contain perturbations of the B-chain α-helix and the C-terminus of the A-chain lend additional support to these interpretations. DAA-insulin was a very poor inhibitor of the interaction between Ni-insulin antibodies and ^{125}I-monoiodoinsulin indicator, but a good inhibitor of the interaction of MC-insulin antibodies with the same indicator. This suggests that the C-terminal Asp is centrally involved in maintaining the integrity of the determinant(s) with which Ni-insulin crystals interact. Evidence for this interpretation is based on the very poor interaction of Ni-insulin antibodies with DAA-insulin where the C-terminal Asp has been removed. Likewise, perturbations of the B13 and B16 residues in the B-chain α-helix result in a poorer interaction with the Ni-insulin antibodies than with those raised against MC-insulin.

These results suggest that the antibodies raised against Ni-insulin crystals interact with determinants comprising the C-terminus of the A-chain, the B-chain loop comprising (B21, 22, 23, 24), portions of the C-terminus of the B-chain (B25, 26, 27), and also the segment of the B-chain α-helix from B10 to B19 (Fig. 3, stippled area). These observations complement each other and are reinforced by the fact that the antibodies raised against MC-insulin are affected to a lesser degree by derivatives with perturbations involving the C-terminus of the A-chain and the α-helix of the B-chain.

A very significant interpretation regarding insulin structure follows from the results obtained with the des-B16-Tyr derivative and also the endo-B-16 Tyr derivative which had the insertion of an extra Tyr. It is likely that the α helix is markedly altered in these two derivatives and in turn, the whole of the insulin molecule is perturbed. This is reinforced by the observation that both of these derivatives are very poor inhibitors of the antibodies in the MC-insulin antiserum and also in the Ni-insulin antiserum, requiring two to three orders of magnitude more of each of these derivatives than the MC-insulin needed for 50% inhibition. This supports the concept that the B-chain α helix must be maintained for the integrity of the insulin molecule.

This interesting observation suggests the possibility that the interactions between the A- and the B-chain involving the A6 to A11 and A7 to B7 disulfides (Fig. 3, vertical lines) affect the spatial relationships of that portion of the molecule but have a relatively minor affect on the remainder of the insulin molecule which includes the C-terminus portion of the A-chain, the α-helix of the B-chain, the B-chain loop and the proximity of the C-terminal B-chain to the core of the molecule (Fig. 3 stippled area). It appears that alterations in the α-helix and the C-terminus of the A-chain affect the interactions involving the C-terminus of the A-chain, the B-chain loop (B21, 22, 23, 24), the α-helix of the B-chain and the C-terminus (B25, 26, 27) of the B-chain. To a certain extent these interactions seem to be independent of the interactions comprising the other portions of the molecule.

Also of interest is the fact that when MC-insulin is used as the antigen, a significantly greater number of antibodies are made against the A-chain loop (A8, 9, 10), the residues in proximity to the A6 to A11 and A7 to B7 disulfides, the N-terminus B-chain and the extreme C-terminus of the B-chain. Conversely, antibodies generated when the Ni-insulin crystals are used as the antigen seem to be primarily directed against those portions of the molecule involving the C-terminus of the A-chain, the B-chain loop (B21, 22, 23, 24), the B-chain α-helix and C-terminal portions of the B-chain (B25, 26, 27) in close proximity to the core of the molecule.

Acknowledgements

This work was supported by grants from United States Public Health Service (AM-13441-11) and from the Kroc Foundation.

We thank Barbara Speaker for her valuable assistance in preparing the manuscript. We appreciate the help of Janice Haymond in the revision of the manuscript.

REFERENCES

1. Kelso, J. M., Tamai, I. Y., Roth, M.D., Valdes, I., Arquilla, E. R.: Diabetes 29, 383-390 (1980).

2. Arquilla, E. R., Dorio, R. J., Brugman, T. M.: Diabetes 25, 397-403 (1976).

3. Hamlin, J. L., Arquilla, E. R.: J. Biol. Chem. 249, 21-32 (1974).

4. Sodoyez, J. C., Sodoyez-Goffaux, F., Goff, M. M., Zimmerman, A. F., Arquilla, E. R.: J. Biol. Chem. 250, 4268-4277 (1975).

5. Schlichtkrull, J.: Acta Chem. Scand. 10, 1455-1458 (1956).

6. Schlichtkrull, J.: Acta Chem. Scand. 10, 1459-1464 (1956).

7. Waugh, D. F.: J. Cell. Comp. Physiol. 49, 145 (1957).

8. Brugman, T. M., Arquilla, E. R.: Biochemistry 12, 727-732 (1973).

9. Arquilla, E. R., Thiene, P., Brugman, T., Ruess. W., Sugiyama, R.: Biochem. J. 175, 289-297 (1978). tt

10. Herbert, V., Kam-Seng, L., Gottlieb, C. W., Bleicher, S. J.: J. Clin. Endocrinol. Metab. 25, 1374-1384 (1965).

11. Arquilla, E. R., Finn, J.: J. Exp. Med. 122, 771-784 (1965).

12. Sieber, P., Eisler, K., Kamber, B., Riniker, B., Rittel, W., Marki, F.: Hoppe-Seyler's Z. Physiol. Chem. 359, 113-123 (1978).

13. Marki, F., deGasparo, M., Eisler, K., Kamber, B. Riniker, B., Rittel, W., Sieber, P.: Hoppe-Seyler's Z. Physiol. Chem. 360, 1619-1632 (1979).

MOUSE HYBRIDOMA ANTIBODY RECOGNITION OF THE INSULIN MOLECULE

J. Schroer
Laboratory of Immunogenetics, Building 8, Room 100,
National Institutes of Health, Bethesda, Maryland 20205

Introduction

Insulin is one of the better physically and chemically characterized proteins (1) of a group of structurally defined proteins (2-5) that have been the object of intense study by immunologists for several years (6-17). The insulin monomer consists of two chains connected by interchain disulfide bonds. The A chain has two helical portions separated by a loop region formed by an intrachain disulfide bond between cysteines 6, 11 and the B chain consists of pleated sheet segments at the amino and carboxy termini, joined by a central helical region intertwined with the carboxy-terminal A chain helical region.

During the past few years in the laboratories of Alan Rosenthal and Richard Asofsky at the National Institutes of Health, I have been searching for antibodies to species variants of insulin that recognize a distinct region of the molecule, the A chain loop of beef insulin. The three amino acids, A 8-10, in this region show considerable evolutionary diversity as can be seen in Figure 1.

Basic and Clinical Aspects of Immunity to Insulin

AMINO ACID SEQUENCES OF INSULIN

INSULIN A CHAIN

	1	2	3	4	5	6	7	8	9	10	11	12	13	14	15	16	17	18	19	20	21
Beef	Gly	Ile	Val	Glu	Gln	Cys	Cys	Ala	Ser	Val	Cys	Ser	Leu	Tyr	Gln	Leu	Glu	Asn	Tyr	Cys	Asn
Sheep									Gly												
Pork								Thr		Ile											
Chicken								His	Asn	Thr											
Rat				Asp				Thr		Ile											
Human								Thr		Ile											
Rabbit								Thr		Ile											
Fish								His	Lys	Pro		Asn	Ile	Phe	Asp		Gln				
Guinea-pig				Asp				Thr	Gly	Thr		Thr	Arg	His			Gln	Ser			

INSULIN B CHAIN

		1	2	3	4	5	6	7	8	9	10	11	12	13	14	15	16	17	18	19	20	21	22	23	24	25	26	27	28	29	30
Beef		Phe	Val	Asn	Gln	His	Leu	Cys	Gly	Ser	His	Leu	Val	Glu	Ala	Leu	Tyr	Leu	Val	Cys	Gly	Glu	Arg	Gly	Phe	Phe	Tyr	Thr	Pro	Lys	Ala
Sheep																															
Pork																															
Chicken		Ala	Ala																									Ser			
Rat				Lys						Pro*																				Met†	Ser
Human																															Thr
Rabbit																															Ser
Fish	Val	Ala	Pro	Pro										Asp								Asp						Asn			‡
Guinea-pig				Ser	Arg						Asn				Thr			Ser			Gln	Asp	Asp					Ile			Asp

*Present only in Rat I.
†Present only in Rat II.
‡Deletion.

Figure 1. The amino acid differences between beef insulin and several species variants of insulin used throughout the study are shown using the three letter amino acid code (18). Identities are shown by solid lines.

I began my search for anti-A chain loop antibodies by isoelectric focusing (IEF) immune sera from st 2 and st 13 guinea pigs and visualizing specific anti-insulin antibodies by binding and subsequent audioradiography with 125I-beef or pork insulin. Our method (19,20) of isoelectric focusing excluded IgM antibodies but examined IgG anti-insulin antibodies. We had hoped to see populations of antibodies from beef insulin immune sera that bound ^{125}I-beef insulin and not ^{125}I-pork isulin. As illustrated in Figure 2, no such A chain loop-specific antibodies were detected in numerous guinea pig sera.

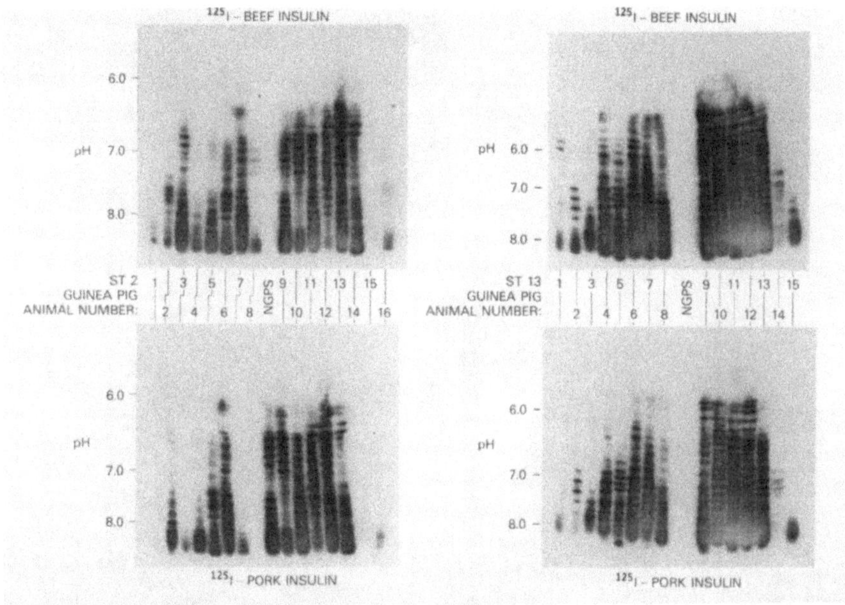

<u>Figure 2.</u> Strain 2 and strain 13 guinea pig anti-beef insulin or anti-pork insulin antibodies binding to ^{125}I-beef or pork insulin

Next, in search of anti-A chain loop antibodies, we turned to similar studies in man using sera from diabetic patients who had taken mixtures of beef or pork insulin. As can be seen in Figure 3, several individuals made antibody bands that bind ^{125}I-beef insulin well and ^{125}I-pork insulin weakly or not at all.

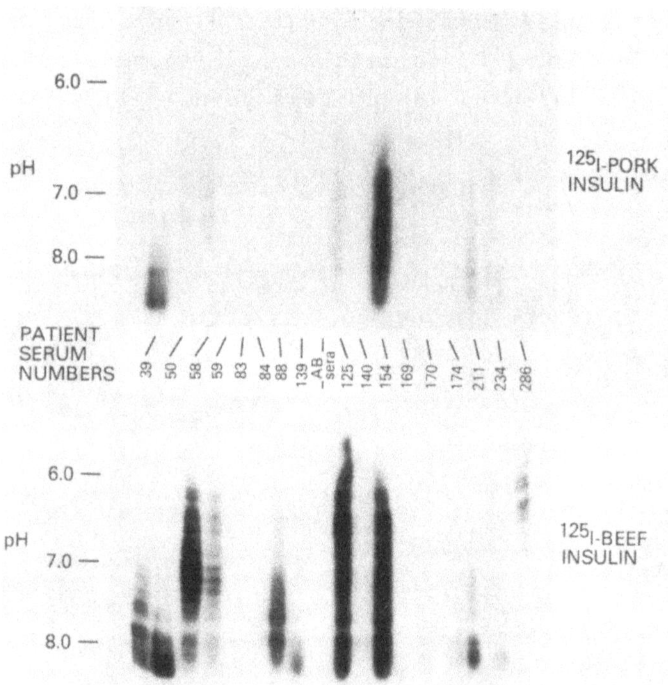

Figure 3. Isoelectric focused human anti-insulin antibodies. Autoradiographs of isoelectric focusing gels of human anti-insulin antibodies binding to ^{125}I-pork insulin or ^{125}I-beef insulin.

Thus, we could detect in man and not in guinea pig A-chain loop specific antibodies. A possible explanation for this finding may be that because a guinea pig's own insulin differ's greatly in amino acid sequence (17a.a.) from beef or pork insulin, many antibodies are made to the multiple regions of the insulin molecule where these exchanges occur. These competing determinants mask in someway the specific response to the A chain loop region of the molecule where beef and pork insulin differ. On the other hand, human insulin differs by only three amino acids from beef and pork insulin. Thus, some individual patients make antibodies directed to the A-chain loop region of beef insulin. Because the titers of antibody in diabetic patients were low, we decided to continue our search for anti-A chain loop antibodies in mice whose insulins (21,22), like human insulin, differ by few amino acids from beef and pork insulin. Using the method of isoelectric focusing described for guinea pig and human anti-insulin sera, we screened anti-insulin immune sera from various strains of mice for anti-A chain loop antibodies. Again as in human, in some individual mice of certain strains (C57 BL10 and not $B10.D_2$, unpublished observation) IEF revealed some antibodies that bind beef insulin and not pork insulin although most individuals make antibodies that cross-react. We were pleased to see that mice made such anti-A chain loop antibodies because we had hoped to use somatic cell fusion (23) to generate large amounts of monoclonal antibodies to defined determinants on the insulin molecule. In our first fusion of lymph node cells from mice immunized with beef insulin and the plasmacytoma cell line NS1/1-Ag-4-1, four hybridoma antibodies were generated. These four anti-insulin antibodies have been compared by IEF, isotyping, affinity and specificity for species variants of insulin.

Results

<u>IEF patterns and isotypes of four anti-insulin hybrid cell antibodies</u>. Four stable anti-insulin antibody-secreting cell lines were obtained from one somatic cell hybridization of beef insulin immune BALB/c lymph node cells with the NS1/1-Ag-4-1 myeloma cell line (details of the hybridization can be found in ref 24). Each cell line grew as ascites producing tumors. When three of the antibodies were specifically purified by affinity chromatography from ascites their concentrations were 2.3 mg/ml, 6.0 mg/ml and 17 mg/ml for AD 2, CB 6 and CB 5 respectively. The IEF patterns of the four anti-insulin hybrid antibodies are shown in figure 4. The upper panel shows an IEF gel after 18% NA_2SO_4 precipitation which visualizes total immunoglobulin excluding IgM of ascites from the hybrid antibodies. The lower panel is an autoradiograph of the same IEF gel after overlay with ^{125}I-beef insulin. Also shown are IEF patterns of a pool of normal BALB/c sera and P3-X63-Ag 8 ascites which both fail to bind ^{125}I-beef insulin.

Ascites from the four anti-insulin antibody secreting cell lines were collected from serial transfers of pools of 3-5 mice over a period of 1-6 months. Each pool of sera obtained from a single transfer was isoelectric focused and shown to be identical before being combined in the pool for determinations of isotype, binding specificity and affinity that follow. Three of the four anti-insulin hybrid antibodies gave identical IEF spectrotypes for 6 months ascites passage while the fourth, CB6, lost five bands after 45 days and 4 more bands at 5 months of passage. The isotype, affinity and specificity of the CB6 antibody was determined on a pool of ascites collected

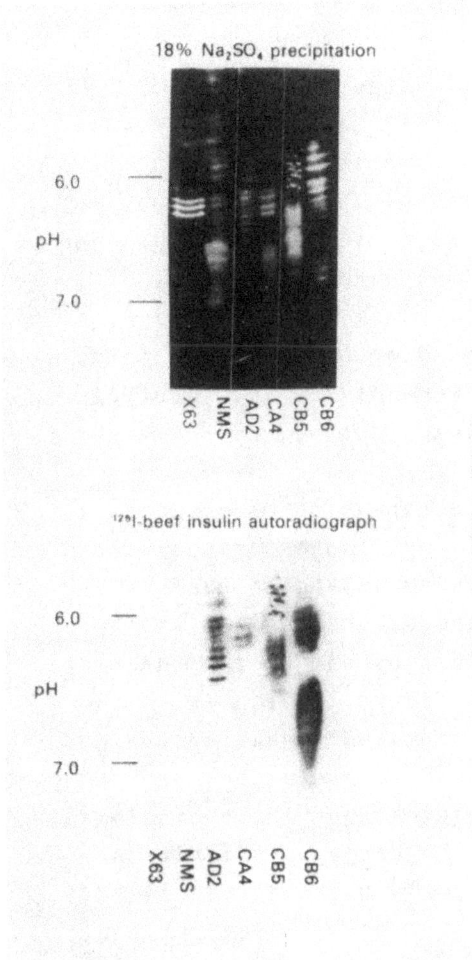

Figure 4. Isoelectric focusing of anti-insulin hybrid antibodies. One to five µl of anti-insulin ascites and 20 µl each of X63 ascites and a pool of normal mouse sera were loaded.

during the first month. From repeated IEF gels the spectrotypes of the four anti-insulin hybrid antibodies were determined: CA4 and CB5 consisted of 5 bands, AD2 gave 11 bands and CB6 consisted of 13 bands which in each case bound ^{125}I-beef insulin. No two spectrotypes appeared to share bands; thus each of the spectrotypes were unique. When ascites from each hybridoma or purified antibody except for CA4 (see below) were isotyped by immunoelectrophoresis using rabbit anti-mouse IgM, IgA, IgG_1, IgG_{2a}, IgG_{2b}, and IgG_3 sera prepared by R. Asofsky, NIH, Bethesda, MD., CB6 and CB5 were of the IgG_1 isotype while AD2 and CA4 were of the IgG_{2b} isotype.

Affinity. Because insulin has no repeating determinants, the affinity of each anti-insulin hybridoma antibody for beef insulin was determined by using unlabeled beef insulin to compete for the binding of the antibody to ^{125}I-beef insulin. Scatchard plots of one of the three or more determinations are shown in figure 5. Each anti-insulin hybridoma antibody repeatedly gave a straight line Scatchard plot (coefficients of correlations between 0.973-0.996) confirming the homogeneity of their binding sites and their monoclonality. The range of affinities from 10^6 to 10^8 L/M though relatively high may be slightly underestimated as serum insulin was not removed from the hybridoma ascites before testing.

Determinant specificty of anti-insulin hybridomas. Using species variants of insulin, the exact localization of the antigenic determinant recognized by one of the four

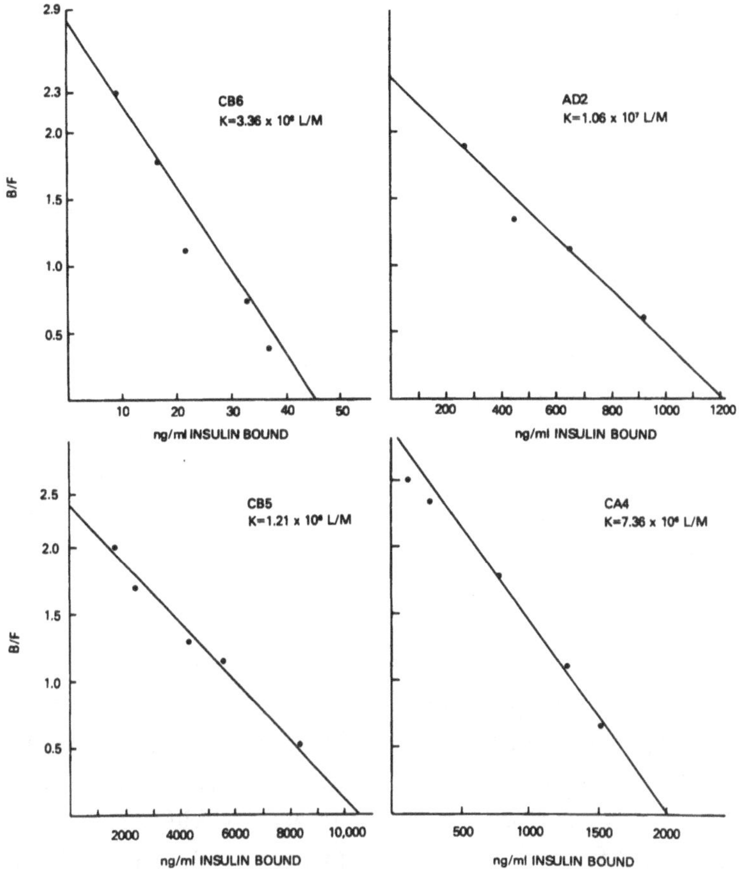

Figure 5. Scatchard analysis of the binding of four anti-insulin hybrid antibodies to ^{125}I-beef insulin:
Upper left panel, CB6 antibody; upper right panel, AD2 antibody, lower left panel, CB5 antibody; lower right panel, CA4 antibody (details of the radioimmunoassay used for affinity measurements are in ref 24).

anti-insulin hybridomas has been determined by comparing the immunological cross reactivities of members of the set. Furthermore, the antibody combining site on the insulin molecule for another of these anti-insulin hybridomas has been tentatively identified using the species variants and chemically modified insulin. The antigenic determinants recognized by the remaining two anti-insulin hybridomas have not yet been elucidated.

The fine specificity of each antibody was studied by using various concentrations of species variants to inhibit the binding of a limiting dilution of each anti-insulin hybridoma to ^{125}I-beef insulin. An example of such a competition assay for each hybridoma is shown in figure 6 where % binding is plotted against concentration (ng/ml) of each species variant.

Table I shows a compilation of data from two or more such competition assays where the results are expressed as the ratio of the concentration of each species variant needed to inhibit 50% of antibody binding to ^{125}I-beef insulin compared to the concentration of unlabeled beef insulin required to give the same inhibition. Low numbers between 1-5 indicate a species of insulin is close to being as good a competitor as beef insulin. High numbers indicate that many times the concentration of a species variant of insulin compared to beef insulin is needed to inhibit the same amount of binding of ^{125}I-beef insulin. Numbers that have $>$ symbols are underestimates as the highest concentrations tested gave less than 50% inhibition. Particularly for CB5 and CA4, the lowest affinity antibodies, higher concentrations for each variant insulin were not available to determine a 50% inhibition.

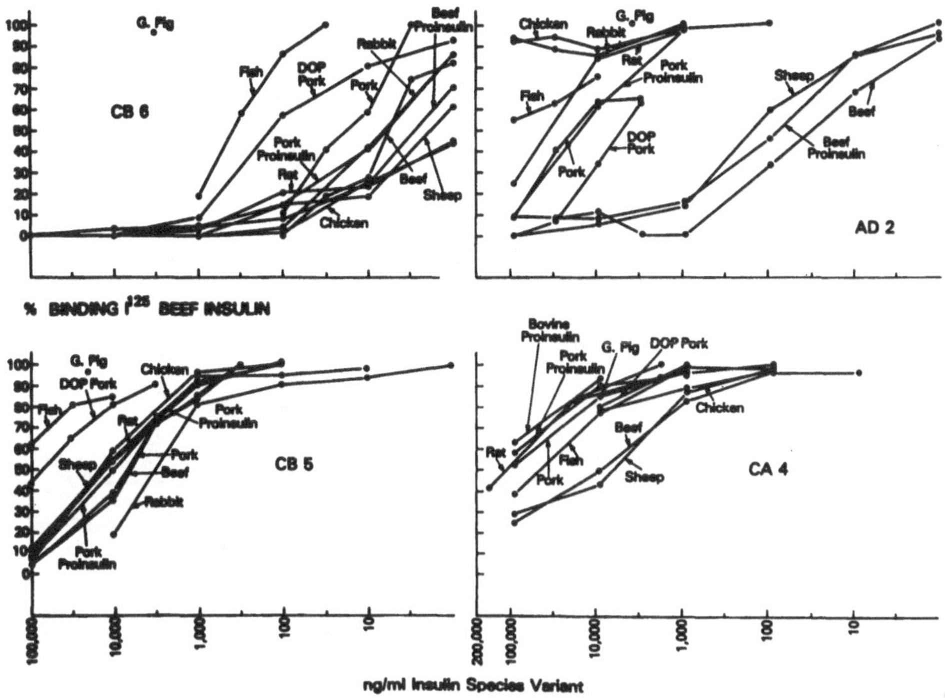

Figure 6. Competition of the binding of anti-insulin hybrid antibodies to ^{125}I-beef insulin with species variants of insulin: upper left panel, CB6 antibody; upper right panel, AD2 antibody; lower left panel, CB5 antibody; lower right panel, CA4 antibody.

The ability of rat and mouse insulin to inhibit the binding of the CB6 antibody to ^{125}I-beef insulin was surprising as we assumed mice would not make antibodies to the parts of the insulin molecule identical to their own insulin. Later the CB5 antibody was also shown to be autoreactive.

AD2 recognizes the A chain loop region of beef insulin. The exact location of the antigenic determinant recognized by AD2 has been identified as the region of A chain residues 8,9,10 of beef insulin. The three species analogues which give low I_{50} ratios are beef, beef

TABLE 1.

I_{50} ratio[a] of insulin species variants to beef insulin

Insulin	CB6	AD2	CB5	CA4
Beef	1	1	1	>1
Beef Proinsulin	1±0.4	4±1	1±0.1	17
Sheep	1±1	7±5	1±0.3	1±0.3
Pork	3±2	324±56	1±0.1	15±3
Pork Proinsulin	2±1	527±163	1±0.5	>17
Rat	3±2	1225±336	1±0.3	23±6
Rat I	9±0.2	>37	>6	>3
Rat II	7±0.3	>37	1±0.1	>3
Mouse	4±1	629±153	4±2	>3
Human	2±0.2	246±27	1±0.1	10±1
Rabbit	1±1	>3,000	1±0.1	12±6
Chicken	1±1	>3,000	2±1	50
Fish	45±8	>3,000	>17	6±1
Guinea Pig	[b]>4,000	>1,000	>3	>3

[a]Ratio of amount (nanograms) of each species variant divided by the amount of beef insulin needed to inhibit 50% of the binding of a limiting dilution (27-75% binding of ^{125}I-beef insulin) of each hybridoma.

[b]Greater than ratios are the highest amount tested which gave less than 20% inhibition divided by the amount of beef insulin needed to inhibit 50% of ^{125}I-beef insulin binding.

proinsulin (identical to beef insulin at A 8-10 residues and said to have the same 3 dimensional configuration as insulin, ref 25) and sheep insulin which differs by 1 amino acid. All other species variants having two (pork, rat, human and rabbit insulin) or three (chicken, fish and guinea pig insulin) different amino acids in the A 8-10 region give much higher ratios of inhibition. Clearly AD2 binds to a 3 dimensional determinant formed around residues 8-10 of the A chain of the insulin molecule and this antibody can distinguish this region of beef insulin from the same region of pork insulin.

CA4 probably recognizes a 3-dimensional determinant formed near residues B29, A4 and A8 of beef insulin. A second antigenic determinant recognized by anti-insulin hybridoma antibody CA4 has also been tentatively identified as near the B29 lysine residue of insulin. There are two lines of evidence supporting this conclusion. The first is that insulin which is covalently conjugated to sepharose (23) via this amino acid cannot be used to affinity purify this antibody as it was for the other three anti-insulin hybridoma antibodies. Using a computer simulated model of insulin based on the x-ray crystallographic data for pork insulin (courtesy of Richard Feldman, Division of Computer Research and Technology, NIH, Bethesda, MD.), one can see that the B29 residue lies on the surface of the insulin molecule in close proximity to residues 8-10 of the A chain with residue A4 between B29 and A8 which lie in a line. A sequence difference from beef insulin at residue A8 like those in pork, human, rat (also differs at A4), chicken and rabbit insulin make these variants poorer inhibitors. While sheep insulin which has a different amino acid at A9 is as good an inhibitor as beef insulin. Further evidence that the residues A9-10 are not important parts of the antigenic determinant recognized by the CA4 antibody is the inhibition by beef proinsulin which retains the determinant seen by AD2 but is a very poor inhibitor of CA4 binding to beef insulin. X-ray crystallography has not been completed for beef proinsulin (1,25) so we do not know the 3 dimensional configuration of the C-peptide portion of this molecule. Other studies of proinsulin indicate that the insulin part of the molecule exists in the same 3-dimensional shape before and after C-peptide removal (1). Thus, the presence of the C-peptide joining the B30 residues to the A1 residues appears to impede beef proinsulin from inhibiting the binding of CA4 antibody to beef insulin.

Only CB5 binds to isolated B chain. The site on the insulin molecule of the binding of CB5 has not yet been identified but this antibody unlike the other three binds to isolated B chain (12.8% binding above background). Furthermore, the CB5 antibody binds (9.4% binding) to a fragment of the B chain, the B1-16 amino acid fragment of this chain. The low but significant binding of CB5 and no binding for the other three anti-insulin antibodies establishes that this binding is not due to slight contamination by intact insulin molecules. The best explanation for less than 100% binding even in great antibody excess (17 mg/ml as recovered by purification on an insulin affinity column) is that only a small percentage of the isolated chains or fragments are in the same 3 dimensional confirmation as that found in the intact molecule (26).

Discussion

Search for antibodies directed to regions of amino acid variation in the insulin molecule. As discussed in the introduction, insulin antibodies from three species, guinea pig, man and mouse were examined by IEF for the presence of antibodies directed to the A chain loop region of insulin. Within the limitations of the IEF technique (detecting IgG antibodies at concentrations greater than 10 µg/ml), guinea pigs failed to make such antibodies while some individual men or mice did. When these experiments were begun, the short term goal was to obtain reasonably high affinity anti-insulin antibodies directed to the A chain loop region of beef insulin that differed from mouse or pork insulin. Such an antibody, the mouse hybridoma antibody AD2, was used to attempt to block macrophage presentation of insulin to T cells (17) in a response where the precise molecule determinants important in triggering T cell proliferation were well documented (11).

The long term goal of generating monoclonal antibodies to insulin is to define the range of molecular determinants seen by B cells for a relatively small (MW 5750), structurally defined protein. Using the insulin immune response we hope to understand more about Ir gene function by contrasting the determinants recognized by B cells with those seen by T cells or macrophages (15,16) attempting to determine whether these populations are mutual, exclusive or overlapping. Like others using another antigen (27), we seek to use the techniques of somatic cell hybridization to help us immortalize and mass produce individual antibodies that will give us greater insights into the humoral response to insulin.

Our results are preliminary in the sense that four unique anti-insulin hybrid antibodies have been produced when perhaps hundreds of antibodies to insulin are made by BALB/c mice. This original fusion also used the NS1 cell that secretes a parental myeloma light chain while subsequent fusion experiments have used only total nonsecretor cell lines in order to simplify immunochemical characterization, i.e. interpretation of anti-idiotype studies, L chain analysis and ultimately amino acid sequencing.

However, our study has revealed several fundamental facts: a) Anti-insulin hybrid antibodies were easily elicited in BALB/c mice because of our previously acquired knowledge of the site (lymph node) and kinetics (near the peak primary PFC response) of anti-insulin secreting B cells (13). b) It is not yet clear whether cell fusion techniques yield results that faithfully mirror the expressed humoral immune response (28) but the four anti-insulin hybrid antibodies compared here are of the predominant isotypes, IgG_1 and IgG_2, found in a primary immune response to insulin. c) The molecular determinant recognized by these four anti-insulin antibodies reveal that some antibodies, like AD2, are directed to regions of amino acid variation in the insulin molecule. Other antibodies, like CB5 and CB6, are directed to determinants common to an animal's own circulating insulin despite the postulate by Jemmerson and Margoliash (29) that few such antibodies would be produced. The ability of mice to make such antibodies, expands the repertoire of determinants seen by anti-insulin antibodies. Studies to generate more anti-insulin hybrid antibodies are underway and the predictive value of our findings with these 4 antibodies will be tested.

Footnotes

*This work was supported by grant F 32 AI 05415 from the National Institutes of Health to J. A. S.

References

1. Blundell, T., Dodson, G., Hodgkin, D., Mercola, D.: Adv. Protein Chem. 26, 279-402 (1972).

2. Crumpton, M.J.: The Antigens, edited by M. Sela, 1-78. Academic Press, Inc., New York (1974).

3. De Weck, A.L.: The Antigens, edited by M. Sela, 141-248. Academic Press, Inc., New York (1974).

4. Reichlin, M.: Adv. Immunol., 20, 71-123 (1975).

5. Atassi, M.Z., Stavitsky, A.B., editors: Immunobiology of Proteins and Peptides I., Plenum Publishing Corp. New York (1978).

6. Attasi, M.A.: Immunochemistry, 12, 423-438 (1975).

7. Hill, S.W., Sercarz, E.E.: Eur. J. Immunol., 5, 317-324 (1975).

8. Urbanski, G.J., Margoliash, E.: Immunochemistry of Enzymes and Their Antibodies, edited by M. Salton, 203-224. John Wiley and Sons, Inc., New York (1976).

9. Keck, K.: Nature, 254, 78-79 (1975).

10. Keck, K.: Eur. J. Immunol., 5, 801-807 (1975).

11. Barcinski, M.A., Rosenthal, A.S.: J. Exp. Med., 145, 726-742 (1977).

12. Kapp, J.A., Strayer, D.S.: J. Immunol., 121, 978-982 (1978).

13. Schroer, J.A., Inman, J.K., Thomas, J.W., Rosenthal, A.S.: J. Immunol., 123, 670-675 (1979).

14. Kapp, J.A., Strayer, D.S., Robbins, P.F., Perlmutter, R.M.: J. Immunol. 123, 109-114 (1979).

15. Rosenwasser, L.J., Barcinski, M.A., Schwartz, R.H., Rosenthal, A.S.: J. Immunol., 123, 471-476 (1979).

16. Schroer, J., Rosenthal, A.S.: Function of Macrophages as Antigen Presenting Cells. Springer Seminars in Immunopathology, K. Eichmann (ed.) West Germany 3(2), 247-264 (1980).

17. Loblay, R.H., Schroer, J., Rosenthal, A.S.: Macrophage Regulation of Immunity, edited by E. Unanue and A.S. Rosenthal, 87-94. Academic Press, New York (1980).

18. Dayhoff, M.O., editor: Atlas of Protein Sequence and Structure. The National Biomedical Research Foundation, Washington, D.C. (1972, 1976, 1978).

19. Briles, D.E., Davie, J.M.: J. Immunol. Methods, 8, 363-372 (1975).

20. Nicolotti, R.A., Briles, D.E., Schroer, J.A., Davie, J.M.: Isoelectric focusing of immunoglobulins.

Improved Methodology J. Immunol. Methods. 33, 101-115 (1980).

21. Markussen, J.: Int. J. Protein Res., 3, 149-155 (1971).

22. Bünzli, H.F., Glatthaar, B., Kunz, P., Humbel, R.E.: Hoppe Seyler's Z. Physiol. Chem., 353, 451-458 (1972).

23. Kohler, G., Milstein, C.: Nature, 256, 495-497 (1975).

24. Schroer, J.A.: Hybridoma antibody recognition of the insulin molecule, Monoclonal antibodies in endocrine research, ed. Fellows, R.E. Raven Press, N.Y. (in press).

25. Fullerton, W.W., Potter, R., Low, B.W.: Proc. Natl. Acad. Sci., U.S.A., 66, 1213-1219 (1970).

26. Sachs, D.H., Schechter, A.N., Eastlake, A., Anfinsen, C.B.: J. Immunol., 109, 1300-1310 (1972).

27. Roth, M., Hammerling, G.J., Rajewsky, K.: Eur. J. Immunol., 8, 393-400 (1978).

28. Schroer, K.R., Kim, K-J., Prescott, B., Baker, P.J.: J. Exp. Med., 150, 698-702 (1979).

29. Jemmerson, R., Margoliash, E.: Nature, 282, 468-471 (1979).

Section II

Clincal Aspects of Immunity to Insulin

CLINICAL ASPECTS OF IMMUNITY TO INSULIN

K. Federlin, H.-G. Velcovsky, E. Mäser

Medizinische Klinik III und Poliklinik, Zentrum für Innere Medizin, Justus-Liebig-Universität, D-6300 Gießen, Germany

Already in 1922 shortly after the introduction of insulin into the treatment of diabetes mellitus a paper was published by JOSLIN, GRAY and ROOT (1) which apart from the great benefit of the new medicament reported about several side effects. The authors described local and generalized allergic reactions of the skin after insulin injections which they suggested to be caused by pancreatic impurities. Indeed the first samples of insulin used for therapy were still a crude mixture of hormones and pancreatic proteins compared to the highly purified products which are available at the present time. However also modern diabetes treatment confronts the physician with immunological side effects as recently summarized in the review articles of KAHN and ROSENTHAL (1979) (2) and KURTZ and NABARRO (1980) (3). The various phenomena can be listed as follows: (Tab. I)

TABLE I:

Immunologic reactions to insulin
Cutaneous reactions
Local (limited to the injection site)
Immediate: IgE-mediated
Intermediate: Arthus reaction
Delayed: T-cell-mediated
Combinations of the above
Lipoatrophy or lipohypertrophy: uncertain role of immune response
Systemic
Urticaria and angioedema with or without shock
Insulin resistance
Serum sickness
Purpura
Thrombocytopenic
Nonthrombocytopenic
Arthus phenomenon with LE cells, eosinophilia, and hyperglobulinemia
Autoimmune insulin syndrome

From: KAHN and ROSENTHAL, 1979

1. Cutaneous reactions to insulin

Skin reactions can be observed as local delayed allergy, as local immediate allergy, as Arthus type reactions and in form of local atrophies of the subcutaneous fat tissue.

a) Local delayed form: the most common immunological reaction to insulin is the delayed allergic reaction. It is expressed by a firm redness and occasionally swelling of an 1 - 5 Ø cm large area accompanied by itching and stinging sensations. The reaction starts about 18-24 hours after the s.c.injection, has its maximum at 24-36 hours and may last until 96 hours.

It occurs mostly at the beginning of an insulin treatment i.e. during the first 8-10 days but may be observed earlier in the case of interrupted or intermittent insulin therapy.

The intensity varies greatly as shown by the following figures: (fig. 1, 2)

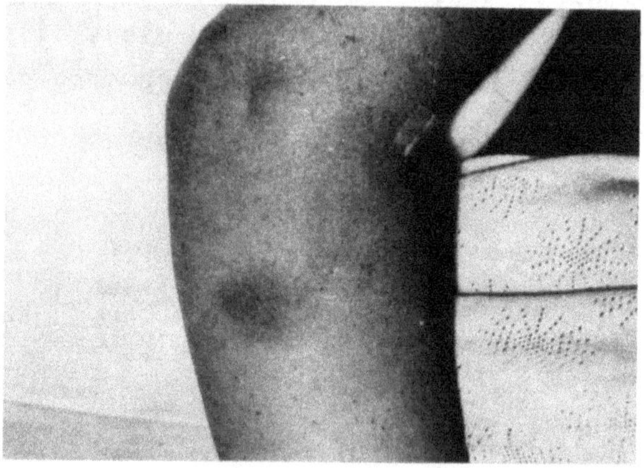

Fig.1: Insulin allergy of the delayed type, mild form. 14 days after beginning of therapy.

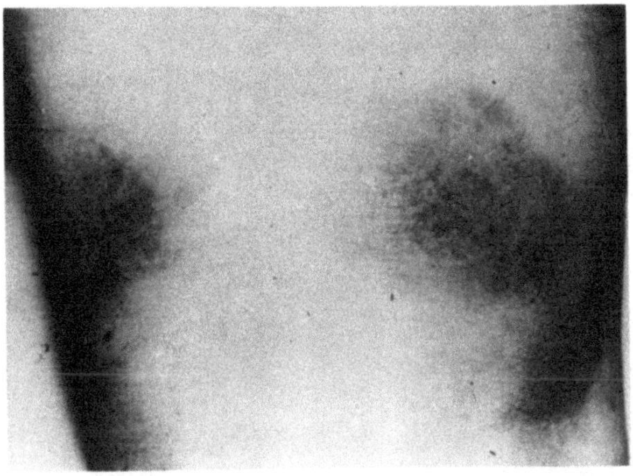

Fig.2: Insulin allergy of the delayed type,severe from 6 days after beginning of a second insulin therapie after interruption of 3 years.

This form of insulin allergy can clearly be defined as a type IV reaction according to GELL and COOMBS (4) because of its clinical picture, the result of the skin test and the histological examination. The following histological pictures demonstrate examples for mild and severe forms of type IV allergy to insulin.

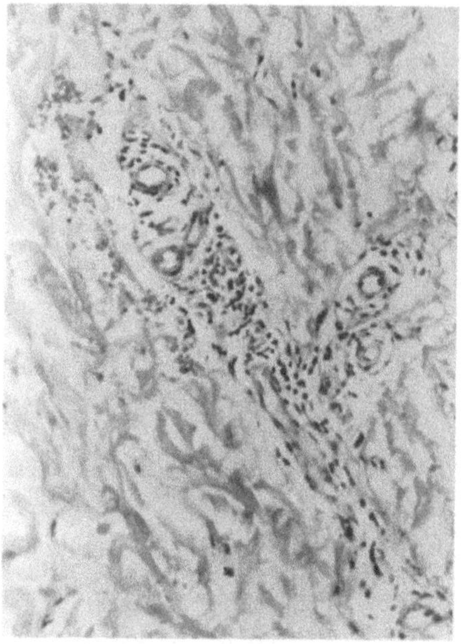

Fig.3: left Skin biopsy of a patient with delayed insulin allergy of the mild form. Scattered round cell infiltrates in the subcutis.-

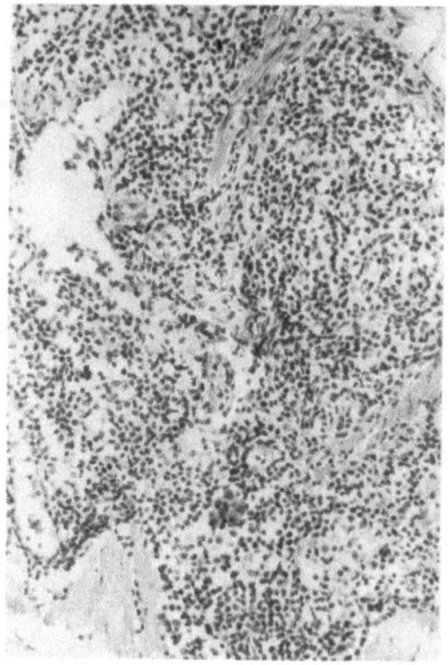

Fig.4: right Skin biopsy of a patient with a severe form of delayed insulin allergy. Massive infiltration of the subcutis with small lymphcytes.-

The frequency of the delayed allergic reaction varies between 35 and 70% depending on the describing author and whether also mild reactions are included which to a great extent are not observed by the patient himself (3). Most of the mild reactions subside after a few days spontaneously provided the injection technique was correctly performed. Otherwise when insulin (and here predominantly acid solutions) are injected in a too flat angle, the tendency to allergic reactions increases. Furthermore non-allergic skin irritations due to the acid pH may follow wich are similar to the true allergic reaction however are lacking inflammatory symptoms as redness, warming and swelling. The typical form of this non-allergic skin change are

small deep nodules which persist over many weeks.
The local allergic reaction of the immediate type is much rarer and can clearly be distinguished from the delayed form. It starts within a few minutes after the injection and is expressed by flare and wheal reaction which may extend to a generalized reaction with anaphylactic symptoms when this first warning signal was neglected and insulin injections were not stopped. The skin test demonstrates this also as a type I reaction. (fig. 5)

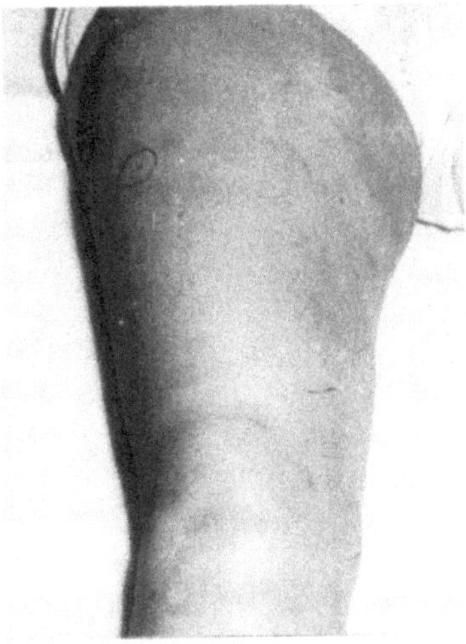

Fig.5: <u>left</u> Local insulin allergy of the immediate type 10' after injection.

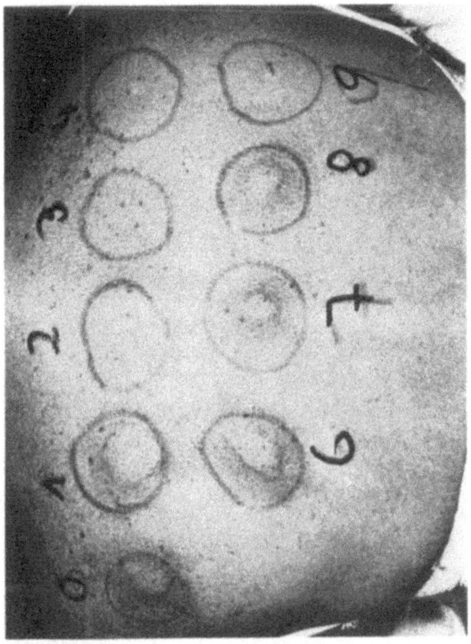

Fig.5: <u>right</u> Skin test in the same patient (wheal and flare reaction to several insulins).

The frequency of the immediate type reactions is about 0,1 - 0,5 % in insulin treated diabetics. In contrast to the delayed reaction the immediate forms occur also after long lasting insulin therapy without former complications. As in delayed allergy interrupted insulin therapy increases the tendency of the organism to develop this form of allergy.

A third type of allergic reactions after insulin injections ranges timely between the both forms already mentioned (6, 7). It appears after 4-6 hours and does not last longer than a few hours until one day. The clinical picture is similar to that of the delayed type namely local redness, itching, swelling, the skin however not being as firm. Local bleeding is not uncommon. Skin biopsies with histological and immunohistological evaluation in our experience support the view of type III reactions on the basis of immune complexes. (fig. 6)

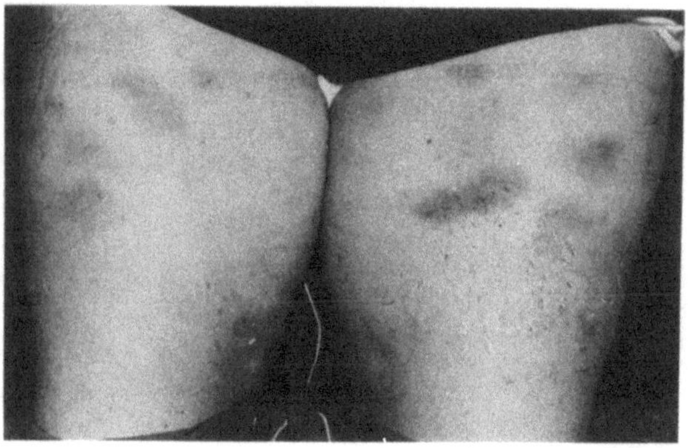

Fig.6:A) Insulin allergy of the Arthus type onset after 6 hours.

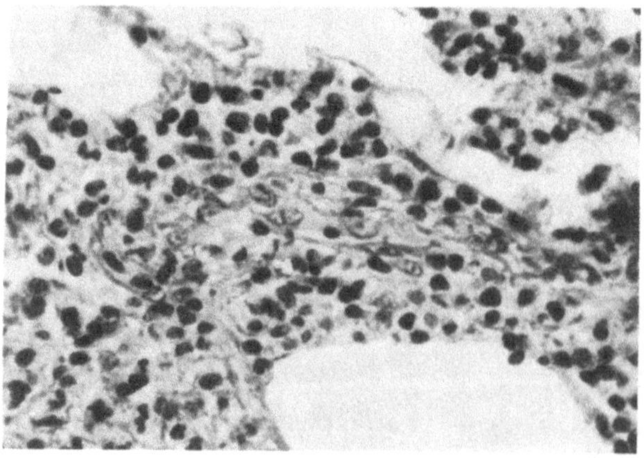

Fig.6:B) Skin biopsy of the same patient.Local infiltrates with a mixture of polymorphonuclear cells and lymphocytes. In the center a small vessel with a swollen wall.

The last skin reaction to be mentioned in this context is lipoatrophy, formerly interpreted as an abnormal metabolic reaction of fat cells to insulin but in mean while clearly defined as the consequence of local inflammatory reactions in the subcutaneous fat tissue. Mostly lipoatrophy is preceeded by skin phenomena (redness, swelling) after 4-6 hours indication Arthus type reactions. Very recently REEVES et al.(1980) (8) described immune complexes in the wall of small vessles of the s.c.tissue in those patients. (fig.7)

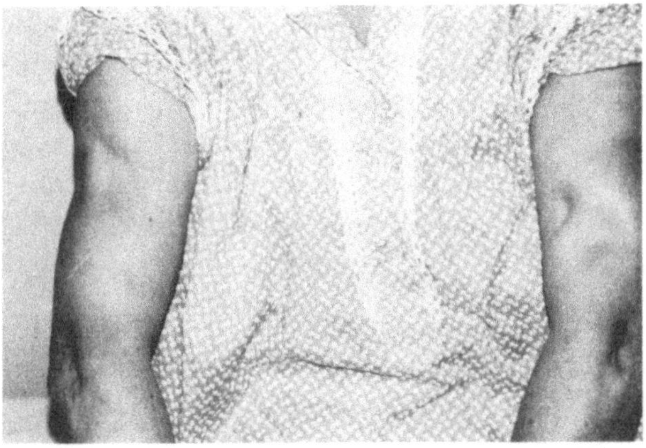

Fig.7:A) Lipoatrophy after insulin treatment

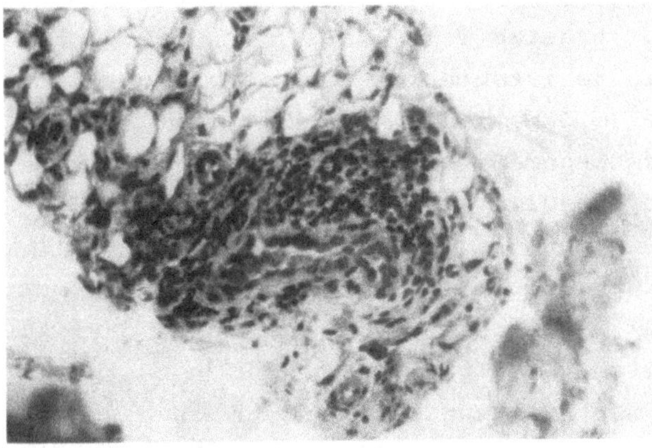

Fig.7: B) Skin biopsy of a patient with lipoatrophy in an earlier state: perivascular mononuclear infiltrate.

It is still unexplained why lipoatrophy occurs more frequently in children than in adults. The tendency to develop these lesions decreases in the young diabetics when they have reached the age of about 20.

Apart from histological studies in these patients the main proval for an immunological basis of lipoatrophy was the introduction of purified insulin into the therapy 10 years ago which very soon was accompanied by a marked decrease of the frequency and intensitiy of lipoatrophy in all countries using the new insulins (9).

In very few cases insulin immunology affects other organs or cell systems than the skin. Thus single cases of thrombocytopenia and anemia have been reported (10, 11). The underlying mechanism was the attachement of insulinantibody complexes onto the surface of the blood cells which than were removed by the clearing mechanism of the spleen. Furthermore serum sickness like symptoms with joint swelling have also been observed. Another rare example was a syndrom including LE cells and hypergammaglobulinemia (17). Such observations however are extremely rare.-

2. Insulin resistance.

As early as insulin allergy insulin resistance was observed among the first diabetics treated with insulin in 1922. In the following decades insulin resistence for the clinician remained a rare condition 1 - 2 / 1000 patients, which however could lead to a long lasting derangement of the metabolism. In some cases enormous amounts of insulin were injected or infused (at that time probably without realizing the very short half life of the hormone in the circulation) e.g. in the report of TUCKER et al. (1956) (12) a total of 156000 units per day. Although the insensitivity of the organism to insulin in those cases was attributed to neutralizing antibodies this was not earlier demonstrated as in 1956 when BERSON and YALOW (13) introduced the radioimmunological method for measuring antibody and hormone. Since that time from many studies it became evident that nearly every diabetic injecting insulin develops antibodies against the foreign insulin. After a short period in which IgM antibodies can be detected IgG antibodies are produced and persist over many years. Having reached a concentration which for the single patient is mostly constant the antibody level frequently remains unchanged. Rarely antibodies of the other Ig-classes as IgA and IgD can be found. Interestingly also IgE antibodies in low concentration are produced in most diabetics regardless whether they exhibit signs of insulin allergy or not (14). This phenomenon represents a much more sensitive indicator for the immunogenicity of purified insulins than antibodies of the other Ig-classes.

Many techniques have been worked out for the measurement of neutralizing antibodies. Their practicability varies however greatly. The total binding capacity for insulin of a given serum can be measured by adding radioactive as well as "cold" insulin and removing the unbound insulin by charcoal or cellulose. CHRISTIANSEN (1970) (15) developed the technique measuring exclusively insulin binding immunoglobulins. From the clinical point of view the titer of the binding capacity of a serum for insulin might be less important than the affinity of the antibody for the hormone a method which was intensively worked out by KERP et al.(1968) (16). While antibodies with strong affinity to the antigen insulin (socalled AK 1) showed a close correlation to the daily insulin requirement, patients containing antibody type AK 2 showed a less close correlation indicating that low binding forces intermittently cause the liberation of insulin from the antibody.- (fig. 8, 9).-

Fig. 8 + 9: Daily insulin requirement (U per 24 h) and concentration of antibody-binding sites for insulin in insulin-treated diabetics. (O insulin-sensitive diabetics, n=91); □ insulin-resistant diabetics, n=7).

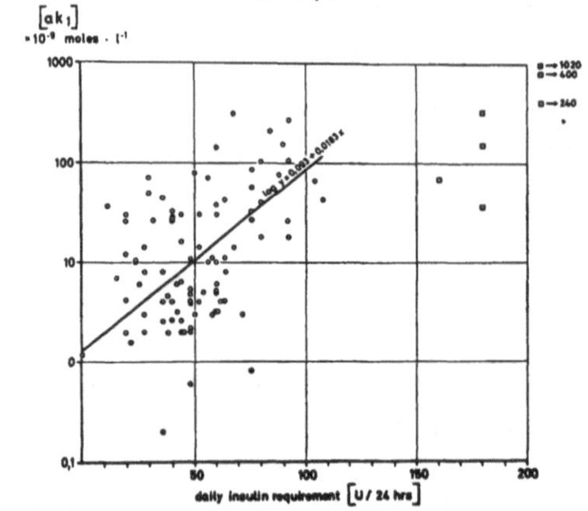

Fig.8: Binding to high-affinity antibody binding sites (Ak_1) r=0.605; $p<0.0005$ (top)

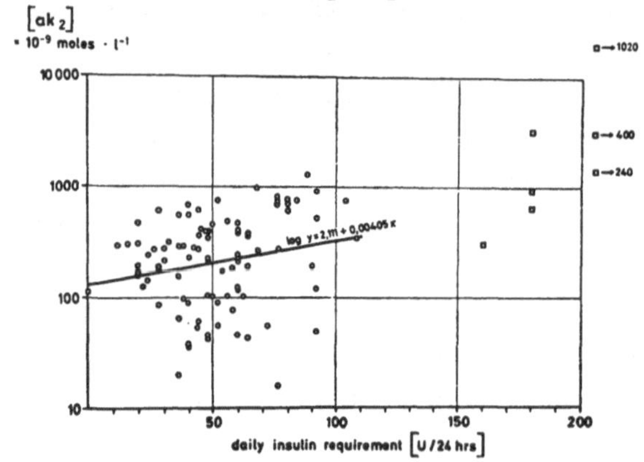

Fig.9: Binding to low-affinity antibody binding sites (AK_2), r=0.33; $p< 0.005$ (bottom)

From: Kerp, L., Henrichs, H., Kasemir, H.: Handbuch d. exp. Pharm XXXII/2, Insulin, part. 2. Eds. A. Hasselblatt, F. v. Bruchhausen Springer, Berl.-Heidelb.-New-York. 1975, p. 595

Measuring antibodies against insulin one has to have in mind that much of the antibody may be bound to insulin in form of a circulating complex. In those cases for determining the total insulin binding capacity it is necessary to split the complexes by lowering the pH (17). Furthermore it is noteworthy to state that rarely antibody titre and daily insulin requirement are in close correlation (18). Another point of interest in insulin therapy is the fact that insulin antibodies might influence the pharmacocinetics of the hormone greatly (19).

True insulin resistance may be diagnosed in cases with increasing insulin requirement reaching amounts of more than 100 units per day although the usual terminus is to postulate 200 units per day over a period of more than 48 hours according to MARTIN et al. (1941) (20). However clinical experience has shown that especially in obese diabetics the diagnosis "immunologically mediated insulin resistance" is made much too often. Future investigations will show that receptor defects or socalled "down regulation" of the number of insulin receptors by too high doses of exogenous insulin are much more common the cause of insulin insentivity than neutralizing antibodies. While formerly insulin resistance was observed in a frequency of about 0,1 % (21) the introduction of chromatographically purified insulin has still reduced the number of allergic patients. Nevertheless insulin resistance is still observed although exact figures of its frequency are lacking.-

Increased insulin requirements due to antibodies can develop for several reasons. Similar as in insulin allergy interrupted or intermittent insulin therapy favour the occurrence of antibodies and may lead to a mostly temporary insulin resistance. Furthermore ketoacidosis may be followed by short periods of insulin resistance although certainly non-immunological factors are included. Infections and some chronic disease may enhance antibody production as measles or liver cirrhosis.
In about one third of the cases of insulin resistance as observed before 1970 (the year of the introduction of purified insulins) preceeding insulin allergy either of the delayed or of the immediate type was reported (22) . However when increasing insulin requirement in a patient is observed other metabolic causes as hyperthyroidism, Cushings disease or hypophyseal-hypothalamic disturbances have to be excluded firstly.

Treatment of insulin allergy and insulin resistance:

The following tables give some rough recommendations how to overcome immunological problems of insulin therapy as allergy or resistance. (Table II + III)

1. **Insulin allergy:**

a) **local delayed form:**
- correct insulin injections
- change bovine/ porcine
- addition of antihistaminics
- addition of cortisone

b) **local or generalized immediate form:**
- interrupt injections!
- attempt with oral treatment
- skin testing with various insulins
- insulin + steroids (s.c. or i.v.)
- boiled insulin
- desensitization

Table II: Therapeutical recommendations in cases of insulin allergy.

2. **Insulin resistance:**

Change bovine/porcine insulin

increased doses (3x40, 3x60, 3x80...) (induction of tolerance?)

insulin intravenously (cave allergic shock)

insulin + steroids

Table III: Therapeutical recommendations in cases with increased insulin requirement (insulin resistance).-

Pathogenetical mechanisms:

Up to the present there is no clearcut definition of the nature of the antigen responsible for the immunological reactions as mentioned above. Apart from the fact that among the patients treated with insulin there are those to be classified immunologically as high and low responder and that genetical inflences surely play an important role in this respect there is no doubt that either the hormone itself because of the species difference acts as immunogen or that insulin related products still induce an antibody response. A remarkable example has been reported recently by SIMMONDS et al. (1980) (23), wehn a patient developed generalized allergic reaction to monocomponent insulins of bovine and of porcine origin. Because this is a separate point of discussion during this symposium from the clinical point of view the following aspects should be mentionend only briefly:

1) For several reasons insulin related proteins as proinsulin, and others must be regarded as potential antigens or immunogens because their removal undoubtedly has greatly reduced the frequency and intensity of insulin allergy, of lipoatrophy and to a lesser degree of insulin resistance.

2) Insulin itself may serve as an antigen because after the change from bovine to porcine insulin the immune reactions may subside.

3) Potentiating effects for the development of immunological reactions can be seen in:

a) frequent with-drawal of insulin treatment
b) the subcutaneous deposition of insulin with easy access of macrophages and following sitmulation of the immune response,
c) the factor of the pH. In patients with increased tendency to allergic reactions acid insulins are less well tolerated than neutral suspensions,
d) adjuvant affects of substances used for a prolonged liberation of the injected hormone as protamin, surfen or even the bigger crystals of insulins which are free from additional carriers for insulin.

While in a few cases it has been shown that the allergic reaction was directed against the insulin coupling material as pro-

tamin or surfen for the overwhelming number of cases exhibiting immunological reactions to insulin a pathogenetic role of these substances seems to be very improbable.
Regarding antibodies to insulin as general statement it must be expressed that in the non allergix patient a reasonable insulin profile over the day is a much more important fact than possible antigenic components and antibodies. Lastly insulin with very slow absorption may also exhibit some adjuvant effects simply by the low solubility. Finally it has been argued by BLOOM and coworkers (1976) (24) that the traces of other islet cell hormones within the commercial insulin and even in the purified commercial preparations as somatostatin, glucagon, VIP and PP could contribute to autoimmune reactions against the resting islet tissue, but this is highly hypothetical and has no clinical relevance up to now.-
In conclusion it can be stated that insulin from cattle and pigs also in its highly purified form in diabetic patients can elicit immune reactions. According to the intensive studies of NEUBAUER and SCHÖNE (1978) (25) in various species with homologous or heterologous insulins antibody production is far more developed due to species specificities than to purity. Future studies using the newly produced human insulins will clarify whether this holds true also for this form of treatment.

1) Joslin,E.,Gray,H.,Root,R.: Insulin in Hospital and Home J.metab.Res.2, 651 (1922)

2) Kahn,C.R., Rosenthal,A.S.: Immunologic Reactions to Insulin:Insulin Allergy,Insulin Resistance and the Autoimmune Insulin Syndrome. Diabetes Care 2, 283 (1979)

3) Kurtz,A.B., Nabarro,J.D.N.: Circulating Insulin-binding Antibodies. Diabetologia 19,329 (1980)

4) Coombs,R.R.A.,Gell,P.G.H.: Classification of allergic reactions responsible for clinical hypersensitivity and diesase. In:Clinical aspects of immunology.Eds.Gell-Coombs-Lachmann, Blackwell,Oxford,London,Edinb. Melbourne,1975, p.761

5) Federlin,K.: Immunopathology of Insulin . Heidelberg-Berlin,Springer-Verlag, p.19 (1971)

6) Schirren,G.C.: Ein ungewöhnlicher Fall von lokaler Insulinanaphylaxie.Hautarzt 4, 531 (1953)

7) Porter,R.D.,Hartmann,C.R.: Arthus reactions form insulin association with lupus erythematosus cell phenomena. JAMA 214, 1884 (1970)

8) Reeves, W.G., Allen,B.R., Tattersall, R.B.: Insulin.induced lipoatrophy:evidence for an immune pathogenesis Brit.Med.J.280 1500 (1980)

9) Yue, D.K., Turtle, J.R.: New forms of insulin and their use in the treatment of diabetes. Diabetes 26, 341 (1977)

10) Constam,G.R.: Thrombocytopenie purpura as a probable manifestation of insulin allergy:report of a case. Diabetes 5, 121 (1956)

11) Faulk,W.P.,Tomsovic,E.J., Fudenberg,H.: Insulin resistance in juvenile diabetes mellitus.Immunologie studies.Amer.J.Med.49,133(1970)

12) Tucker,W.R.,Klink,D.,Goetz,F., Zalme,E., Knowles,H.C.: Insulin resistance and acanthosis nigricans. Diabetes 13,395 (1964)

13) Berson,S.A.,Yalow,R.S.,Bauman,A., Rothchild,M.A., Newerly,K.: Insulin-J^{131} metabolism in human subjects:demonstration of insulin binding globulin in circulalation of insulin treated subjects. J.Clin.Inves.35,170 (1956)

14) Federlin,K.,Velcovsky,H.G.: IgE-Antikörper bei Patienten mit Insulinallergie.Verh.Dtsch. Ges.Inn.Med.80, 1613 (1974)

15) Christiansen,A.H.: A new method for determination of insulin-binding immunolobulins in insulin-treated diabetic patents.Horm.Metab.Res.2, 187 (1970)

16) Kerp,E.,Kasemir,H.,Kieling,F.: Insulinbindende Antikörper und Insulin-bedarf bei Diabetikern. Klin.Wschr.46, 376 (1968)

17) Jayarao,K.S.,Faulk,W.P.,Karam,J.H., Grodsky,G.M., Forsham,P.H.: Measurement of immune complexes in insulin-treated diabetics. J.Immunol.Methods 3, 337 (1973)

18) Asplin,C.M.,Hartog.M.,Goldie,D.J., Alberti,K.G.M.M.,Smythe,P.: A comparison between diabetics receiving a high or low daily insulin dosage.Horm.Metab.Res. 10, 365 (1978)

19) Bollinger,R.E.,Morris,J.H., McKnight,F.G., Diederich,D.A.: Disappearance of 131 I labeled insulin from plasma as a guide to management of diabetes. N.Engl.J.Med.270,767(1964)

20) Martin,W.P.,Martin,H.E.,Lyster,R.W., Strouse,S.: Insulin resistance.Critical survey of the literature with the report of a case.J.clin. Endcr.1,387(1941)

21) Daweke,,H.: Klinik der Insulinresistenz, Dtsch.med.Wschr.91, 973(1966)

22) Shipp,J.C.,Cunningham,R.W.,Russell,R.O, Marble,A.: Insulin resistance:clinical features, natural course and effects of adrenal steroid treatment. Medicine(Baltimore)44,165 (1965)

23) Simmonds,J.P.,Russell,G.I.,Cowley,A.J., Sewell, H.F., Hearnshaw: Generalized allergy to porcine and bovine monocomponent insulins.Brit.Med.J. 2, 355 (1980)

24) Bloom,S.R.,Adrian,R.E.,Mitchell,S.J., Barnes,A.J., Kohner,E.M.: Dirty insulin, a stimulant to autoimmunity.Diabetologia 12, 381 (1976)

25) Neubauer,H.P., Schöne, H.H.: The Immunogenicity of Different Insulins in Several Animal Species. Diabetes 27, 8 (1978)

ANTIBODY PRODUCTION DURING INSULIN THERAPY - PATTERNS OF RESPONSE AND CLINICAL SEQUELS

W. G. Reeves
Department of Immunology, University Hospital, Nottingham, NG7 2UH, U.K.

Most patients develop insulin antibodies within 1-2 months of commencing treatment with sub-cutaneous injections of bovine insulin. There are five broad categories of bovine insulin preparation in current use (table 1). Most regimes consist of twice daily injections of a short acting soluble form combined with a longer acting preparation. Prolongation of the metabolic effect is usually achieved by the addition of fish protamine (e.g. isophane insulin), increasing the zinc concentration (e.g. lente insulin) or both (i.e. protamine zinc insulin - PZI). Some patients with a modest insulin requirement are adequately controlled on a single daily injection of a longer acting insulin e.g. isophane or lente. Traditionally, insulins have been purified by sequential recrystallization but the equivalent forms of porcine insulin are now prepared by chromatographic techniques. These highly purified porcine preparations are much less immunogenic and transfer to such preparations can produce a marked fall in circulating insulin antibody in patients previously treated with bovine insulins (figure 1) (1).

Many methodological approaches have been used to quantitate insulin antibodies (1). Few methods include removal of insulin (endogenous or exogenous) from samples prior to assay. Many fail to document the binding substance as immunochemical antibody and precision has often been poor. We have used a second antibody co-precipitation assay specific for IgG anti-

Basic and Clinical Aspects of Immunity to Insulin

Table 1. Insulin preparations in current use. RC = recrystallized. HP = highly purified.

Preparation	Examples	Species	Purity	pH	Physical state	[Zn]*
SOLUBLE	Soluble	Beef	RC	Acid	Solution	⩽ 40
NEUTRAL	Neutral soluble (nuso)	Beef	RC	Neutral	Solution	⩽ 20
	Actrapid	Pork	HP	Neutral	Solution	⩽ 20
	Leo Neutral	Pork	HP	Neutral	Solution	⩽ 20
ISOPHANE	Isophane (NPH)	Beef	RC	Neutral	Crystalline Suspension	⩽ 40
	Leo Retard	Pork	HP	Neutral	Crystalline Suspension	⩽ 40
INSULIN ZINC SUSPENSION	Lente	Beef	RC	Neutral	30% amorphous 70% crystalline	c.100
	Monotard	Pork	HP	Neutral	30% amorphous 70% crystalline	c.100
PROTAMINE ZINC INSULIN	PZI	Beef	RC	Neutral	Amorphous Suspension	c.200

* Zinc concentration in μg/100 U insulin.

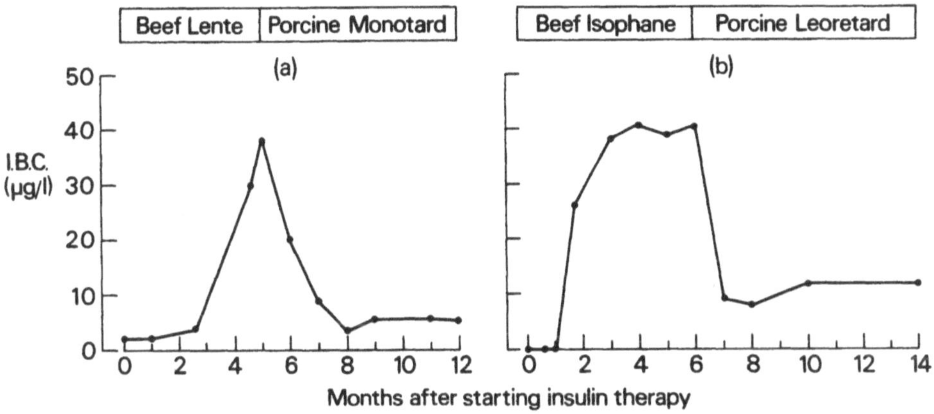

Figure 1. Changes in antibody reactive with recrystallized bovine insulin seen in two patients switched from conventional bovine to equivalent forms of highly purified porcine insulins (1).

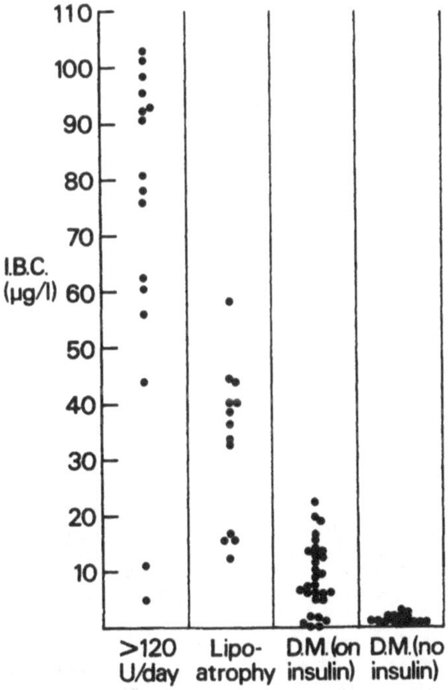

Figure 2. Levels of IgG antibody reactive with recrystallized bovine insulin in the sera of patients requiring more than 120 units insulin daily; patients with lipo-atrophy; well-controlled diabetics on conventional soluble and isophane insulins, and diabetic patients prior to insulin therapy (2).

body with the concentration of anti-IgG adjusted to give "optimal proportions". Insulin is removed from sera prior to assay by adsorption with dextran-coated charcoal at acid pH and ^{22}Na is used as a volume marker to avoid washing precipitates and to improve precision (2). The IgG insulin binding capacity (IBC) is expressed as μg ^{125}I-insulin bound per litre of test serum or as % bound (2). The levels found in different patient groups are shown in figure 2.

Specificity of Response

Although much of our work has involved the use of labelled recrystallized bovine insulin as antigen (which resembles the material injected into patients receiving conventional bovine insulins), the levels of antibody reactive with highly purified (i.e. monocomponent) bovine or porcine insulins are broadly similar (figure 3).

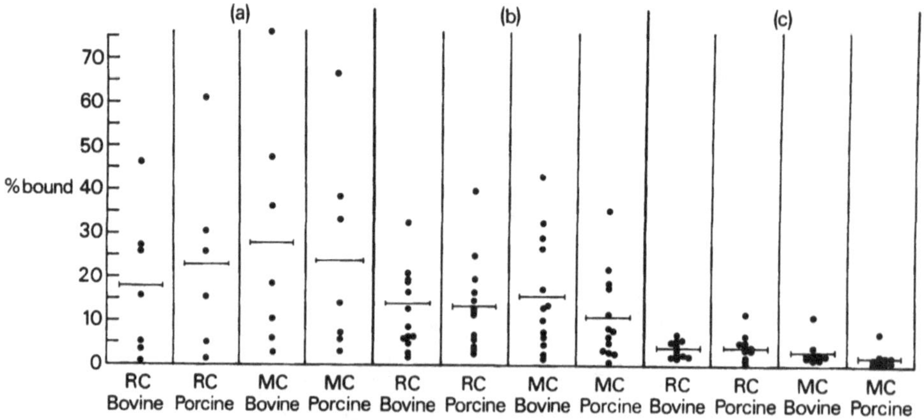

Figure 3. Levels of IgG antibody in the sera of three groups of patients after treatment with (a) beef lente, (b) beef isophane and (c) pork isophane insulin for six months. Each serum was assayed against labelled recrystallised (RC) and monocomponent (MC) bovine and porcine insulins and the results expressed as percentage bound to give comparability between the different labelled antigens (1).

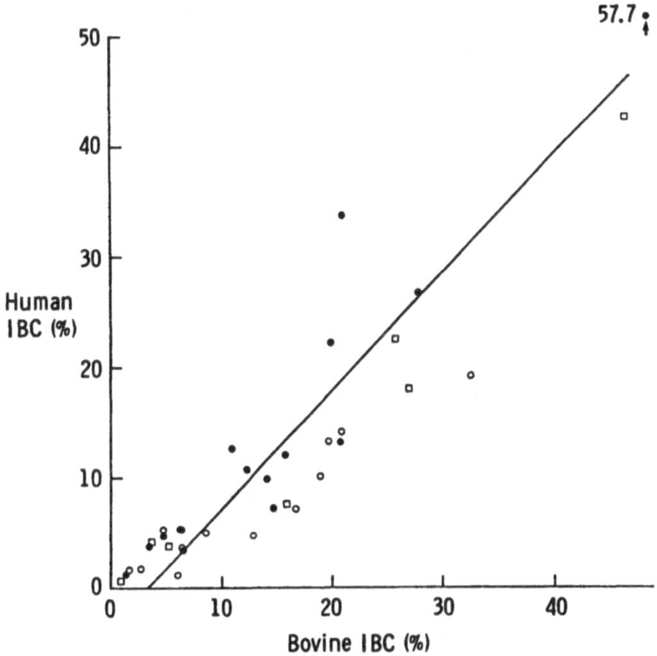

Figure 4. Correlation (r = 0.917) between antibody levels reactive with human and bovine insulins in sera from 35 patients receiving bovine insulin therapy (● - PZI + soluble, □ - lente, and o - isophane) expressed as percentage bound (26).

The greater immunogenicity of bovine insulin preparations has often been regarded as a consequence of the three amino acid residue differences (as between human and bovine insulins in contrast to the single residue difference (as between human and porcine insulins). However, it seemed important to establish whether these antibodies react with shared determinants also present on the human molecule. The international reference preparation of human insulin (66/304 - obtained from the National Institute for Biological Standards and Control, Hampstead, U.K.) was used for most of this work and the correlation between the reactivity of 35 insulin antibody containing sera in terms of bovine and human monomer binding is shown in figure 4. This close correlation holds for almost all sera that we have examined from patients maintained on conventional bovine insulin and solid-phase adsorption experiments using human insulin linked to CH-sepharose confirm that most antibodies reactive with bovine insulin cross-react with the human insulin molecule (4).

Antibodies reactive with the connecting or C-peptide of the bovine pro-insulin molecule have been quantitated using labelled bovine pro-insulin as antigen. Anti-monomer antibodies are removed before assay by adsorption with sepharose-linked monocomponent bovine insulin. The data presented in figure 5 indicates that most patients with insulin resistance or injection site lipo-atrophy, as well as most patients on bovine insulin regimes which include soluble insulin, possess high levels of circulating C-peptide antibody, in contrast to patients receiving bovine lente or isophane insulins even though

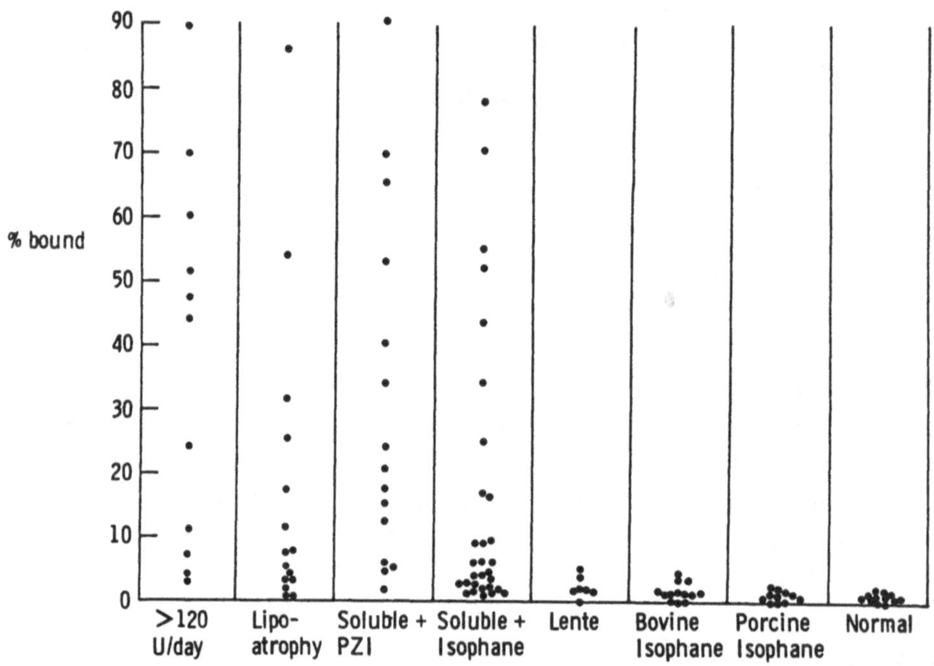

Figure 5. C-peptide antibody levels in seven groups of patients receiving insulin therapy and normal individuals expressed as percentage bound (26).

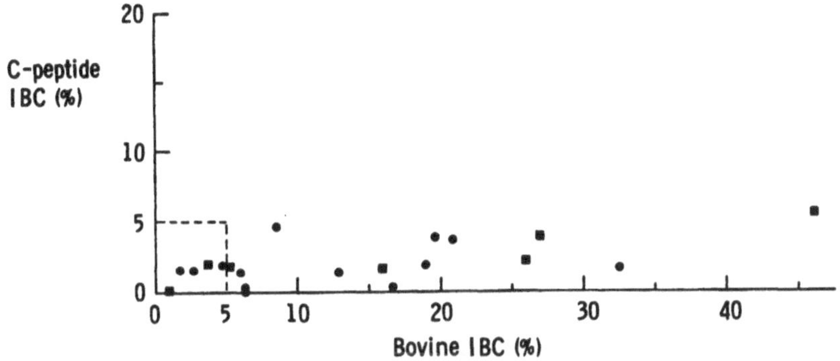

Figure 6. Correlation between antibodies reactive with bovine C-peptide and bovine insulin monomer in 20 sera from patients receiving conventional lente (■) and isophane (●) insulins. The broken line indicates the upper limit of normal (26).

these latter patients usually produce plentiful antibody reactive with the insulin monomer (figure 6). Thus, there is not such a close correlation, overall, between C-peptide and insulin monomer responsiveness and these two kinds of antibody may behave differently when patients are switched from conventional bovine to highly purified porcine insulin and vice versa (e.g. figure 7).

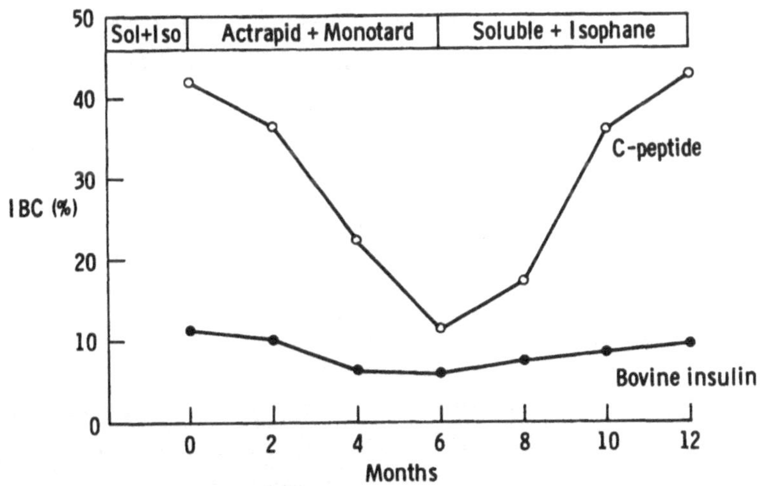

Figure 7. Patient S.D.: changes in C-peptide and bovine insulin monomer antibody levels during alternation between bovine soluble and isophane and porcine actrapid and monotard insulin regimes (26).

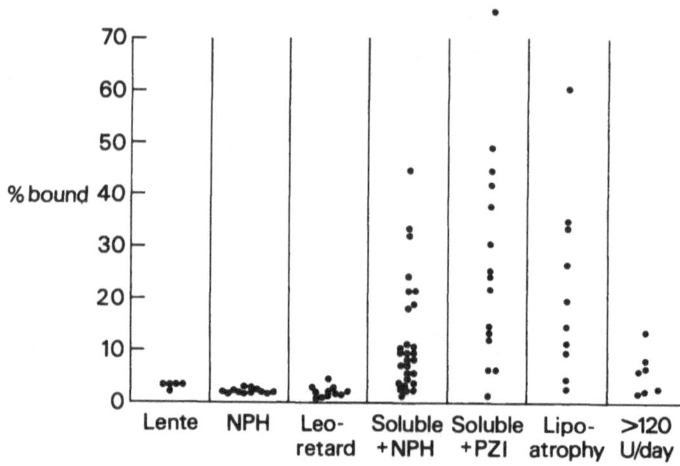

Figure 8. Levels of IgG antibody reactive with pancreatic polypeptide in seven groups of sera expressed as percentage bound. Lente, NPH and leo-retard refer to sera obtained six months after commencement of treatment with these insulins. Soluble + NPH and soluble + PZI refer to sera from patients established on these bovine insulins (1).

Significant amounts of other islet hormones e.g. glucagon, pancreatic polypeptide (PP), vaso-active intestinal peptide (VIP) and somatostatin, are often present in preparations of conventional bovine insulin (5,6) and antibodies can be demonstrated against some of these contaminants (notably PP) (figure 8). Once more, it is of interest that bovine regimes containing soluble insulin are more effective in inducing such antibodies. This is in keeping with the finding that soluble insulins contain rather more contaminating PP than isophane or lente preparations (5).

Factors Affecting Immunogenicity

Table 2 lists various factors which may play a part in determining the immunogenicity of individual insulin preparations. Acid preparations of soluble insulin are more immunogenic than those maintained at neutral pH (7,8). The intrinsic solubility of the insulin variety used may be an important factor and manipulation of the zinc concentration extends the time course of absorption from sub-cutaneous sites via its effect on crystallization. However, variation in the zinc concentration can have a marked effect on the antigenicity of insulin via alterations in its tertiary structure (9). The higher concentrations of zinc used in both lente and protamine zinc insulin (PZI) preparations may explain the higher levels of insulin antibody which develop following their administration (1). Bovine insulin is inherently less soluble than its porcine equivalent and this may partially explain any species difference in antigenicity.

pH
Solubility and [Zn]
Retarding agents
Species of origin
Purity
Mode of administration
Age
Sex
Infection
Constitutional variation (Ir genes)

Table 2. Factors affecting the immunogenicity of insulin preparations.

The use of fish protamine as a retarding agent is also likely to enhance the immune response to insulin which complexes with it in preparations such as isophane and PZI (1). Both protamine and zinc itself can activate the complement system (10,11); zinc can also induce lymphocyte stimulation (12) and protamine is a powerful adjuvant in mice (13).

It is possible that the A chain loop differences which are present in the bovine insulin molecule may be important in determining its greater immunogenicity when injected into man even though the antibody produced cross-reacts with both porcine and human molecules. Nevertheless, when conventional bovine preparations contaminated with pro-insulin are used, C-peptide is present with its 30 or so amino acid residues, 14 of which differ between the bovine and human molecules. It is not surprising, therefore, that antibodies do develop against the insulin monomer itself (possibly via a carrier effect) and that antibodies specific for the C-peptide are often detectable. Thus, purity of the preparation - whatever its species of origin - is of major importance and highly purified porcine insulins containing less than 1 p.p.m. proinsulin rarely induce insulin antibodies.

The regularity and frequency of insulin injections for the control of diabetes may explain why antibody production is not more of a problem for, experimentally, small frequent doses of heterologous insulin can produce a state of tolerance (14,15) and one of the commonest causes of antibody-mediated insulin resistance is that of intermittent therapy with immunogenic preparations. Injection site lipo-atrophy is more commonly seen in women although, this apart, there is little evidence to indicate a major difference in the sexes in terms of antibody production to insulin preparations. Likewise, there is little evidence to invoke concurrent infection as a factor in insulin antibody production.

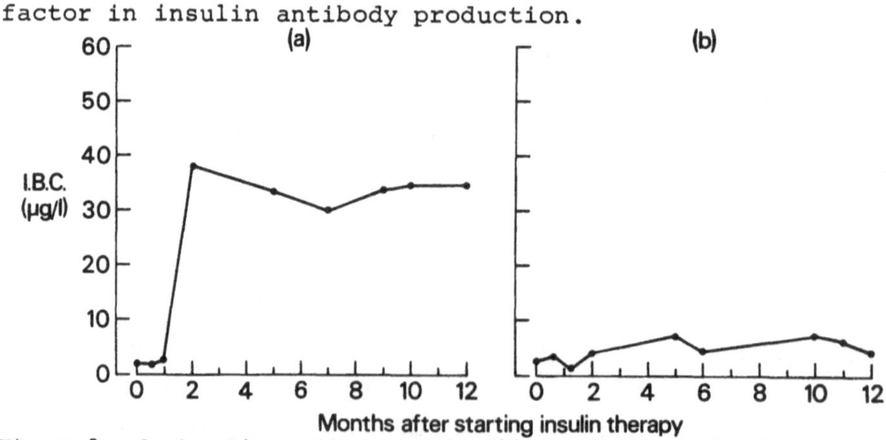

Figure 9. Contrasting patterns of insulin antibody production in two patients each treated with bovine lente insulin once daily (1).

There is, however, considerable constitutional variation in the ability of patients to produce insulin antibodies: patients possessing the HLA-B8/DRw3 phenotype produce lower levels whereas those with the B15/DRw4 phenotype produce higher levels of insulin antibody (16). Figure 9 demonstrates the marked difference seen during the first twelve months of therapy with once daily bovine insulin given to two diabetic males (1).

Sequels to Antibody Production

Insulin resistance is currently defined as a daily insulin requirement in excess of 120 units. A number of studies have confirmed the presence of markedly elevated levels of insulin antibody in most patients developing resistance without any other primary cause (figure 2) and the sera taken from such patients are able to neutralise the metabolic effect of insulin (1). Insulin resistance is rare but often develops in patients who have had intermittent therapy with bovine insulins.

Mild local reactions at injection sites are not uncommon during the initial period of insulin therapy but serious allergic manifestations are extremely rare. IgE antibody has been implicated in some allergic patients and desensitization has been successful in alleviating their symptoms. Switching to highly purified insulins may also improve the situation although once patients have been sensitized by more immunogenic preparations, highly purified material may still elicit acute allergic manifestations (1). One group has suggested that the zinc component of the insulin preparation may cause "allergic" problems which can be remedied by the use of zinc-free insulin (17).

Injection site lipo-atrophy (figure 10) is a common complication of treatment with bovine insulins affecting between 10 and 55% of patients treated (18). Lipo-atrophy is almost

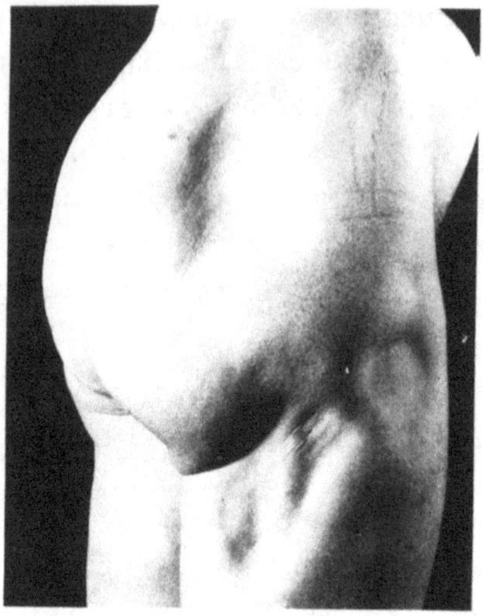

Figure 10. Woman aged 39. Appearance of lipo-atrophy at injection sites.

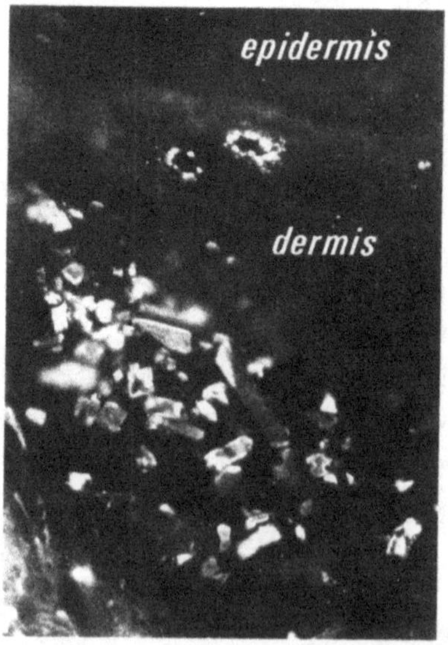

Figure 11. Deposition of C3 in vessel walls in superficial dermis and presence of crystals (independently shown to react with anti-insulin serum) in deeper dermis in biopsy sample from edge of lipo-atrophic area, demonstrated by a direct immunofluorescent technique (18).

Case No.	IgM	C3	Fibrin
	Patients with lipoatrophy		
1	+++	++	+
2	+	++	+
3	+	+	-
4	+	+	-
5	+	-	++
6	+	-	+
7	+	-	+
8	+	-	-
	Controls		
15	-	-	-
16	-	-	-
17	-	-	-
18	-	-	-
19	-	-	-

Table 3. Dermal blood vessel deposition of immunological components in biopsy samples taken from the edge of lipo-atrophic areas in eight patients and from injection-sites in five control patients (18).

unknown in patients treated exclusively with highly purified porcine insulin and has been described following injection of relatively impure preparations of vasopressin and human growth hormone.

Patients with lipo-atrophy show higher levels of circulating insulin antibody (figure 2) and immunofluorescent examination of tissue taken from the edge of lipo-atrophic areas shows the deposition of immunological components (notably IgM, C3 and fibrin) in the walls of dermal blood vessels (figure 11, table 3) (18). It seems likely, therefore, that insulin induced lipo-atrophy results from the local formation of immune complexes, complement fixation and release of inflammatory mediators from the cellular infiltrate.

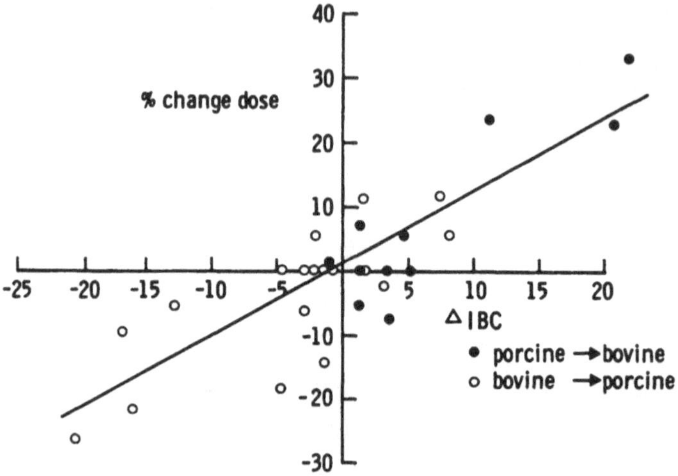

Figure 12. Correlation (r = 0.81) between percentage change in insulin dose and change in IgG insulin binding capacity observed during a randomized cross-over study between conventional bovine and highly purified porcine insulin regimes (20).

Debate continues concerning the significance of circulating insulin antibodies in patients who do not show insulin resistance, insulin allergy or injection site lipo-atrophy (19). The presence of a relationship between insulin antibody levels and insulin dose and/or diabetic control has been disputed (1). A recent cross-over study of patients switched from twice daily bovine soluble and isophane insulins to actrapid and monotard insulins has demonstrated that changes in insulin antibody correlate with pecentage change in dose whether the switch is from ordinary bovine to highly purified porcine insulin or vice versa (figure 12) (20). Such a clear relationship is obscured if the patients studied are not stratified to exclude those who experience marked changes in diabetic control as measured by glycosylated haemoglobin (HbA_1) levels and those who possess very low levels of insulin antibody (20).

The period of "remission" experienced by some diabetics when first started on insulin therapy - often called the "honeymoon period" - may be less prolonged in those patients producing significant levels of antibody (21). Whether this is because insulin antibody hastens the exhaustion of endogenous insulin reserves or because those patients who tend to produce more antibody present later or with more severe disease is not clear.

Perhaps the most important aspect of all is the possible link between antibody production and the aggravation of diabetic vascular disease affecting large vessels (macro-angiopathy) or small vessels (micro-angiopathy) - the latter causing disease predominantly in the eyes and kidneys (1). Immune complexes can be detected within the circulation of insulin-treated diabetics (22,23) and in some instances these have been shown to contain insulin and insulin antibody (22,24). One study found a correlation between high levels of insulin antibody and circulating immune complexes (22) and higher antibody levels have been corrélated with an increased incidence of diabetic retinopathy (25). Analogy with classical models of serum sickness and immune complex mediated injury encourages the view that circulating IC may well be harmful to the diabetic patient but it will be important to determine what proportion of the total immune complex load is relevant to immunogenic insulin therapy in carefully matched groups of patients with and without documented vascular disease before conclusions are drawn about any definitive link between such therapy and the vascular complications of diabetes.

Conclusion

Insulin is the most common heterologous protein to be injected into patients. When non-highly purified material of bovine origin is used, most patients develop a detectable immune response dependent partly on their genetic background but also on various aspects of the form and mode of insulin administration. The development of sensitive assays and highly purified antigens has enabled us to learn a lot about the specificity of this response. Various sequels to insulin antibody production have been described e.g. insulin resistance, insulin allergy and lipo-atrophy. Further work is required before a definitive answer can be given to the possibility that circulating insulin antibodies and immune complexes are an important factor in the pathogenesis of the vascular complications of diabetes.

Acknowledgements: I thank Una Kelly for expert technical assistance; Mr. Geoffrey Lythe for preparing the figures; Anne Willington for typing the manuscript and many clinical colleagues for their helpful collaboration. It is also a pleasure to thank Novo Laboratories Ltd. (Dr. David Owens) for their valuable assistance and the Novo Research Institute, Copenhagen (Dr. Lise Heding) for help with the provision of highly purified insulins. Development of the antibody assay methods was supported by a grant from the British Diabetic Association.

References

1. Reeves, W. G.: Recent Advances in Clinical Immunology 2, 183-220 (1980).
2. Reeves, W. G., Kelly, U.: J. Immunol. Methods 34, 329-338 (1980).
3. Bristow, A. F.: Personal communication (1980).
4. Reeves, W. G.: In preparation (1980).
5. Bloom, S. R., Adrian, T. E., Barnes, A. J., Polak, J. M.: Lancet 1, 14-17 (1979).
6. Villalpando, S., Drash, A.: Diabetes 28, 294-299 (1979).
7. Deckert, T., Grundahl, E.: Diabetologia 6, 15-20 (1970).
8. Andersen, O. O.: Acta. Endocrinologica 72, 33-45 (1973).

9. Arquilla, E. R., Thiene, P., Brugman, T., Ruess, W., Sugiyama, R.: Biochem. J. 175, 289-297 (1978).

10. Montgomery, D. W., Chvapil, M., Zukoski, C. F.: Infection and Immunity 23, 424-431 (1979).

11. Claus, D. R., Siegal, J., Petras, K., Skor, D., Osmand, A. P., Gewurz, H.: J. Immunol. 118, 83-87 (1977).

12. Hart, D. A.: Exp. Cell. Res. 121, 419-425 (1979).

13. Huget, R., Opitz, H. G., Flad, H. D.: Z. Immun.-Forsch. 152, 190-199 (1976).

14. Kerp, L., Kasemir, H., Langer, J., Steinhilber, S.: Diabetologia 6, 51 (1970).

15. Menzel, R., Knospe, S., Ziegler, M., Wilke, W., Michael, R.: Diabetologia 7, 386-390 (1971).

16. Irvine, W. J., DiMario, U., Feek, C. M., Ting, A., Morris, P. J., Gray, R. S., Duncan, L. J. P.: J. Clin. Lab. Immunol. 1, 111-114 (1978).

17. Feinglos, M. N., Jegasothy, B. Y.: Lancet 1, 122-124 (1979).

18. Reeves, W. G., Allen, B. R., Tattersall, R. B.: Brit. Med. J. 280, 1500-1503 (1980).

19. Lancet Editorial:Lancet 1, 363-364 (1979).

20. Walford, S., Allison, S. P., Kelly, U., Deverill, I., Reeves, W. G.: Diabetologia 19, 10-11 (1980).

21. Andersen, O. O.: Acta. Endocrinologica 205S, 231-238 (1976).

22. Irvine, W. J., Al-Khateeb, S. S., DiMario, U. et al.: Clin. Exp. Immunol. 30, 16-21 (1977).

23. Kilpatrick, J. M., Virella, G.: Clin. Exp. Immunol. 40, 445-452 (1980).

24. Følling, I.: Acta. Endocrinologica 205S, 199-207 (1975).

25. Andersen, O. O., Egeberg, J.: Acta. Paed. Scand. 270S, 63-68 (1977).

26. Reeves, W. G. et al: In preparation (1980).

STUDIES OF THE IMMUNOGENICITY OF CHROMATOGRAPHICALLY PURIFIED INSULINS IN TYPE-I AND TYPE-II DIABETICS

H.-G. Velcovsky, E. Mäser, K. Federlin

Medizinische Klinik III und Poliklinik, Zentrum für Innere Medizin, Justus-Liebig-Universität, D-6300 Gießen, Germany

Following insulin therapy, circulating insulin antibodies are frequently observed in many diabetics. The insulin itself is the specific antigen. To test the immunogenicity of various chromatographically purified insulins, we wanted to investigate the response of patients with different types of diabetes mellitus (type I or type II) and the effect of preliminary treatment.

Patients and methods

For this reason we investigated the sera of 98 type I - diabetics and 34 patients with a type I - diabetes from the beginning of the insulin therapy. Furthermore 118 patients with a type II - diabetes were observed. Additionally 13 diabetics with an immediate or delayed type of allergy to insulin were examined. In all these groups some patients were observed during many months from the beginning of the insulin therapy.

The insulin binding capacity in the serum or the anti-insulin antibodies were measured with the following methods:
a) cellulose absorption method by KERP et al. 1966 (1),
b) radio-immunoelectrophoresis described by CHRISTIANSEN (2),
c) insulin specific IgE measurement (3, 4, 5).
The sera were obtained from the patients in the morning before the daily dose of insulin was administered. Free insulin was removed from serum aliquots by means of absorption with antibody coated tubes. The individual groups of patients were

Basic and Clinical Aspects of Immunity to Insulin

treated with various insulins: highly purified or monocomponent bovine and porcine insulins or a monocomponent mixed insulin (Depot-Insulin CR Hoechst, Depot-Insulin CS Hoechst, Optisulin Hoe 03R Hoechst, Optisulin Hoe 03S Hoechst, Optisulin Hoe 05S long Hoechst, Monotard MC Novo, Rapitard MC Novo).

Results

The results obtained from the 98 type I - diabetics are shown in table 1. The mean age of the various groups lay between 16 and 32 years, the mean values of the IgG-insulin antibodies differed from 7.9 to 12.4 mU/ml. The number of the positive patients fluctuated from 0 per cent of the Hoe 03R-Insulin group to 40.2 per cent of the Monotard MC group. The mean values of the positive antibody levels were between 25.2 and 31.1 mU/ml some with a high SEM. The levels of specific IgE-antibody to insulin were very low: between 1.3 and 3.2 U/ml. The number of the positive patients was between 27.3 and 43.7 per cent in the individual groups with mean levels between 4 and 8.3 U/ml. The 3 patients of the Hoe 03R group showed no IgG-antibodies to insulin and one patient only showed specific IgE-antibodies.

Additionally 34 patients with a type I - diabetes were controlled from the beginning of the insulin therapy. The mean age of this group was 10.7 years, the mean dose of insulin per day 19.8 U. Most patients of this group were treated with a porcine insulin, 4 diabetics with a bovine insulin only (s. fig. 1). The antibody levels of the individual patients were partly controlled during two years. 18 of 34 patients or 52 per cent however partly showed high titers of neutralizing antibodies to insulin after a short time. The data from the individual patients are shown in figure 1. Specific IgE-antibodies to insulin were found in 12 patients or 35.2 per cent in this group with a mean value of 2.16 U/ml.

Insulin - antibodies / type I - diabetics

table 1

insulin	n	age	IgG - a. b. total (mU / ml)	IgG - a. b. % positive (mU / ml)	IgE - a. b. total (U / ml)	IgE - a. b. % positive (U / ml)	insulin U. p.d.
CR	3o	25,7 ± 2,2	12,4 ± 3,9	4o,2 % 31,1 ± 6,9	2,8 ± o,8	33,4 % 8,3 ± o,9	4o,9 ± 2,4
CS	44	16,o ± 1,5	11,2 ± 2,9	36,5 % 3o,7 ± 5,2	1,8 ± o,5	27,3 % 6,8 ± o,9	38,3 ± 3,4
Rapi-tard	16	31,1 ± 2,6	7,9 ± 4,9	31,2 % 25,2 ±11,5	3,2 ± 1,1	43,7 % 7,4 ± 1,3	45,o ± 3,4
Mono-tard	5	26,2 ± 4,9	12,4 ±1o,5	4o,o % 31,o ±22,9	2,o ± 1,4	4o,o % 5,o ± 1,9	36,8 ± 8,9
Hoe O3 R	3	32,o ± o,9	o	o	1,3 ± 1,3	33,3 % 4,o	38,6 + 4,8

mean values with SEM

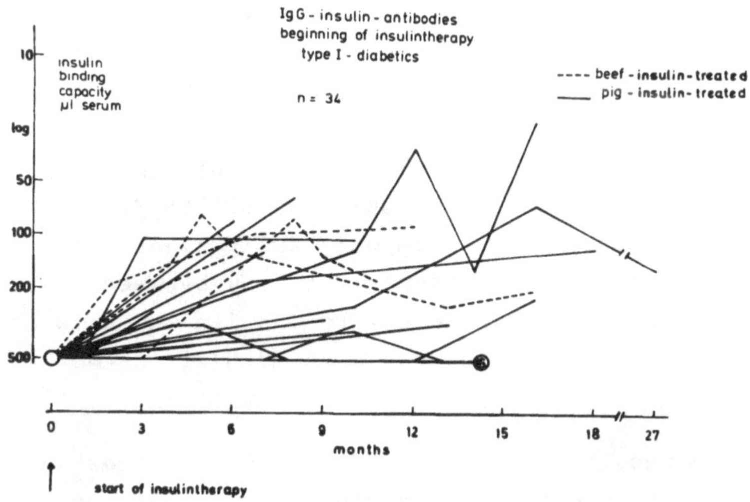

figure 1

Insulin - antibodies / type II - diabetics

insulin	n	age	IgG - a. b. total mU / ml	IgG - a. b. % positive mU / ml	IgE - a. b. total U / ml	IgE - a. b. % positive U / ml	insulin U. p.d
CR	41	67,1 ± 1,1	5,8 ± 2,3	22,1 % 26,3 ± 7,3	1,7 ± o,5	26,3 % 6,4 ± 1,o	52,o + 2,9
CS	2o	64,3 ± 2,1	11,2 ± 4,9	3o,4 % 37,3 ±11,o	1,6 ± o,8	2o,1 % 8,o ± 1,8	59,9 + 4,8
Rapi-tard	16	63,5 ± 2,6	9,4 ± 4,3	41,2 % 25,2 ± 8,3	1,9 ± o,9	29,5 % 7,5 ± 1,7	41,6 ± 4,5
Mono-tard	11	63,3 ± 3,4	12,6 ± 6,8	36,5 % 34,7 ±13,1	1,8 ± o,9	27,8 % 6,7 ± o,7	45,6 ± 5,5
Hoe 03 R	16	62,8 ± 2,4	1,7 ± 1,2	12,6 % 14,o ± 2,9	1,3 ± o,7	18,7 % 6,7 + 1,5	59,1 ± 6,4
Hoe 03 S	2	62,o ± 2,9	17,o ±16,9	5o,o % 34,o	1,5 ± 1,5	5o,o % 3,o	74,o ±21,9
Hoe 05 S	12	66,8 ± 1,7	1,3 ± 1,2	8,3 % 15,o	o	o	33,6 ± 3,7

table 2

mean values with SEM

Furthermore 118 patients with a type II - diabetes were investigated. Table 2 summarizes the results. In the various insulin groups the mean age was between 62 and 67.1 year. The levels of the IgG-antibodies were from 1.3 mU/ml of the Des-phe-insulin Hoe 05S to 17 mU/ml of the Des-phe-insulin group Hoe 03 S. The number of positive patients was 8.3 to 50 per cent. In the Hoe 03S group there were only two patients. The IgG-antibody levels in the positive patients lay between 14 and 37.3 mU/ml. The specific IgE levels to insulin lay between 0 and 1.9 U/ml in general, but between 3 and 8 U/ml in the positive patients.

Figure 2 shows the results of 12 type II - diabetics treated with a Des-phe-insulin Hoe 05S, a long insulin (30 per cent Des-phe-insulin, 70 per cent normal Depot-Insulin CR).Only in

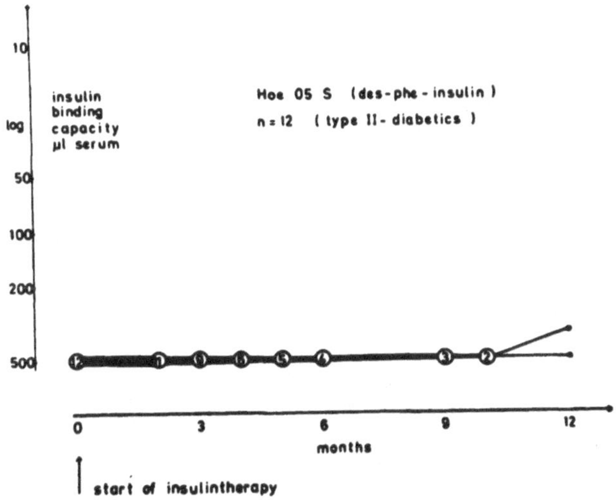

figure 2

one case were IgG-antibodies to insulin found after a 12 months' treatment with insulin. IgE-antibodies could not be found in these patients. This group of patients will be further observed.

Moreover 13 diabetics with an insulin allergy were examined. Six patients had an immediate type of allergy (3 patients to CR-Insulin, one to CS-Insulin, one to Hoe 03S-Insulin and one to

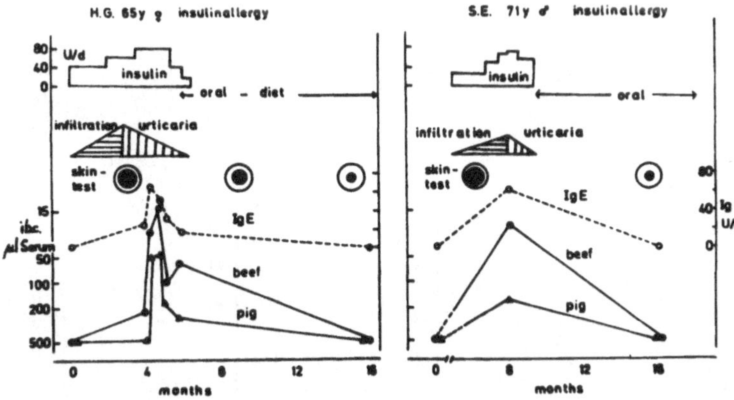

figure 3

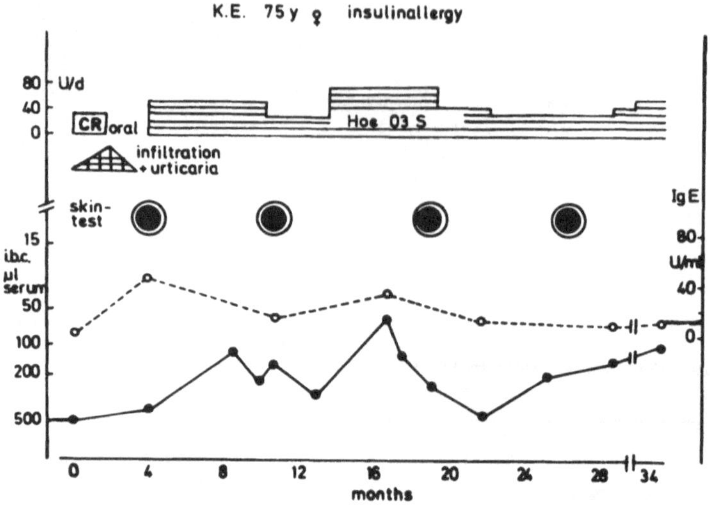

figure 4

Monotard), 7 diabetics a delayed type of allergy (3 to CR-Insulin, 2 to CS-Insulin, one to Hoe 03R and one to Rapitard). The figures 3 and 4 show the courses of the disease of 3 patients with an immediate type of allergy to insulin.The therapy of the diabetes mellitus of two patients (s. fig. 3) could be continued with oral antidiabetica and diet after the acute allergic reaction. During the allergic reactions an increase of the specific IgG- and IgE-antibodies in the serum of pa-

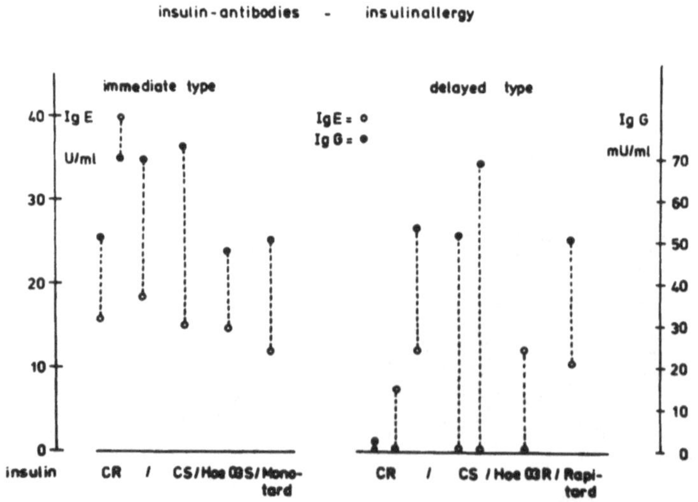

figure 5

tients could be observed. After the insulin therapy was finished the antibody levels decreased. The treatment of another patient with an immediate allergic reaction to CR-Insulin (s. fig. 4) could be continued with a porcine Des-phe-insulin Hoe 03S. Under this therapy no local skin reactions were observed after the daily insulin injection. But in the skintest the patient still showed strong positive reactions of the immediate type to all insulins. In the lower part of this figure the courses of the specific IgG- and IgE-antibody levels can be seen. These examples show, that high titers of insulin specific IgE were found only in patients with allergic skin reactions to the insulin injection. In figure 5 the specific IgE- and IgG-antibody levels of all 13 allergic diabetics are represented. It demonstrates that some patients with allergic reactions of the delayed type also show specific IgE- and IgG-antibodies in low concentrations.

Furthermore the antibodies to insulin of the other Ig-classes were measured in 44 of 98 type I - diabetics. In all groups, only 7 patients with antibodies of the IgA-class were found; IgM-antibodies to insulin could be found in 9 children in the first phase of the diabetes mellitus after the treatment with insulin. In all groups the daily dose of insulin was given in normal quantity. No correlation between the development of insulin antibodies and the dose of insulin per day was found.

Summary of findings and discussion

In 28.7 per cent of the investigated sera of the type I - diabetics and in 33.3 per cent of the type II - diabetics we found neutralizing insulin antibodies of the IgG-class (s. table 1 and 2). Insulin specific IgE-antibodies could be measured in 36.6 per cent of the sera of the type I - diabetics and in 24.6 per cent of the type II - diabetics. Antibodies to insulin of the other Ig-classes could be found only in some patients of all groups, especially in some children after the beginning of the treatment with insulin. This result demonstrates that fewer type II - diabetics than type I - diabetics develop antibodies to insulin. In the examination of the various insulin types, the patients of both groups treated with the Des-phe-insulins Hoe 03R (a neutral bovine Des-phe-insulin) and Hoe 05S (a neutral porcine Des-phe-insulin) rarely show specific insulin antibodies of the IgG- or IgE-class. The group of patients treated with Hoe 03S is an exception, because only two patients without allergic reactions were treated with this insulin. The levels of the antibody titers in all groups of patients were very similar; significant differences could not be found (s. fig. 6 and 7). In contrast to diabetics treated with highly purified insulins, patients treated with "conventional" insulins on the average showed IgG-antibodies to insulin of 42.3 $\pm$ 4.8 mU/ml and IgE-antibodies of 21.6 $\pm$ 3.7 U/ml. These results have already been published earlier (3, 5). Insulin specific IgE was also noted in low concentrations in many investigated diabetics who had no symptoms of allergy after the

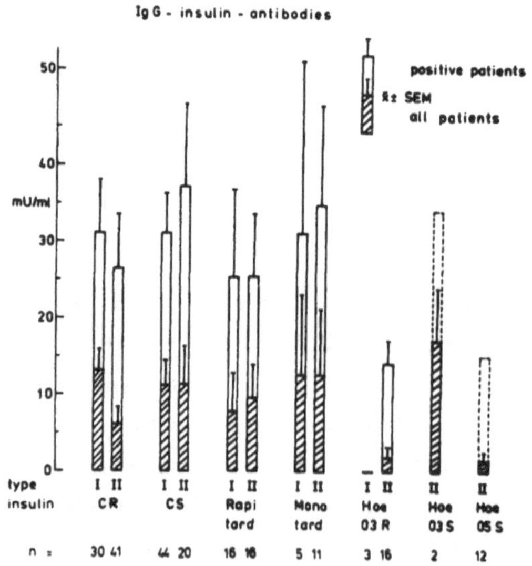

figure 6

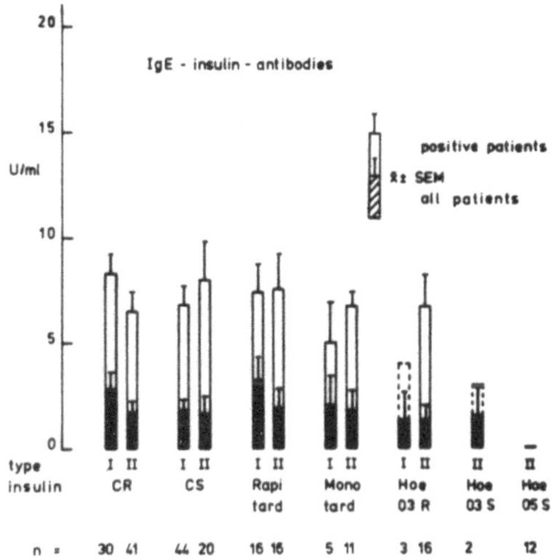

figure 7

therapeutic application of insulin. High titers of insulin-specific IgE were found in patients with allergic skin reactions after an insulin injection. This phenomenon has already been described by PATTERSON et al. (6) and NAKAGAWA et al. (7). No correlation to the preliminary therapy of the diabetes mellitus with the development of insulin antibodies could be found. So we conclude that the development of antibodies to insulin in each diabetic patient is influenced by genetic and individual factors.

References

1. Kerp, L., Steinmüller, S., Kieling, H.: Klin. Wschr. 44, 560 (1966).
2. Christiansen, A.H.: Horm. Metabol. Res. 5, 147 (1973).
3. Federlin, K., Velcovsky, H.-G.: Verh. Dtsch. Ges. Inn. Med.

80, 1613 (1974).

4. Velčovsky, H.-G., Federlin, K.: Wien. Klin. Wschr. 88, 36 (1976).

5. Velčovsky, H.-G., Beringhoff, B., Federlin, K.: Immun. Infekt. 6, 146 (1978).

6. Patterson, R., Mellies, C.J., Roberts, M.: J. Immunol. 110, 1135 (1973).

7. Nakagawa, S., Saito, N., Nakayama, H., Sasaki, T., Watanabe, T., Aoiki, N.: Diabetologia 14, 33 (1978).

Genetic Control Of The IgE Response To Insulin

I. Kallenberger and K. Keck

Universität Konstanz
D-775 Konstanz

As mentioned by several speakers during this symposium, the production of the two classes of antibodies (IgG and IgM) is controlled by H-2 linked Ir genes. In the case of IgM antibodies, we have an additional control by genes coding for the heavy chain of the immunoglobulins (allotype linked genes). We here report results demonstrating that the production of antibody of the IgE class (responsible for immediate type hypersensitivity) is controlled by at least two genes: H-2 linked Ir genes control the response of all three classes of antibody: IgE, IgG and IgM. A second gene, present in the background, influences the level and kinetics of IgE antibody production.

The animals were immunized intraperitoneally with insulin in aluminum hydroxide and Bordetella Pertussis. Sera were pooled and levels of IgE antibody were determined by passive cutaneous anaphylaxis in the rat, by the method of Ovary (1). IgG antibodies were measured with the Farr test as described previously (2).

This work was supported by the Deutsche Forschungsgemeinschaft, Sonderforschungsbereich 138, "Biologische Grenzflächen und Spezifität".

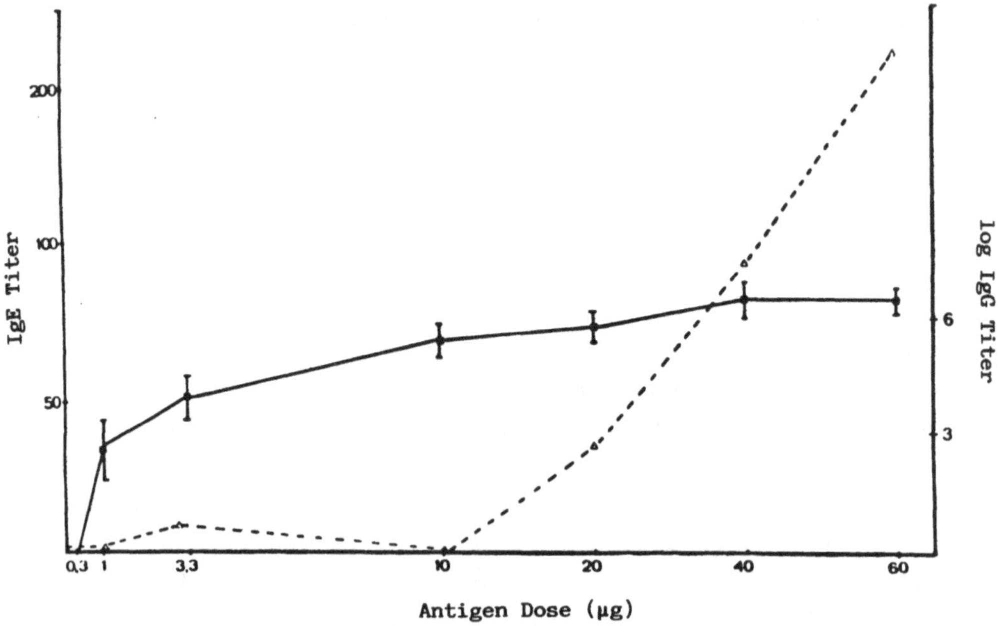

Fig. 1 Dose Response Curves in BALB/c mice to bovine insulin

- - - IgE antibody

――― IgG antibody

Fig. 1 shows a dose response curve for IgG and IgE antibody obtained with BALB/c mice. The IgG response starts at a dose level of 1µg antigen, whereas at least 20µg were needed to induce the production of IgE antibody. The IgG titer reaches a maximum at about 60µg. Such a maximum is not observed for the IgE antibody production in the dose range tested.

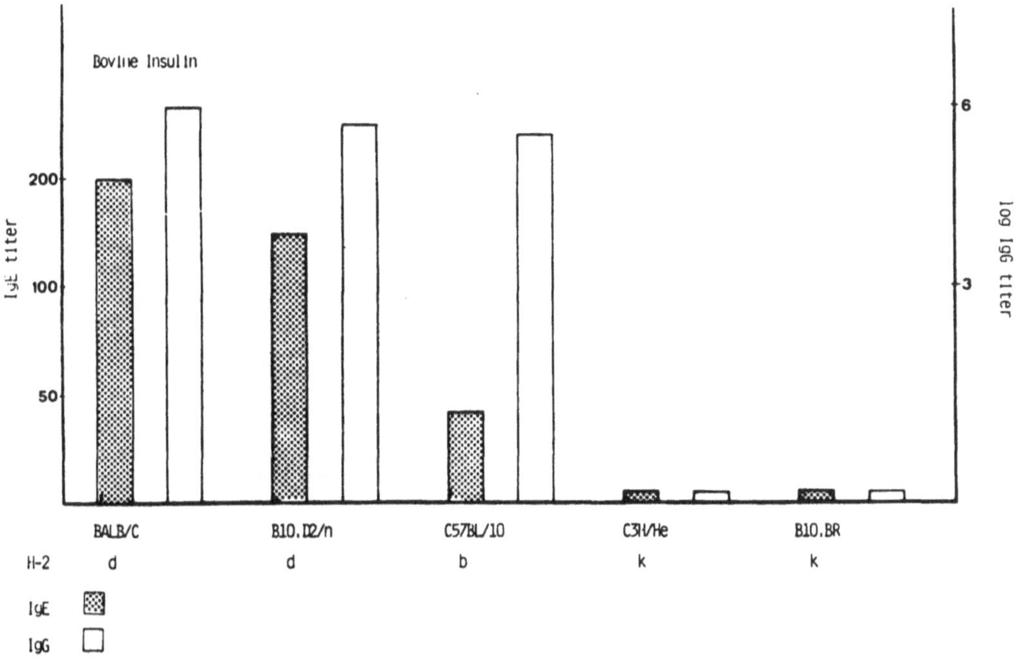

Fig. 2 IgE and IgG response of different strains of mice to bovine insulin

In Fig. 2 the IgE and IgG response to bovine insulin in different strains of mice is shown. All strains were immunized with 20µg of bovine insulin.The strains BALB/c,B10.D2/n and C57BL/10 are responders to bovine insulin with respect to the production of IgE and IgG antibody. The strains C3H/He and B10.BR are nonresponders with respect to both antibody classes. This result shows that the production of IgE antibody is controlled by the same H-2 linked Ir genes as the production of IgG antibody.

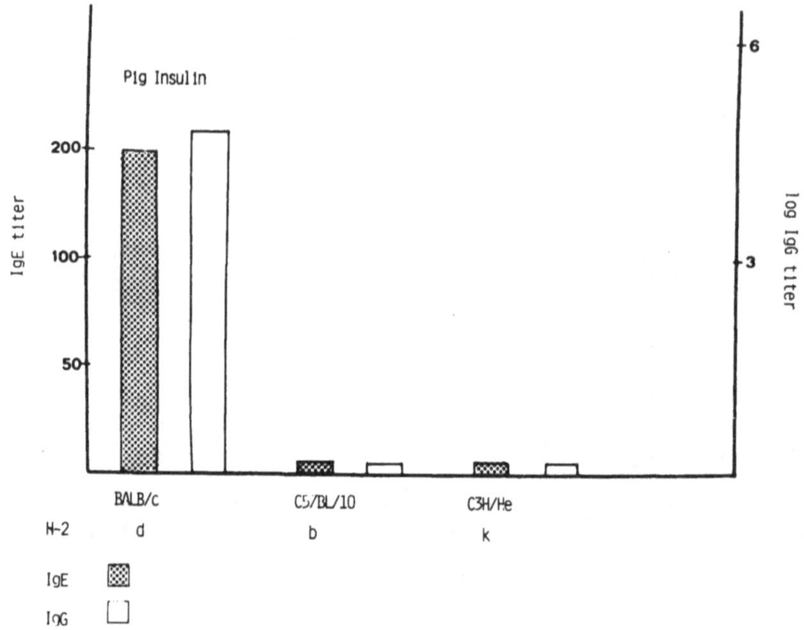

If pig insulin, which has the same A-chain loop sequences as mouse insulin, is used as an antigen, only BALB/c mice with the H-2 haplotype respond with the production of IgG and IgE antibody. The strains C57BL/10 and C3H/He are nonresponders. This demonstrates, as shown earlier, that the strain C57BL ($H-2^b$) needs the A-chain loop of bovine insulin as a carrier determinant for the production of IgG and IgM antibody. Fig.3 shows that the same type of regulation is found when IgE antibodies are measured. C3H/He mice ($H-2^k$), however, can respond to sheep insulin. Table 1 demonstrates the parallel regulation found for both classes of antibody, depending on the A-chain loop sequences of the insulin used for immunization.

Table 1. IgG and IgE response of BALB/c and C3H/He mice to sheep insulin

Strain	IgG (log antibody)	IgE (PCA-titer)
BALB/c	6,2	200
C3H/He	6,1	50

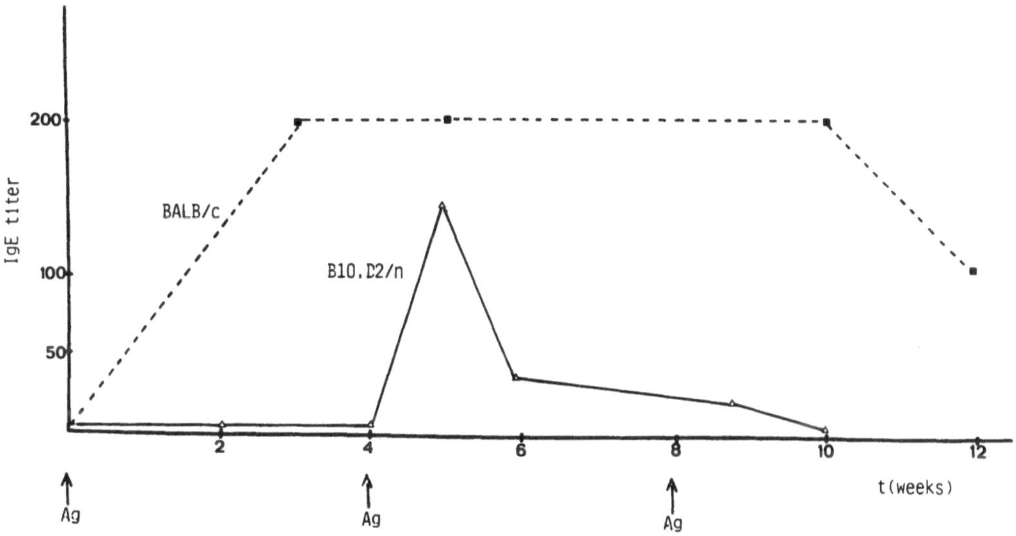

Fig. 4 Kinetic of the IgE response to bovine insulin in the strains BALB/c and B10.D2/n

The production of IgE antibody is not only influenced by H-2 linked Ir genes, but also by the genetic background of the mice. (Fig. 4). The strain B10.D2 carries the same H-2 haplotype as the strain BALB/c but the genetic background of C57BL. In contrast to BALB/c, the IgE response to insulin in this strain is strikingly transient; it begins late and falls rapidly. These results suggest that the background genes control the kinetics and the amount of IgE antibodies produced.

The data suggest that the production of IgE antibody is regulated (a) by the same H-2 linked Ir genes as those involved in the production of IgG antibody and (b) background genes not yet identified seem to influence the amount of IgE antibody and the kinetics of production.

References:

1. Ovary, Z.
   Int. Arch. Allergy appl. Immun. 3, 293 (1952).
2. Desbuquois, B. and Aurbach, G.D.
   J. Clin. Endocrinol. 33, 732-738 (1971).

HLA-DR ASSOCIATION OF HUMORAL IMMUNORESPONSIVENESS TO INSULIN IN INSULIN-DEPENDENT (TYPE I) DIABETES MELLITUS*

J. Bertrams

Abteilung für Laboratoriumsmedizin
St. Elisabeth Krankenhaus
(Akademisches Lehrkrankenhaus der Universität Essen)
D-4300 Essen 1

D. Grüneklee

Diabetes Forschungsinstitut
Universität Düsseldorf
D-4000 Düsseldorf 1

Introduction

The immune response to insulin, both in mouse and guinea pig, has been shown to be under control of major histocompatibility complex (MHC)-linked immune response(Ir) genes (1-5). Because of the great analogy between the MHC of mice (H-2) and men (HLA) it was not very surprising to find an association between the immunoresponsiveness to insulin and HLA antigens in patients with insulin-dependent (type I) diabetes mellitus. In 1976 we could demonstrate a significant association between the insulin antibody production and HLA-B15, while non-responder patients showed an association with HLA-B8 (6). These findings could be confirmed later by other investigators (7-9). Since HLA-DR antigens most probably are the gene products of

---

*Supported by Deutsche Forschungsgemeinschaft SFB 113, B3 and B4

human immune response(Ir) genes, we analyzed the HLA-DR phenotypes in relation to the humoral immune response to insulin in order to find an association between certain HLA-DR antigens and a negative or positive immune response to insulin, respectively. Since both in normal controls and in type I diabetes a positive linkage disequilibrium exists between HLA-B8 and DR3 on the one side and between B15 and DR4 on the other side, an association between responders and DR4 and between non-responders and DR3 could be expected.

Material and Methods

Insulin antibodies were determined in the sera of 86 Caucasoid patients with insulin-dependent diabetes mellitus, typed for HLA-A,B,C, and DR antigens as part of an international study on the genetics of diabetes, which was performed during the "8th International Histocompatibility Workshop" in 1980 (10). HLA-A,B,C, and DR antigens were determined by standard microlymphocytotoxicity techniques (11,12). B lymphocytes for DR typing were isolated after rosetting the T lymphocytes with AET (=2-Aminoaethylisothiuroniumbromid)-treated sheep erythrocytes and separation of B lymphocytes and rosetted T lymphocytes by density gradient centrifugation.

Quantification of serum antibodies to insulin was performed by radioimmunoassay with the cellulose-adsorption method (13).

According to the level of insulin binding the patient group was subdivided into three classes: (a) 17 non-responders with less than 25% fixation of 1mU/ml radioactive insulin at a serum dilution of 1:2, (b) 47 doubtful responders with more than 25% but less than 50% fixation of 1mU/ml radioactive insulin at a serum dilution of 1:2 ("grey area"), and (c) 22 definite responders with more than 50% fixation of 1mU/ml radioactive insulin at a serum dilution of 1:2. Group (c) included 8 high responders to insulin with more than 50% fixation of 1mU/ml radioactive insulin even in a serum dilution of 1:5.

Control frequencies for HLA-A,B,C antigens were taken from (14) and for DR antigens from (15).

Results

As could be expected from previous studies (10,16) type I diabetes is primarily positive associated with HLA-DR3 and DR4.

HLA association of type I diabetes mellitus

HLA antigen	All(n=86) Patients	Normal Controls*	P-value	Relative Risk
B7	16 (18.6%)	118 (22.0%)	n.s.	0.8
DR2	4 (4.7%)	793 (24.9%)	$<10^{-4}$	0.1
B18	21 (24.4%)	62 (11.6%)	<0.005	2.5
B8	32 (37.2%)	99 (18.5%)	$<10^{-4}$	2.6
DR3	43 (50.0%)	665 (20.9%)	$<10^{-6}$	3.8
Cw3	16 (18.6%)	117 (21.8%)	n.s.	0.8
B15	14 (16.3%)	69 (12.9%)	n.s.	1.3
DR4	44 (51.2%)	686 (21.6%)	$<10^{-6}$	3.8

*n= 536 for HLA-A,B,C (14) and 3184 for HLA-DR antigens (15)

According to a strong linkage disequilibrium, which normally exists in Caucasians between single HLA-A,B,C, and DR alleles, B8 and B18 are increased secondary to DR3, and B15 secondary to DR4. The strongest negative association was found for HLA-DR2 and secondarily for B7. Disease susceptibility genes as well as protective genes for type I diabetes thus are located in the HLA-DR region of the HLA-complex. The relative risk for both DR3 and DR4 is 3.8. Individuals being positive for one or the other of these disease markers have a 3.8-fold chance to get type I diabetes in comparison to DR3- or DR4-negative persons. Vice versa DR2-positive individuals have only a tenth of the disease risk of a DR2-negative proband.

A totally different distribution of HLA antigens was obtained, when responder and non-responder patients were compared.

HLA antigen frequencies in non-responder and responder patients

HLA antigen	Non-responders n=17	Responders n=22	P-value	All Pat. n=86
B7	3 (17.6%)	7 (31.8%)	n.s.	16 (18.6%)
DR2	0	1 (4.5%)	n.s.	4 (4.7%)
B18	2 (11.8%)	5 (22.7%)	n.s.	21 (24.4%)
B8	10 (58.8%)	3 (13.6%)	<0.01	32 (37.2%)
DR3	11 (64.7%)	7 (31.8%)	= 0.06	43 (50.0%)
Cw3	2 (11.8%)	5 (22.7%)	n.s.	16 (18.6%)
B15	1 (5.9%)	6 (27.3%)	n.s.	14 (16.3%)
DR4	4 (23.5%)	16 (72.7%)	<0.01	44 (51.2%)

In agreement with our previous published data non-response to insulin is associated with HLA-B8 and in addition with DR3. While all patients showed a B8 frequency of 37.3%, insulin non-responders had a B8 increase (58.8%) and responders a B8 decrease (13.6%). HLA-DR3, both in normal controls and type I diabetes linked to HLA-B8, similarily was increased in non-responders (64.7%) and decreased in responder patients (31.8%).

Opposite results were obtained, when the immune response to insulin was related to the HLA-B15,DR4 linkage group. In comparison to a B15 frequency of 16.3% among all patients, B15 was decreased to 5.9% in non-responders, but increased to 27.3% in responders. Likewise DR4 was decreased in non-responders (23.4%) and increased in responders (72.7%), when compared to the frequency among all patients (51.2%). The association of the humoral response to insulin with the HLA-B15,DR4 linkage group and of the non-response to insulin with the HLA-B8,DR3 linkage group is especially impressive when graphically presented. The patient group with a doubtful response to insulin is included in the figure.

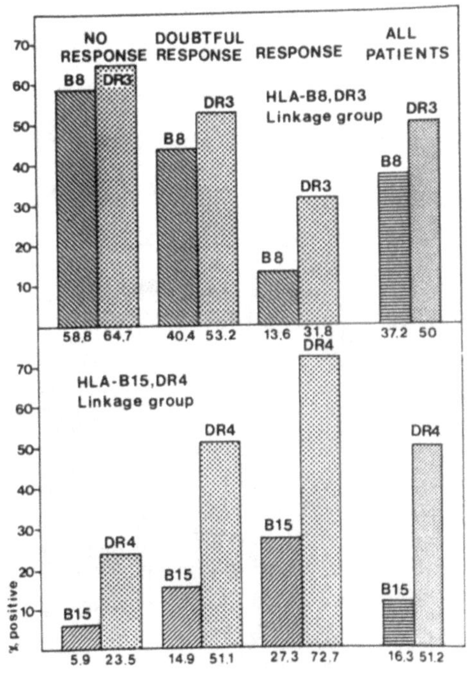

According to these data the immune response to insulin shows a significant association with the same HLA-antigens, which are associated with type I diabetes in most populations (10).

The HLA association of the immune responsiveness to insulin can be expressed by the relative risk value of DR4-positive patients to develop insulin antibodies, which is 2.5 higher than in DR4-negative patients. For B15-positive patients the risk is 1.9 times increased. The risk to develop no antibodies to insulin is 2.5 in B8-positive and 1.8 in DR3-positive patients. The position of the Ir gene(s) for insulin thus may be between the HLA-B and DR loci.

Concerning the association of the non-response to insulin with the HLA-B8,DR3 linkage group the existence of lacking Ir genes or of suppressor genes may be discussed. As shown in the figure, the frequency of HLA-DR3,DR4 heterozygotes is very low in non-responder patients (5.9%) and increased in responder patients (15.1%). This is not compatible with the existence of a DR3-associated immune suppression gene but with a lacking immune response gene for insulin.

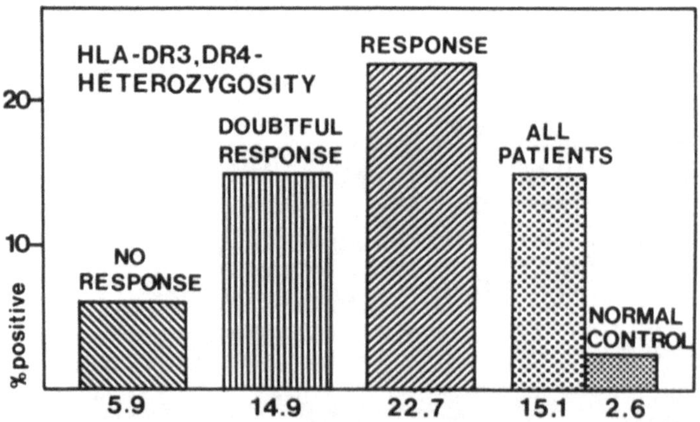

In vitro crossreactivity of the insulin antibodies with pork and beef insulin was observed in our study in 49 of 69 patients (=71%). No significant results were obtained, when different patterns of in vitro reactivity of the insulin antibodies were related to the HLA patterns of the patients.

Discussion

The findings of the present paper demonstrate a significant association between the humoral immune response to insulin and HLA-B15 and DR4. Type I diabetes patients being positive for B15 or DR4 have a 1.9 or 2.5 times higher risk to develop insulin antibodies than patients without these antigens.

Previous published data (16.17) and the present study furthermore emphasize, that there are at least two distinct high risk genes (Ir genes?) operative in tpye I diabetes. One of these high risk genes is closely linked to B8 and DR3 and associated with persistent islet cell antibodies and other clinical autoimmune disorders (18). It has been shown that such patients with Ir genes for organ-specific autoimmunity are non-responders to exogenous antigens like insulin. The second diabetes high risk gene is in linkage disequilibrium with B15 and DR4 and associated with high titres of antibody against exogenous antigens like Coxsackie viruses (19) and insulin, as could be shown by the present study. It would thus appear, that the HLA-B8,DR3-linked high risk gene(s) may be Ir gene(s) for endogenous antigens, while the HLA-B15,DR4-linked high risk gene(s) may be Ir gene(s) for exogenous antigens. Thus the association between HLA-antigens and humoral immunoresponsiveness to insulin contributes not only to a better understanding of the immunity to insulin but also of the pathogenesis which results in the clinical picture of type I diabetes.

Summary

Insulin antibodies and HLA-A,B,C, and DR antigens have been determined in 86 Caucasoid patients with insulin-dependent (type I) diabetes mellitus. The whole patient group showed a significant positive association with the HLA-B8,DR3 as well as the HLA-B15,DR4 linkage group. Patients with antibodies to insulin (responders) were significantly positive associated only with HLA-B15 and DR4, while non-responder patients exhibited a significant positive association with HLA-B8 and DR3. The B15,DR4- linked high risk genes for type I diabetes may be Ir genes for exogenous antigens, while the B8,DR3- linked diabetes high risk genes may be Ir genes for endogenous antigens.

Acknowledgements

The authors wish to thank M. Wronski, W. Wiers, A. Köster, U. Hintzen and E. Lackmann for excellent technical assistance and A. Frankenstein for excellent typing of the manuscript

Reference

1. Keck, K.: Nature 254, 78-79 (1975).
2. Keck, K.: Eur. J. Immunol. 5, 801-807 (1975).
3. Bareinski, M.A., Rosenthal, A.S.: J. exp. Med. 145, 726-731 (1977).
4. Rosenthal, A.S.: Immunol. Rev. 40, 135-151 (1978).
5. Schroer, J.A., Inman, J.K., Thomas, J.W., Rosenthal, A.S.: J. Immunol. 123, 670-675 (1979).
6. Bertrams, J., Jansen, F.K., Grüneklee, D., Reis, H.E., Drost, H., Beyer, J., Gries, F.A., Kuwert, E.: Tissue Antigens 8, 13-19 (1976).
7. Ludwig, H., Schernthaner, G., Mayr, W.R., Willvonseder, R.: Diabetologia 12, 407 (1976).
8. Ludvigsson, J., Säfwenberg, J., Heding, L.G.: Diabetologia 13, 13-17 (1977).
9. Irvine, W.J., Di Mario, U., Feek, C.M., Ting, A., Morris, P.J., Gray, R.S., Duncan, J.P.: J. Clin. Labor. Immunol. 1, 111-114 (1978).
10. Svejgaard, A., Platz, P., Ryder, L.P.: Histocompatibility Testing 1980 (in press).
11. Ray, J.G., Hare, D.B., Pedersen, P.D., Mullally, D.I.: Manual of Tissue Typing Techniques, DHEW Publication No. (NIH) 76-545, 1976, pp. 22-24.
12. Singal, D.P., Naipaul, N., Hidalgo, R.: Manual of Tissue Typing Techniques, DHEW Publication No. (NIH) 76-545, 1976, pp. 107-109.
13. Kerp, L., Steinhilber, S., Kasemir,H.: Klin. Wschr. 44, 560-567 (1966).
14. Bertrams, J., Baur, M.P.: Tissue Antigens 14, 317-324 (1979).
15. Baur, M.P., Danilovs, J.A.: Histocompatibility Testing 1980 (in press).
16. Bertrams, J., Sodomann, P., Gries, F.A., Sachsse, B., Jahnke, K.: Dtsch. med. Wschr. 1980 (in press).
17. Rittner, Ch., Bertrams, J.: Hum. Genet. 1980 (in press).
18. Irvine, W.J., Di Mario, U., Feek, E.M., Gray, R.S., Ting, A., Morris, P.J., Duncan, L.G.P.: J. clin. Lab. Immunol. 1, 109-110 (1978).
19. Cudworth, A.G., Gamble, D.R., White, G.B.B., Lendrum, R., Woodrow, J.C., Bloom, A.: Lancet 1, 385-388 (1977).

INSULIN ANTIBODY FORMATION FOLLOWING CONVENTIONAL OR MONOCOMPONENT INSULIN TREATMENT IS INFLUENCED BY GENES OF THE HLA-DR LOCUS

G. Schernthaner

Department of Medicine II, University of Vienna, Ludwig Boltzmann Institute for Clinical Endocrinology, Vienna, Austria

W.R. Mayr

Institute for Blood Group Serology, University of Vienna, Vienna, Austria

Introduction

During the last 10 years it could be clearly shown, that antibody formation against insulin preparations depends on a variety of factors (table 1). In addition to species specificity, physical state (pH, solubility, Zn, retarding agents) and purity of insulin preparations, mechanisms inherent in the individual patient influencing insulin antibody formation have been suspected for a long time.

TABLE 1

FACTORS INFLUENCING INSULIN ANTIBODY FORMATION IN MAN

age
sex
pH
solubility and [Zn]
retarding agents
species specificity (beef, pork, human)
purity of insulin preparations
constitutional factors (Ir genes, HLA-DR)

In animal studies, evidence for the essential role of immune response (Ir) genes controlling humoral anti-insulin immunity has already been obtained (1,2). During the last 6 years, it could be shown that certain genes of the HLA complex (B8, B15, Cw3, DR3, DR4) increase the susceptibility (3-9) to juvenile-onset insulin-dependent diabetes mellitus (IDD) - now called

Basic and Clinical Aspects of Immunity to Insulin

type-I diabetes - and influence immune responsiveness. In this respect, it seems to be of special interest that type-I diabetes associated HLA antigens play a significant role in the humoral immune response to insulin. Four years ago, we were able to show (10) an influence of type-I diabetes associated HLA-B and C locus antigens on insulin antibody formation (figure 1). HLA-B7 and B8 frequencies were considerably higher in patients with low insulin-antibody titers following conventional insulin treatment for many years, whereas B15 and Cw3 were higher in patients with formation of high insulin-antibody titers. These preliminary data were confirmed by consecutive studies of our own group (11,12) and by three other groups (13-15).

IgG-Insulin-Binding Capacity (mU/mL)	No. of Patients	HLA B8		HLA BW15	HLA CW3	HLA B7	
Group 1: <0.05	9	3 (33)%		1 (11%)	3 (33%)	4 (44%)†‡	
Group 2: 0.06 - 3.0	38	21 (55%)	24 (51%)* (Groups 1 & 2)	8 (21%)	13 (34%)	3 (8%)†	
Group 3: >3.0	20	5 (25%)		6 (30%)	8 (40%)	3 (15%)†	6 (10%) (Groups 2 & 3)

*P<0.05 vs Group 3.

‡P<0.05 vs Groups 2 & 3.

†Heterogeneity within 3 groups, P<0.025.

FIGURE 1

ANTI-INSULIN IMMUNE RESPONSE AND HLA ANTIGENS IN 67 PATIENTS WITH JUVENILE-ONSET DIABETES (reproduced from Schernthaner at al. (10))

Further progress in HLA typing showed that type-I diabetes is primarily associated with HLA antigens of the D/DR locus (7-9,16) and that the previously described B and C loci associations are only secondary to the D/DR locus associations (figure 2).

FIGURE 2

HLA RISK-AXES WHICH CORRELATE WITH SUSCEPTIBILITY OR RESISTANCE TO THE DEVELOPMENT OF TYPE-I DIABETES

Risk of developing type-I diabetes	HLA genes
High	DR3/Dw3 —— B8 —— A1
High	DR4/Dw4 —— B15 — Cw3 —— A2
Low	DR2/Dw2 —— B7 —— A3

Therefore it seems to be of interest to study the influence of the HLA-DR status on insulin-antibody formation in type-I diabetics treated with either conventional or monocomponent (MC) insulin preparations.

Patients and methods

Determination of insulin antibodies and HLA-DR typing were performed in two groups of type-I diabetics. One group of patients was treated with conventional insulins over a relatively long period of time, whereas the other patients were on MC insulins from the onset of their disease and were followed up prospectively.
In all patients HLA-DR typing was performed by using the two colour-fluorescence technique described by van Rood et al. (17). In addition, HLA antigens of the A, B and C loci were determined by using the NIH-microlymphocytotoxicity technique in all patients. Insulin-antibodies were assayed by the method of Christiansen (18) employing immune-electrophoresis in agar-gel based on binding of ^{125}I ox insulin by serum IgG or IgM. Commercialy obtained (Behring-Werke, Marburg/Lahn) rabbit antibodies to human IgG or IgM (H-chain specific) were used. Monospecific reactivity of these antisera was tested by immunofluorescence on monoclonal bone marrow preparations (19). Nonspecific binding of insulin to IgG or IgM was less than 0.05 U/l in 75 non-diabetic subjects selected at random. ^{125}I ox insulin (20-25 U/l; SA = 20 mCi/mg) was supplied by the Novo Research Institute. The degree of metabolic control was evaluated by measuring the 24 hour-glucosuria and the concentrations of hemoglobin A1 by micro-column chromatography (20).

Results

Retrospective study (therapy with conventional insulins)

The IgG insulin-antibody titers and the clinical data of the 50 patients, who had used conventional insulins for a long time, are shown on table 2. The mean age at onset of the patients was 18.8 years, the mean duration of disease was 11.0 years. All patients were treated with long-acting insulins, namely Lente-Insulin from the Novo Company. In 39 diabetics, two daily doses were administered. No patient had received MC or RI (rare immunogenic) insulin before or at the time of the study. A significant insulin-antibody formation (insulin-binding capacity IBC > 0.05 U/l) was found in 45 (86%) out of the 50 IDD patients treated with conventional insulins. Patients were divided into four groups (table 2) according to the IBC: group I, non-responders (IBC < 0.05 U/l); group II, low-responders (IBC = 0.06 - 1.0 U/l); group III, moderate-responders (IBC = 1.01 - 3.0 U/l); and group IV, high-responders (IBC > 3.0 U/l).

TABLE 2

IgG INSULIN BINDING CAPACITY IN IDD PATIENTS (reproduced from Schernthaner et al. (12))

Group no.	IBC (U/liter)	No. of patients (%)	IBC (mean ± SEM)	Age at onset (yr; mean ± SEM)	Duration of disease (yr; mean ± SEM)	24-h Glucosuria (mean ± SEM)[a]
I	(Nonresponder) <0.05	7 (14)	0.02 ± 0.01	19.6 ± 3.3	10.1 ± 0.9	29.3 ± 6.4
II	(Low responder) 0.06–1.0	23 (46)	0.31 ± 0.04	17.6 ± 1.6	11.3 ± 1.8	33.2 ± 5.7
III	(Moderate responder) 1.01–3.0	7 (14)	1.82 ± 0.16	18.0 ± 3.3	11.6 ± 3.1	31.8 ± 7.8
IV	(High responder) >3.0	13 (26)	6.54 ± 0.86	21.1 ± 2.7	10.7 ± 4.2	35.2 ± 4.6

Insulin-dependent diabetics were treated with conventional insulins.
[a] Mean of 3 consecutive days.

The insulin dosage needed for adequate metabolic control (figure 3) was similar in groups I, II and III, however in patients with high IBC (> 3.0 U/l), insulin-requirement was significantly increased (IV vs. I, $p < 0.001$; IV vs. II, $p < 0.001$; IV vs. III, $p < 0.005$). Duration of disease, age at onset of diabetes manifestations, and mean 24 hour-glucosuria did not significantly differ among the four groups studied.

The insulin antibody titers according to the presence or absence of HLA-DR3 in type-I diabetics treated with conventional insulins are shown in figure 4. IgG insulin-antibody titers were significantly lower in DR3 positive compared to DR3 negative patients, yielding a mean of 0.74 U/l in DR3 positives and 2.24 U/l in DR3 negatives ($p < 0.02$). In this study (12), IgG insulin-antibody titers did not differ significantly between DR4 positive and DR4 negative patients; however, an accurate definition of this antigen was not available at that time.

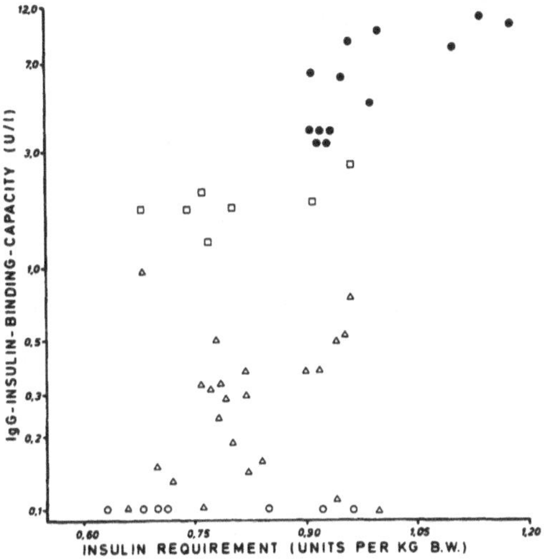

FIGURE 3

IgG IBC AND DAILY INSULIN REQUIREMENT (UNITS / kg BW).

○ diabetics without significant IBC (< 0.05 U/l): group I
△ diabetics with low IBC (0.06-1.0 U/l): group II
□ diabetics with moderate IBC (1.01-3.0 U/l): group III
● diabetics with high IBC (> 3.0 U/l): group IV

(reproduced from Schernthaner et al. (12))

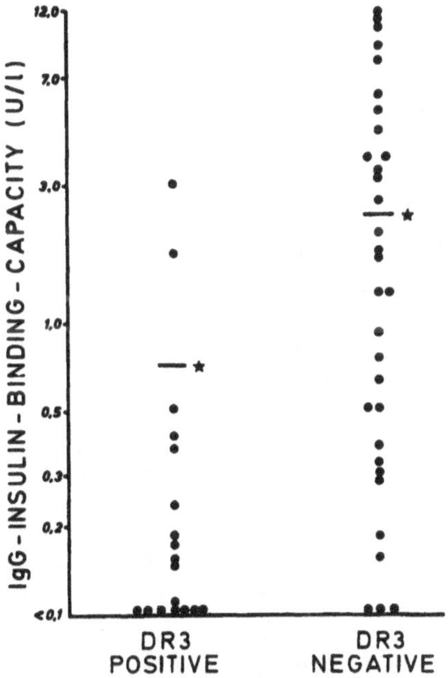

FIGURE 4

IgG INSULIN ANTIBODIES IN DR3 POSITIVE (n=18) AND DR3 NEGATIVE (n=32) INSULIN-DEPENDENT DIABETICS.

The mean values (★) are significantly different ($p < 0.02$)

(reproduced from Schernthaner et al. (12))

Prospective study (therapy with pork monocomponent insulins)

The clinical data of the 48 patients treated with MC insulins from the onset of their disease and followed up in two-monthly intervals are presented in table 3. In 9 of the 48 patients, IgM insulin-antibodies could be detected after 10 days of treatment (mean level in patients with detectable IgM insulin-antibodies: 0.17 ± 0.08 U/l). IgG insulin-antibodies in only low titers could be found in 14 of the 48 patients after treatment with Monotard MC and Actrapid MC insulins over a period of at least one year (mean level of patients with detectable IgG insulin-antibodies: 0.47 ± 0.23 U/l).

TABLE 3

CLINICAL AND IMMUNOLOGICAL DATA OF IDD PATIENTS TREATED WITH MONOCOMPONENT INSULIN PREPARATIONS

number of patients:	n = 48	
mean age at onset:	18.1 ± 3.1 years	
duration of treatment:	1.4 ± 0.4 years	
IgM insulin-antibodies:	9 /48	(0.17 ± 0.08 U/l)
IgG insulin-antibodies:	14/48	(0.47 ± 0.23 U/l)

The analysis of the HLA-DR antigen frequencies in diabetics with and without detectable IgM insulin-antibodies after 10 days of treatment is shown in table 4. There was no significant influence of HLA-DR3 or DR4 on the production of IgM insulin-antibodies. Remarkably, the incidence of DR3 was somewhat higher in the patients without IgM insulin-antibody formation after 10 days of insulin therapy.

TABLE 4

IgM INSULIN-ANTIBODY FORMATION AND HLA-DR ANTIGENS (DR3, DR4) IN TYPE-I DIABETICS TREATED WITH MONOCOMPONENT INSULINS (DURATION OF TREATMENT: 10 DAYS)

IgM insulin-antibodies	type-I diabetics n=48	DR3 positive n=23 (48%)	DR4 positive n=32 (67%)
Detectable (<0.05 U/l)	n= 9	n= 3 (33%)[a]	n= 7 (78%)[b]
Not detectable	n=39	n=20 (51%)[a]	n=25 (64%)[b]

a : n.s. b : n.s.

The analysis of DR3 or DR4 incidence in patients with IgG insulin-antibody formation in comparison with patients without IgG insulin-antibodies after at least one year of treatment with MC insulins is shown on figure 5. Patients with IgG insulin-antibody formation showed a high prevalence of DR4 and a relatively low frequency of DR3, whereas patients without insulin-antibody formation were in 56% HLA-DR3 positive. The degree of metabolic control (24 hour-glucosuria, HbA1) did not differ between patients with or without insulin antibodies.

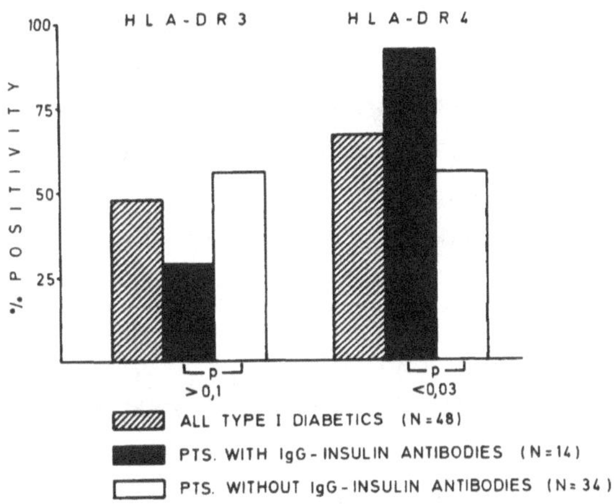

FIGURE 5

IgG INSULIN-ANTIBODY FORMATION AND HLA-DR ANTIGENS (DR3, DR4) IN TYPE-I DIABETICS TREATED WITH MONOCOMPONENT INSULINS (DURATION OF TREATMENT: 1.4 YEARS)

Discussion

Summarizing the present findings and the data reported in the literature (10-15), it seems now well established that HLA-DR associated factors indeed influence insulin-antibody formation in man. As demonstrated in table 5, there is a high degree of correspondence in the data published by various groups regarding insulin-antibody formation and HLA suggesting the existence of at least two immune response risk-axes influencing insulin-antibody formation. HLA-DR4-B15-Cw3 positive patients respond with relatively high insulin-antibody titers following heterologous insulin administration, whereas insulin-antibody production is relatively low in DR3 positive diabetics. This is also true for those patients who from the onset of their disease were treated exclusively with MC insulin. Interestingly, those HLA-DR antigens not associated with type-I diabetes do not influence the humoral responsiveness against heterologous insulin. An influence of the patients age on the extent of insulin-antibody production has been reported in previous investigations (21-23). Andersen et al. (21) showed that insulin-antibody formation declines with increasing age in patients treated with porcine isophane insulin. Akerblom et al. (22,23) reported a high incidence of insulin-antibody production to highly purified insulins in diabetic children in contrast to previous experience in adult IDD patients. Recently, it has been observed that DR4 shows a significantly higher frequency in patients with onset of disease before 15 years of age compared to diabetics with a later onset (16). It might well be, that the high prevalence of DR4 in IDD patients with early onset of disease is the explanation, at least partially, for the increased susceptibility of children in producing insulin-antibodies to highly purified preparations.

TABLE 5

HLA AND INSULIN-ANTIBODY FORMATION (COMPARISON OF DATA REPORTED BY VARIOUS GROUPS)

	Non/low responder		High responder		
Schernthaner et al. (10)	B7↑	B8↑	B8↓	B15↑(?)	Cw3↑(?)
Bertrams et al. (13)		B8↑	B7↑	B15↑	
Ludvigsson et al. (14)	B7↑			B15↑	
Irvine et al. (15)		B8↑		B15↑	Cw3↑
Schernthaner et al. (12) *and present findings		DR3↑		DR4↑*	

The existence of an influence of type-I diabetes associated HLA antigens on the immune response in insulin-dependent diabetics is supported by various data (table 6). DR3-B8 positive patients, low insulin-antibody responders, show a persistent antibody formation against antigens of the Langerhans' islets (24,25). In addition, formation of circulating immune-complexes seems to be increased in those patients (26,27). On the other hand, the risk-axis DR4-B15-Cw3 has no influence on islet-cell antibody persistence or on circulating immune-complex production. Antibody formation against another exogeneous antigen, namely Coxsackie B4 virus, seems to be increased in the DR4-B15 positive IDD patients as reported by Cudworth et al. (28).

TABLE 6

IMMUNE RESPONSE, CLINICAL FINDINGS AND HLA IN IDD

Parameters	HLA-DR3-B8	HLA-DR4-B15-Cw3
Insulin-antibody formation	decreased	increased
Islet-cell antibodies	persistent	transient
Immune-complex formation	associated	not associated
Viral antibody formation	?	increased ?
Residual B-cell function (duration <5 years)	increased	decreased
Proliferative retinopathy	decreased	increased

There are conflicting data concerning the clinical importance of antibodies to insulin and other substances in commercial insulin preparations (12,29,30). Certain data support the possibility that insulin antibodies do reduce by some mechanism the secretion or effect of endogenous insulin (31). For instance, in type-I diabetes, increased serum titers of antibodies to insulin have been reported to be associated with unmeasurable fasting concentrations of human C-peptide, suggesting a significant influence of the insulin-antibody on B-cell function (31). A prospective study (32) regarding residual B-cell function and HLA-DR status in type-I diabetics with recent onset of disease supports the observations of Ludvigsson et al. (31). DR3 positive patients, low insulin-antibody responders, showed considerable amounts of endogenous insulin secretion following carbohydrate intake, whereas DR4 positive diabetics, high insulin-antibody responders, presented with low C-peptide levels after a mean diabetes duration of 3.2 years (32). In a study of insulin treated diabetics, there was no correlation between metabolic control and association constants of high and low affinity antibodies, total insulin-antibody titer, or IBC (33). At the present time we do not know whether insulin-antibodies play any role in the outcome or progression of late diabetes manifestations. The data available to clarify this important question are extremely limited and do not allow a conclusive answer at this time.

Irrespective of these considerations it seems to be of interest that there are some reports in the literature indicating that proliferative retinopathy occurs with increased frequency in DR4-B15 (32,34-37) positive diabetic patients, who are also high insulin-antibody responders. Incidence of the severe form of retinopathy is decreased in patients with DR3-B8 (32,35,38) or DR2-B7 (36), patients, who respond with low antibody titers against heterologous insulin. Although it might be possible that these two findings are only coincidental and independent of each other, a relationship not known at this time cannot be excluded with absolute certainty.

In further studies, patients followed up over many years starting with the onset of the disease and treatment should be checked for HLA-DR type insulin-antibody formation, circulating immune-complexes and degree of microvessel disease. Because of many unanswered questions, a double-blind clinical study has been started in order to ascertain the importance of insulin purity and species source concerning the complications of insulin therapy including immunogenicity, preservation of B-cell function and plasma glucose (30). Finally, a group of patients treated from the onset of disease with human insulin - most likely available in the near future - should also be included in these considerations.

References

1. Keck, K.: Nature 254, 78 (1975).
2. Kapp, J.A., Strayer, D.S.: J. Immunol. 121, 978 (1978).
3. Nerup, J., Platz, P., Andersen, O.O., Christy, M., Lyngsøe, J., Poulsen, J.E., Ryder, L.P., Thomsen, M., Staub Nielsen, L., Svejgaard, A.: Lancet 2, 864 (1974).
4. Cudworth, A.G., Woodrow, J.C.: Brit. Med. J. 3, 133 (1975).
5. Schernthaner, G., Mayr, W.R., Pacher, M., Ludwig, H., Erd, W., Eibl, M.: Horm. Metab. Res. 7, 521 (1975).
6. Thomsen, M., Platz, P., Andersen, O.O., Christy, M., Lyngsøe, L., Nerup, J., Rasmussen, S.K., Ryder, L.P., Staub Nielsen, L., Svejgaard, A.: Transplant. Rev. 22, 148 (1975).

7. Schernthaner, G., Ludwig, H., Mayr, W.R.: Lancet 2, 1128 (1977).

8. Mayr, W.R., Ludwig, H., Schernthaner, G., Bartova, A., Menzel, G.R., Richter, K.V., Ceppellini, R.: In Histocompatibility Testing 1977, Bodmer, W.F., Batchelor, J.R., Bodmer, J.G., Festenstein, H., Morris, P.J., eds., Munksgaard, Copenhagen, p. 391 (1978).

9. Deschamps, I., Lestradet, H., Bonaiti, C., Schmid, M., Busson, M., Benajam, A., Marcelli-Barge, A., Hors, J.: Diabetologia 19, 189 (1980).

10. Schernthaner, G., Ludwig, H., Mayr, W.R., Willvonseder, R.: New Engl. J. Med. 295, 622 (1976).

11. Schernthaner, G., Ludwig, H., Mayr, W.R., Frisch, H.: Diab. Metab. 3, 117 (1977).

12. Schernthaner, G., Ludwig, H., Mayr, W.R.: J. Clin. Endocrin. Metab. 48, 403 (1979).

13. Bertrams, J., Jansen, F.K., Grüneklee, D., Reis, H.E., Drost, H., Beyer, J., Gries, F.A., Kuwert, E.: Tissue Antigens 8, 13 (1976).

14. Ludvigsson, J., Safvenberg, J., Heding, L.G.: Diabetologia 13, 13 (1977).

15. Irvine, W.J., DiMario, U., Feek, C.M., Ting, A., Morris, P.J., Gray, R. S., Dunçan, L.J.P.: J. Clin. Lab. Immunol. 1, 111 (1978).

16. Svejgaard, A., Platz, P., Ryder, L.P.: Insulin-dependent diabetes mellitus. In Histocompatibility Testing 1980, Terasaki, P.I., ed., UCLA, Los Angeles, in press (1980).

17. Rood, J.J.v., Leeuwen, A.v., Ploem, J.S.: Nature 262, 795 (1976).

18. Christiansen, A.H.: Horm. Metab. Res. 5, 147 (1973).

19. Hijmans, W., Schuit, H.R.E., Hulsing-Hesselingk, E.: Ann.N.Y.Acad.Sci. 177, 290 (1971).

20. Welch, S.G., Boucher, B.J.: Diabetologia 14, 209 (1978).

21. Andersen, O.O., Brunfelt, K., Abildgaard, F.: Acta Endocrinol. 69, 195 (1972).

22. Akerblom, H.K., Mäkelä, A.L.: Acta Paed. Scand. 270, 69 (1977).

23. Akerblom, H.K., Mäkelä, A.L., Käär, M.L.: Diabetologia 19, 252 (1980).

24. Irvine, W.J., McCallum, C.J., Gray, R.S., Campbell, C.J., Duncan, L. J.P., Farquhar, J.W., Vaughan, H., Morris, P.J.: Diabetes 26, 138 (1977).

25. Ludwig, H., Schernthaner, G., Mayr, W.R.: Metabolism 28, 797 (1979).

26. Ludwig, H., Schernthaner, G., Tappeiner, G., Mayr, W.R., Freyler, H.: Circulating Immune Complexes in Insulin-Dependent Diabetes Mellitus: Analysis According to Incidence of Islet-Cell Antibodies, Insulin-Antibodies, HLA Antigens, Duration of Disease and Stages of Diabetic Retinopathy. In Autoimmune Aspects of Endocrine Disorders, Pinchera, A., Doniach, D., Fenzi, G.F., Baschieri, L., eds., Academic Press, London, in press (1980).

27. Schernthaner, G.: Wien. klin. Wschr. 92, Suppl. 114 (1980).

28. Cudworth, A.G., Gamble, D.R., White, G.B.B., Lendrum, R., Woodrow, J.C., Bloom, A.: Lancet 1, 385 (1977).

29. Kurtz, A.B., Nabarro, J.D.N.: Diabetologia 19, 329 (1980).

30. Galloway, J.A.: Diabetes Care 3, 615 (1980).

31. Ludvigsson, J., Heding, L.G.: Diabetologia 12, 627 (1976).

32. Schernthaner, G., Heding, L.G., Freyler, H., Mayr, W.R., Tappeiner, G.: Diabetologia 18, 313 (1980).

33. Gonen, B., Goldmann, J., Baldwin, D., Goldberg, R.B., Ryan, W.G., Blix, P.M., Schanzlin, D., Fritz, K.J., Rubenstein, A.H.: Diabetes 28, 749 (1979).

34. Cudworth, A.G., Festenstein, H.: Brit. Med. Bull. 34, 285 (1978).

35. Deckert, T., Egeberg, J., Frimodt-Møller, C., Sanders, E., Svejgaard, A.: Diabetologia 17, 91 (1979).

36. Barbosa, J., Ramsay, R.C., Knobloch, W.H., Cantrill, H.L., Noreen, H., King, R., Yunis, E.: Am. J. Ophthalm. 90, 148 (1980).

37. Bertrams, J., Dewald, G., Spitznas, M., Rittner, C.: HLA-A,B,C,DR,Bf and C2 Alleles in Insulin Dependent Diabetes Mellitus with Proliferative Retinopathy. Immunobiology, in press (1980).

38. Becker, B., Shin, D.H., Burgess, D., Kilo, C., Miller, W.W.: Diabetes 26, 997 (1977).

A STUDY OF HLA ALLOANTIGEN FREQUENCIES IN INSULIN ALLERGIC AND NON-ALLERGIC DIABETICS

D.L. Mann, A.S. Rosenthal, R. Kahn

National Cancer Institute, National Institute of Allergy and Infectious Diseases, and National Institute of Arthritis, Metabolism and Digestive Diseases, National Institutes of Health, Bethesda, MD 20205

A.H. Johnson and N. Mendell

Division of Immunology, Duke University School of Medicine, Durham, NC 27710

Introduction

The immunologic response to insulin has been clearly demonstrated to be under Ir gene control in both mice and guinea pigs (1, 2). These genes map within the major histocompatibility complex of these two species. There is inferential evidence that immune response genes map in the major histocompatibility complex of man. This complex controls the expression of the HLA-A, B, C, and DRw alloantigens which can be detected on peripheral blood lymphocytes or subpopulations thereof. The major histocompatibility antigens in man and mouse are analogous in many respects. This is particularly true of the human DRw antigens and murine Ia antigens where serologic crossreactions have been observed (3). It has been clearly demonstrated that immune response genes, that is, the capability to mount a particular response to an antigen, in mice maps to those regions controlling the expression of the Ia antigens (4).

Basic and Clinical Aspects of Immunity to Insulin

Insulin is an immunogen that is given to humans as a therapeutic modality. Some diabetic patients receiving insulin develop adverse immunologic reactions to the insulin or insulin components. A study was undertaken to examine the nature of the immunologic response to insulin or insulin components in man and to attempt to correlate these responses to the presence or absence of certain HLA alloantigenic determinants and thus attempt to identify immune response genes in man. One hundred sixteen patients with a history of allergic reactions to insulin and 94 patients with no demonstrable allergic reactions were studied by a variety of parameters. The subject of this report is the documentation of the altered HLA alloantigenic frequencies in these two patient groups.

Methods and Materials

The patient groups as well as a control population were typed for 17 alloantigens controlled by the A locus, 31 alloantigens controlled by the B locus, 6 alloantigens controlled by the C locus, and 9 alloantigens controlled by the DRw locus. The typing was performed by the standard microcytotoxicity technique as modified by Amos (5). The DRw alloantigens were determined by the assessment of cytotoxic reactions of alloantisera detecting the DRw specificities, as defined by the 7th International Histocompatibility Workshop. The B cells were isolated by a technique described by Mann et al. Individual alloantigen frequencies were determined in each group and compared for significant differences by Chi-square analysis using the Fisher exact test (two-tailed) with the Yates correction. There was a total of 87 females and 29 males in the allergic diabetic patient population studied. Ninety-one of the patients were Caucasians and 25 were Blacks. The age range of the patients studied was 13-75 years. These patients were studied in response to intradermal skin tests, serum anti-insulin antibodies, and lymphocyte proliferation tests to insulin and insulin components. Of the total of 94 patients with diabetes who had no history or clinical manifestations of allergies, 64 were Caucasians and 30 were Blacks. The age distribution of onset of insulin was similar to that of the allergic patient population.

Results

In the assessment of the frequencies of the HLA alloantigens at the HLA-A, HLA-B, and HLA-C loci, no significant differences were noted between the normal and total diabetic populations studied. Two differences in frequencies that reached a significance level of $p < 0.05$ were DRw1, which occurred in 22% of the diabetic population and in 8% of the normal population studied. A decrease in DRw6 was noted in that this antigen occurred in 15% of the diabetic population and in 27% of the normal population. In comparing HLA alloantigen frequencies in the insulin allergic diabetic population, the non-allergic diabetic population and the normal population, certain antigens at all four loci were noted to be different in frequency. These results are shown in Table I. They represent the data pooled from both races. In the insulin allergic population, HLA-Aw24, Cw1, and DRw6 antigens decreased significantly compared to the normal population. In comparing the non-allergic population to the normal group, DRw6 and 7 again appeared to be decreased in frequency while DRw1 was increased. HLA-Aw24, Cw1, Cw6, and Bw6 were found less frequently in the insulin allergic population compared to in the non-allergic group. HLA-Bw44 was the only antigen that was increased in frequency in this population. Thus, the most remarkable finding was a generalized decrease in the frequencies of certain HLA alloantigens in the allergic diabetic population as compared to the non-allergic group and the normals.

TABLE I

ALTERED HLA ALLOANTIGEN FREQUENCY IN INSULIN ALLERGIC AND NON-ALLERGIC DIABETICS

HLA Alloantigen	Normal	Allergic	Non-allergic
	(75)[a]	(116)	(94)
Aw24	15[b]	4*f	13
Bw44	23	29f	16
Bw6	78	66f	82
Cw6	12	5ff	22
Cw1	9	2*f	10
DRw1	8	19	25**
DRw6	29	16*	10*
DRw7	27	29	11*
DRw9	7	3	0

(a) Total number of individuals in each group
(b) Results expressed as percent; races pooled
* Frequency difference from normal: $p < 0.05$
** Frequency difference from normal: $p < 0.01$
f Frequency difference from non-allergic diabetics: $p < 0.05$
ff Frequency difference from non-allergic diabetics: $p < 0.01$

A comparison was made of the frequencies of HLA alloantigens based on race. Significant differences were noted between the frequencies of certain of the HLA alloantigens. These differences in frequency were based entirely on race and were not reflected at all in the disease state. Thus, analysis of the data could be carried out using Caucasians and Blacks.

The lack of striking differences in frequencies of the HLA antigenic determinants in these populations led us to further analysis of the data. There is a well-known observation that certain of the HLA alloantigens appear in linkage disequilibrium, that is, certain of the antigens controlled by the different loci appear to occur together more frequently than one would expect based on random distribution of these antigens in the normal population. Table II details the results of analysis of the data wherein the association of antigens controlled by the different loci were found together at significance levels of $p \leq 0.001$. Certain of the HLA alloantigens appear to be associated in all groups. These associations reflect the associations generally seen in the normal population as established by other studies. The results of this analysis revealed new antigen associations in the non-allergic diabetic population and the allergic diabetic population which were exclusive to that population. These results suggest the possibility that certain combinations of antigens are contributory

TABLE II

OBSERVED HLA LOCUS DISEQUILIBRIA* IN NORMAL, INSULIN ALLERGIC AND NON-ALLERGIC DIABETICS

All Groups	Normal	Diabetics	Insulin Allergic Diabetics
A1, B8	Aw30, Bw45	Aw34, Bw52	Aw28, B14
B15, Cw3	Aw36, Bw42	A29, Bw49	Aw30, B18
Bw35, Cw4	A29, B12	Aw24, B37	A19, Bw4
Bw44, Cw5	A19, B12	B8, Cx	A3, B7
Bw40, Cw3	A11, Bw35	Bw21, Cw4	Aw33, Bw15a
B7, DRw2	Bw22, Cw3	B45, DRw8	A2, Bw44
B8, DRw3	B13, Cw6	B14, DRw8	Bw44, DRw7
	B40, DRw8		Bw15b, DRw1
	Bw4, DRw7		
	B13, DRw7		
	B17, DRw7		

* Associations of antigens of different HLA loci, to the significance level $p \leq 0.001$

to the disease state and to the manifestation of allergy to insulin or insulin components.

Another method of analysis is to examine the frequency of antigens that are controlled by genes at the same locus appearing together. These allelic antigens would be expected to have a negative correlation. All combinations of antigens were analyzed, and the most significant changes in correlations were observed with the DRw antigens. These results are shown in Table III. The only significant positive association was found with DRw5 and DRw6 in the allergic population. Thus, certain combinations of DRw antigens appeared in both the insulin allergic and the non-allergic population which tended to differ

TABLE III

CORRELATION OF DRw ANTIGENS IN NORMAL, INSULIN ALLERGIC AND NON-ALLERGIC DIABETICS

DRw	Normal	Insulin Allergic	Non-allergic
	(75)	(113)	(81)
DRw1 with DRw3	-0.04	-0.20*	-0.17
DRw2 with DRw3	-0.02	-0.23**	-0.33**
DRw2 with DRw4	-0.18	-0.31*	-0.24
DRw3 with DRw6	-0.18	-0.09*ff	-0.24
DRw4 with DRw7	-0.02	-0.21*	-0.22*
DRw5 with DRw6	-0.06	+0.21**ff	-0.14
DRw5 with DRw7	-0.17	-0.20f	-0.04
DRw6 with DRw7	-0.26	-0.21f	-0.06*

$p < 0.05$ level of significant difference in allergic and/or non-allergic vs. normal

** $p < 0.01$ level of significant difference in allergic and/or non-allergic vs. normal

f $p < 0.05$ level of significant difference in allergic vs. non-allergic

ff $p < 0.01$ level of significant difference in allergic vs. non-allergic between the two groups as well as between either of the two groups and the normal population.

The observation that certain of the antigens controlled by the A locus were associated more often with the B locus and that certain B locus antigens were associated with DRw antigens led to a further analysis of the data obtained from HLA typing of these individuals. The association of HLA-A2, Bw44 and Bw44, DRw7 suggested that this total combination of antigens might differ significantly in the insulin allergic diabetic population compared to the non-allergic diabetics. The frequency of these antigen combinations was determined and is shown in Table IV.

In the insulin allergic population, Bw44 was associated with A2 and/or DRw7 in all of those individuals where it was detected. In the normal population, these associations were less frequent and, in the non-allergic population, essentially absent, save for the 3% association of A2--Bw44. Thus, it appears that combinations of these antigens add a significant risk in the development of allergic reactions to insulin in the diabetic population.

TABLE IV

ASSOCIATION OF HLA-A2, Bw44, AND DRw7 IN NORMAL, INSULIN ALLERGIC AND NON-ALLERGIC DIABETICS

HLA Alloantigen Combination	Normal	% in Non-allergic	Allergic
A2--Bw44	8	3	14
Bw44--DRw7	5	0	11
A2--Bw44--DRw7	5	0	5
A2---------DRw7[(a)]	5	0	9

(a) Analysis includes any B locus antigen other than Bw44

Discussion

The study of the associations of HLA alloantigens with allergic responses to insulin components seemed to us to be a logical approach to the exploration or examination of the association of the human major histocompatibility complex with the specific immune response. The small differences in amino acid composition between the most commonly used insulins, beef, pork and human insulins, provide the basis for assessment of immune response to a limited immunogen.

The data detailed above indicated that the specific HLA alloantigens were not associated with the disease state itself. Since the population of diabetics contained both the juvenile onset and maturity onset diabetics, this in a sense is not surprising. It has been previously reported that DRw2 is decreased and DRw3 and 4 are elevated in the juvenile onset group (7, 8). This was not reflected in the total patient population studied. There were no striking differences in the frequencies of individual antigens comparing the insulin allergic population to the non-allergic diabetics. The alterations that were observed were mainly a decrease in the frequency of particular HLA alloantigens in the insulin allergic population compared to the normal and non-allergic diabetics. It is difficult to ascribe any particular correlation of immunologic function to the decrease of antigenic determinants controlled by the human MHC. The results suggest that combinations of antigens may be more important than individual alloantigenic determinants. This was indeed found when we examined combinations of antigens controlled by genes at the different loci and also combinations of antigens which are allelic, that is, controlled by the same locus. These associations were more pronounced in the DRw locus. This might be expected since this is the portion of the major histocompatibility complex where one might expect control of the immune response to be specifically determined. The changes in the observed HLA locus equilibria in the three populations also suggested that the overall allergic response requires more than one particular gene and thus a combination of genetic factors in order for allergic phenomena to be manifest. The contention is supported by the observation that three of the HLA alloantigens (or combinations thereof), HLA-A2, Bw44, and DRw7, appeared more frequently in the insulin allergic groups than in the non-allergic diabetics. One might predict that in any individual who has combinations of HLA-A2--Bw44 or Bw44--DRw7, has diabetes and is receiving insulin, the chances of developing some type of an allergic reaction to the insulin or insulin components would be far greater than having one of these antigenic determinants. Further analysis of these data is underway in an attempt to determine the relationship of combinations of HLA alloantigens to specific immunologic response (i.e., cutaneous reactions, lymphocyte proliferation, antibody production) to beef and pork insulin, proinsulin and protamine.

In summary, the alteration of frequencies of individual HLA alloantigens in insulin allergic and non-allergic diabetic populations appears to not differ to any great extent from normals or from the frequency of these antigens in the two disease groups. However, the association of particular antigens in the total disease group and in the diabetic populations with allergic manifestations to insulin or insulin components appears to be quite significant. Thus, the immune response in man to insulin or insulin components appears to be quite complicated. It may be difficult to dissect or determine the nature of specific immune response genes in man where many portions of the major histocompatibility complex may attenuate or augment a particular type of immune response and thus a clinical allergic manifestation.

References

1. Keck, K.: Nature (Lond.) 254, 78-79 (1975).
2. Barcinski, M.A., Rosenthal, A.S.: J. Exp. Med. 145, 726-742 (1977).
3. Lunney, J.K., Mann, D.L., Sachs, D.H.: Scand. J. Immunol. 10, 403 (1979).
4. Shreffler, D.C., David, C.: Adv. Immunol. 20, 125-195 (1975).
5. Amos, D.B., Pool, P., In Manual of Clinical Immunology. N.R. Rose and H. Friedman, editors. American Society for Microbiology, Washington, D.C., p 797 (1976).
6. Mann, D.L., Abelson, L., Henkart, P., Harris, S., Amos, D.B., In Histocompatibility Testing, 1975. Kissmeyer-Nielsen, editor. Munksgaard, Copenhagen, pp 705-707 (1975).
7. Salow, H., Hidalgo, R., Singal, D.D.: Diabetes 28, 1-4 (1978).
8. Ilonen, J., Herva, E., Tiilikainen, A.: Tissue Antigens 11, 144-146 (1978).

MORPHOLOGIC CHANGES IN PANCREAS ISLETS AFTER ACTIVE OR PASSIVE IMMUNIZATION AGAINST INSULIN. A REVIEW 1)

G. Freytag 2)
Pathologisches Institut der Universität Münster
Westring 17, D-4400 Münster (F.R.G.)

In diabetes research particular interest has been focused on the morphology of islet changes induced by insulin antibodies on account of their analogy to the early manifestations of type I human diabetes (1).

A. Active Immunization

Active immunization of guinea pigs against bovine or porcine insulin leads to the production of very high titers of insulin-precipitating antibodies (Fig.1).

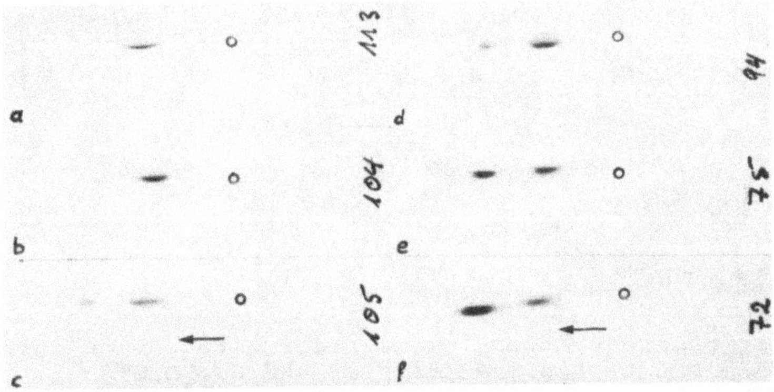

Fig.1: Immune electrophoresis, guinea pig serum against bovine insulin. 2 precipitation lines a) after 2 weeks, f) after 16 weeks of immunization.

---

1) Supported by Sonderforschungsbereich 113, Düsseldorf

2) Dedicated to Prof.Dr.Gerhard Seifert /Hamburg in honour of his 60th birthday.

1 ml of guine pig serum can precipitate 10 to 16 insulin units. The animals will not become diabetic although the insulin antibodies produced have been shown to bind endogenous guinea pig insulin in vivo. Long-term immunization regularly leads to islet hyperplasia and the appearance of the so-called mini islets (Fig.2). An increase in the α : ß cell ratio is also frequently observed. Intraperitoneal injection of 100 U insulin, well tolerated by hyperimmunized guinea pigs, results in extreme degranulation of ß cells. Inflammatory reactions, however, will not develop in the islet areas of these guinea pigs.

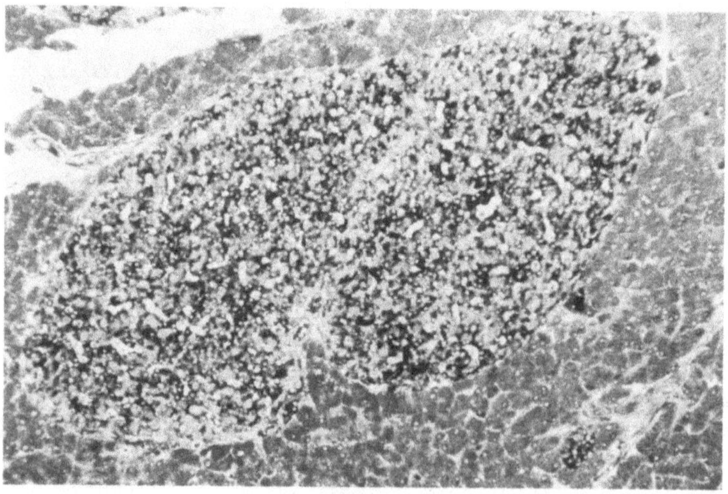

Fig.2: Guinea pig pancreas after immunization with bovine insulin (6 months). Result of i.p.injection of 100 U : Degranulated ß cells in hyperplastic islet. "Mini islet" in right bottom (Aldehyd fuchsin, x 150)

In contrast, lymphoid cellular infiltration of the islets of Langerhans after immunization against insulin, was observed in cattle (2) and, later, in sheep (3) and rabbits (4). Fig.3 shows a typical immune insultis of lymphoidcellular type in a rabbit's pancreas following immunization with bovine insulin and Freund's adjuvant.

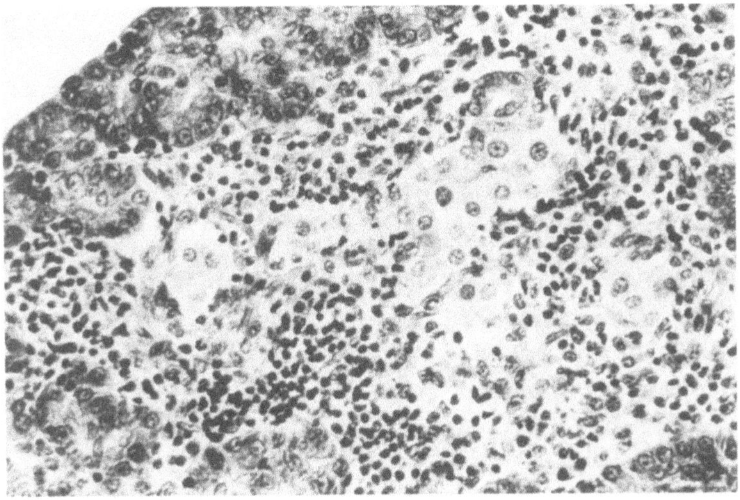

Fig.3a: Rabbit pancreas after weekly immunization with insulin (4th week). Marked round cell infiltration of islets.(PAS,x 500)

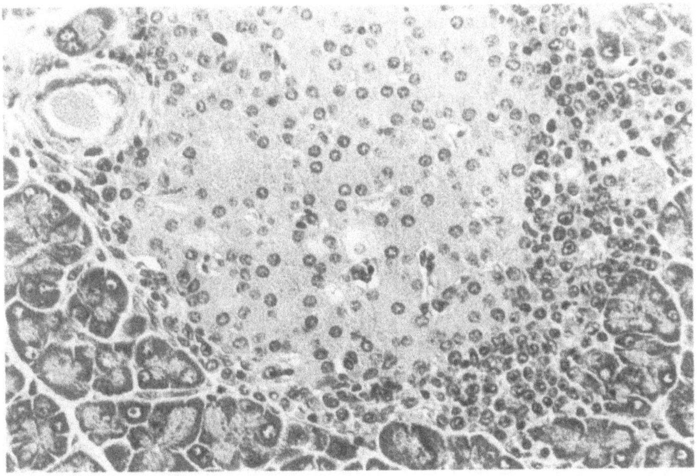

Fig.3b: Pancreas of NMRI mouse after immunization with bovine insulin (12 weeks): slight periinsular round cell infiltration (HE, x 500)

Immune insulitis can be induced only in rabbits of the New Zealand white strain, but not in outbred black NMRI rabbits. Lymphocytic infiltration into rabbit islets was called "insulitis" in analogy to v.MEYENBURG's (5) description of similar morphologic changes seen in diabetics dying shortly after the onset of the disease (6).

The occurrence of insulitis after immunization with insulin suggested that autoaggressive immune processes might be involved in the pathogenesis of human diabetes mellitus. We therefore studied the effect of different immunization protocols on the development of insulin-induced insulitis, and the eventual onset of diabetes. 6 groups of 10 - 13 rabbits were immunized with insulin (10-20 mg/kg), various adjuvants (either complete or incomplete) over different periods of time (4-16 weeks), and with different numbers of insulin injections (for detail see (7).

The strongest expression of insulitis with marked destruction of the islets, was found after 4 weeks irrespective of the mode of immunization. Two animals with severe insulitis developed manifest diabetes mellitus during the fourth week. The mode and duration of immunization did affect, however, the remission of insulitis in these animals: Insulitis was still found after 16 weeks in 60% of those rabbits that received 16 consecutive injections at weekly intervals, in 40% of those that were immunized 7 times at irregular intervals, and in 10% of the animals that were given only 4 consecutive injections at the beginning of the assay.

So far, we have been unable to identify a mouse strain that would develop insulitis in consequence of active immunization against insulin, to the same extent as do the white NZ rabbits. Fig.4 summarizes the results of an experimental assay with 96 NMRI mice receiving bovine insulin at different dosage (1-100 µg/kg) over 12 weeks. Injections were given 3 times a week. One half of the animals received insulin alone, the other Insulin together with Freund's adjuvant. In the animals treated with insulin alone, insulitis is an extremely rare finding. In those treated with insulin-plus adjuvant, insulitis would occasionally occur in both groups. One pathological effect of the insulin antibodies seen in all the mice, was the degranulation of ß cells, resulting in an increasing number of islets

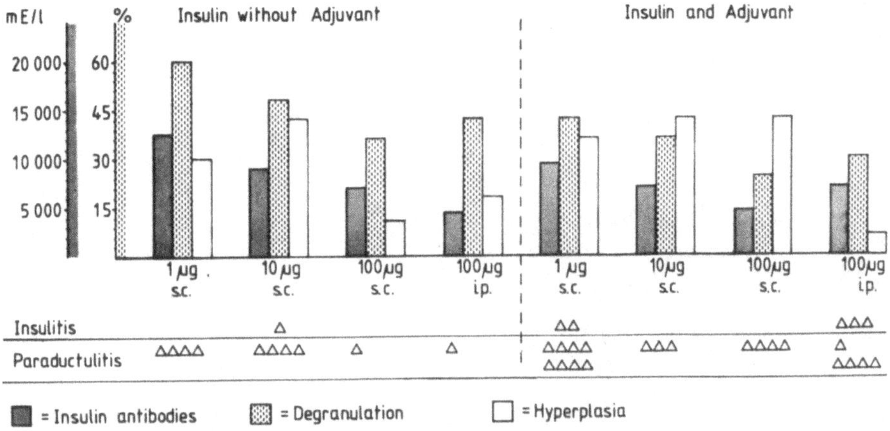

Fig.4: Synopsis of findings in NMRI mice after immunization with bovine insulin.

with oversized diameters. A criterium for islet hyperplasia was the presence of at least 25% enlarged cells with a diameter over 300 µ. ß cell degranulation as well as islet hyperplasia reflect an increased secretory activity of islet cells. NMRI mice with insulitis show fewer lymphocytic infiltrations than did the rabbits of the previous assay. Insulitis in mice is slight, but distinct, there were some 10 - 15 lymphoid or mononuclear cells to be found around each islet or within its periphery (Fig.3b).

Surprising findings were recorded in the pancreas of NMRI mice which, after active immunization with bovine insulin alone at different doses for 12 weeks (single doses ranging from 1 ng to 100 µg), had received two injections of 100 µg Insulin plus Freund's adjuvant. A marked insulitis was observed in these animals (Fig.5). With a dosage of 1 ng to 10 ng of Insulin, 7 out of 13 animals (54%) were positive. Using monocomponent insulin for immunization, insulitis was observed in the high dose range (1 µg, 10 µg, and 100 µg). Correlations between the antibody titer and the appearance of insulitis were individually

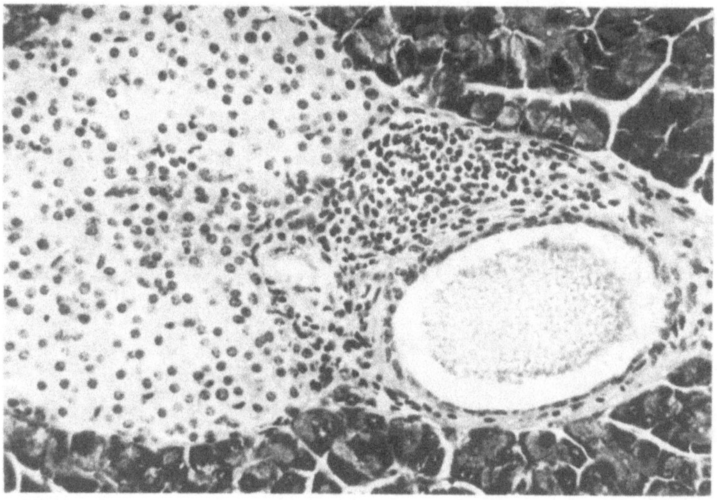

Fig.5: Pancreas of NMRI mouse after second booster injection of 100 μ insulin + adjuvant, 20 weeks aftér preimmunization: Marked parainsular and paraductular infiltration (PAS, x 300)

calculated in 37 animals after the second test immunization,revealing a complete lack of correlation, in contrast to the positive results described in sheep regarding the correlation of antibody titers and insulitis (3). (For details see 8)

B. Transfer of Insulin Antibodies

The passive transfer of antibody leads to an acute type of insulitis in mice and rats (9). Polymorphonuclear cells, especially eosinophilic granulocytes, migrate intro intra- and periinsular spaces (Fig.6a), an inflammatory reaction that depends on the presence of precipitated immune complexes in the islet. Acute insulitis is therefore thought to be an immune reaction of intermediate type (1). Focal islet necrosis (Fig.6b) is rarely induced by high concentrations of antiporcine insulin, and so the full development of a passively induced Arthus phenomenon (10) is an equally exceptional result. Antigen-antibody complexes were not observed at venule walls in the pattern

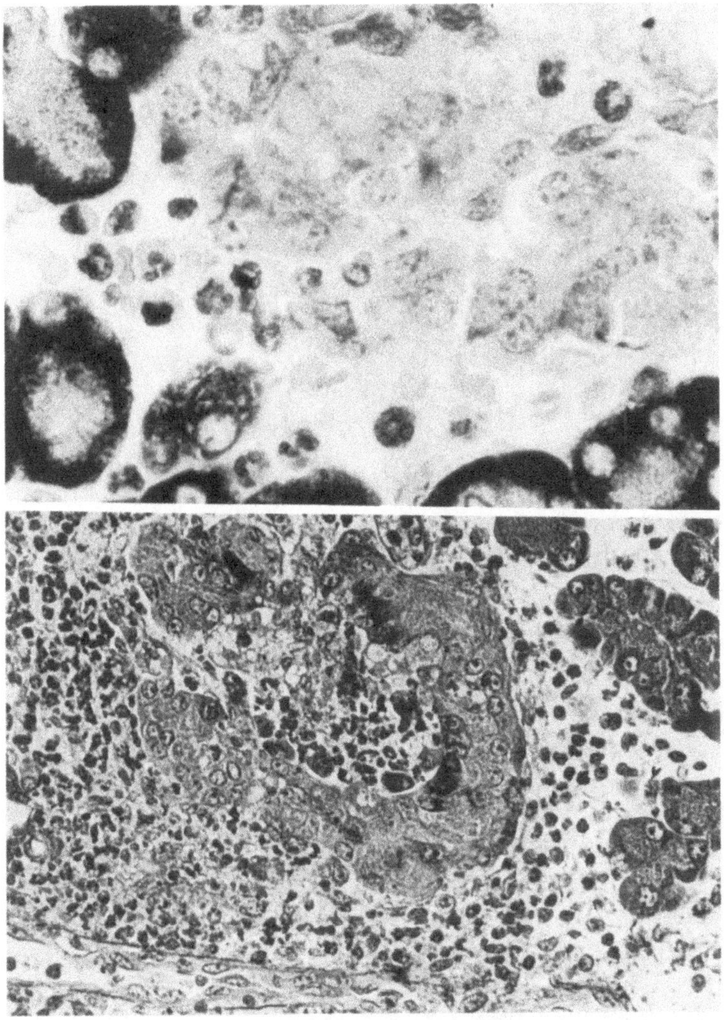

Fig.6: Mouse pancreas 48 hrs after transfer of g.p. anti-insulin serum. a) "Acute insulitis": polymorphonuclear granulocytes infiltrating the islet (Giemsa,x 1200). b) Focal islet necrosis and polymorphocellular infiltration (Ald.-fuchsin,x 600)

typical of the classical Arthus phenomenon.

Repeated injections of antibodies are paralleled by reiterated rises of blood sugar, but no permanent diabetic change was observed. Histologically, a chronic type of insulitis develops (11). Infiltration is mainly seen between smaller veins and the

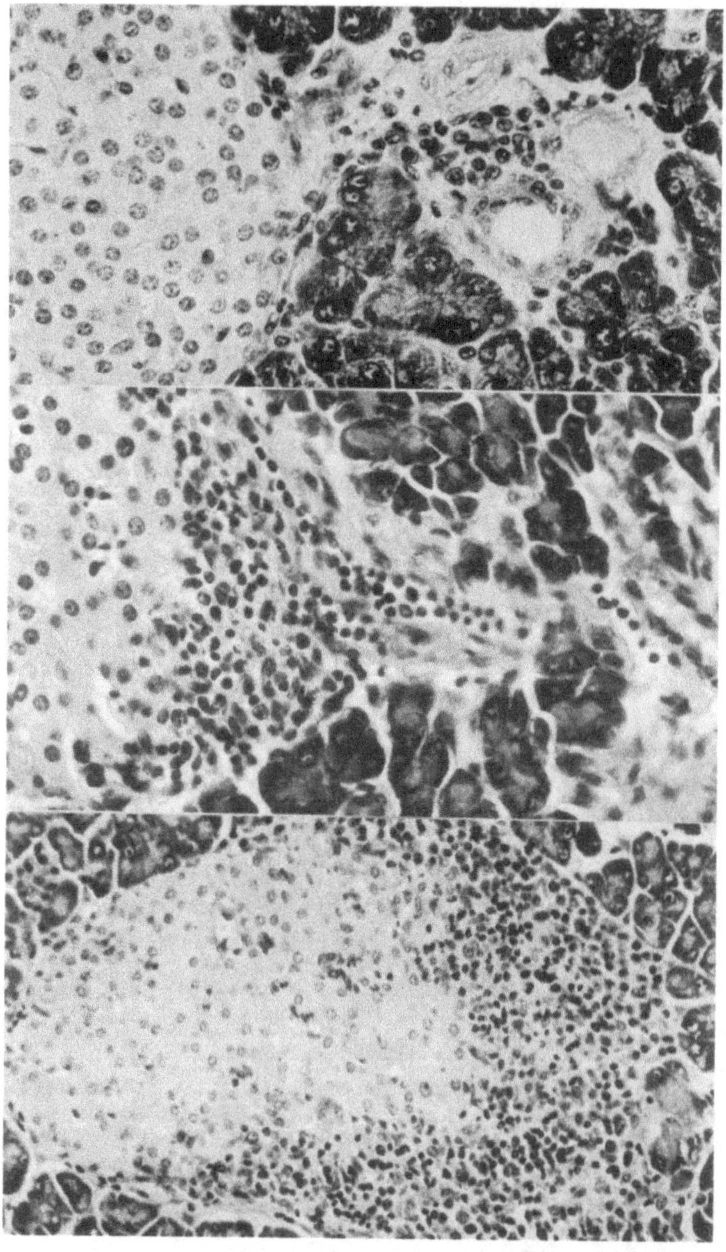

Fig.7: Mouse islets after repeated injection (once daily) of g.p. anti-insulin serum (1-6 weeks) resulting in "chronic insulitis": Infiltration front developing at the ductular pole of the islet (HE, x 500 in a + b, x 300 in c).

adjacent islets (Fig.7a). After the fourth day the infiltrate may increase extending well into the islet area (Fig.7b). Sometimes a typical crescent shape is observed (Fig.7c). Cytologically, large immunoblastic cells with pyroninophilic nucleolus predominate within the infiltrate, leucocytes are less frequent (Fig. 8a).

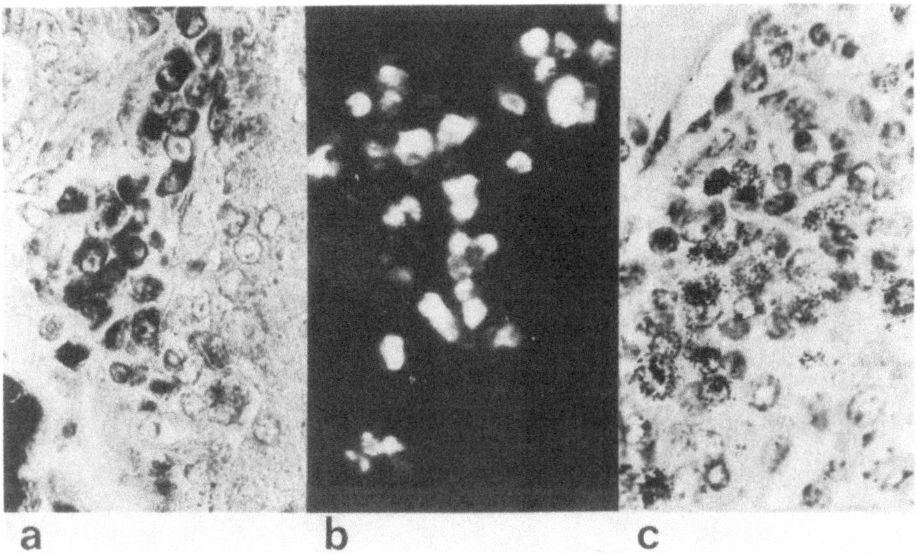

Fig.8: Mouse islet in chronic insulitis. Cytologic characterization of infiltrating blast cells: a) Strong protein synthesis with pyroninophilic nucleoli (Giemsa, x 1200). b) Production of anti-guinea pig serum antibodies (Immunofluorescence, slide coated with labeled g.p. serum). c) Strong mitotic activity (^{3}H thymidine autoradiography).

The intense proliferative activity of these mononucleate cells can be demonstrated autoradiographically: After injection of tritiated thymidine, most of the mononucleat cells were found to incorporate the radioactive aminoacid, thus indicating a high mitotic activity of these immunoblastic cells (Fig.8b). Studies with fluorescine-labeled g.p. gammaglobuline show fluorescence over several infiltrating cells, probably plasma cells, a finding suggestive of cellular immune reaction against foreign (i.e. guinea pig) protein (Fig.8c).

We recently studied the responsiveness of inbred mouse strains against anti-insulin serum (12). The results on table 1 show strain differences in the ability to develop insulitis. Development of chronic insulitis was observed in 55% of DBA/2 mice and in 26% of C57BL/6 mice, and in 38% of BALB/c mice.

Table 1

Mouse Strain	Insulitis Day 15	Insulitis Day 25	Control NaCl Insulitis Day 25	Control G.P.Serum Insulitis Day 25
BALB/c	- -	10/26 (38%)	0/12	1/12
C57Bl/6	- -	6/23 (26%)	1/11	1/11
DBA/2	0/8	6/11 (55%)	1/11	1/ 9

According to the immune histochemical findings mentioned (see Fig. 8 c) we tried to enhance the pathogenic effect of passive insulin antibody transfers by preimmunizing the recipient mice with normal g.p. serum (13).

C. Preimmunization

The experiment was carried out with 50 adult NMRI mice. All the animals were immunized against guinea pig serum prior to the start of the main assay, by 3 injections of g.p.serum plus complete Freund's adjuvant at weekly intervals. 40 of these preimmunized mice were then injected i.p. at 12 hrs intervals either with g.p.antibovine insulin serum, or with its lyophilized globulin fraction. The assay lasted 8 days, then the animals were killed successively at different intervals from their respective last antibody injections.

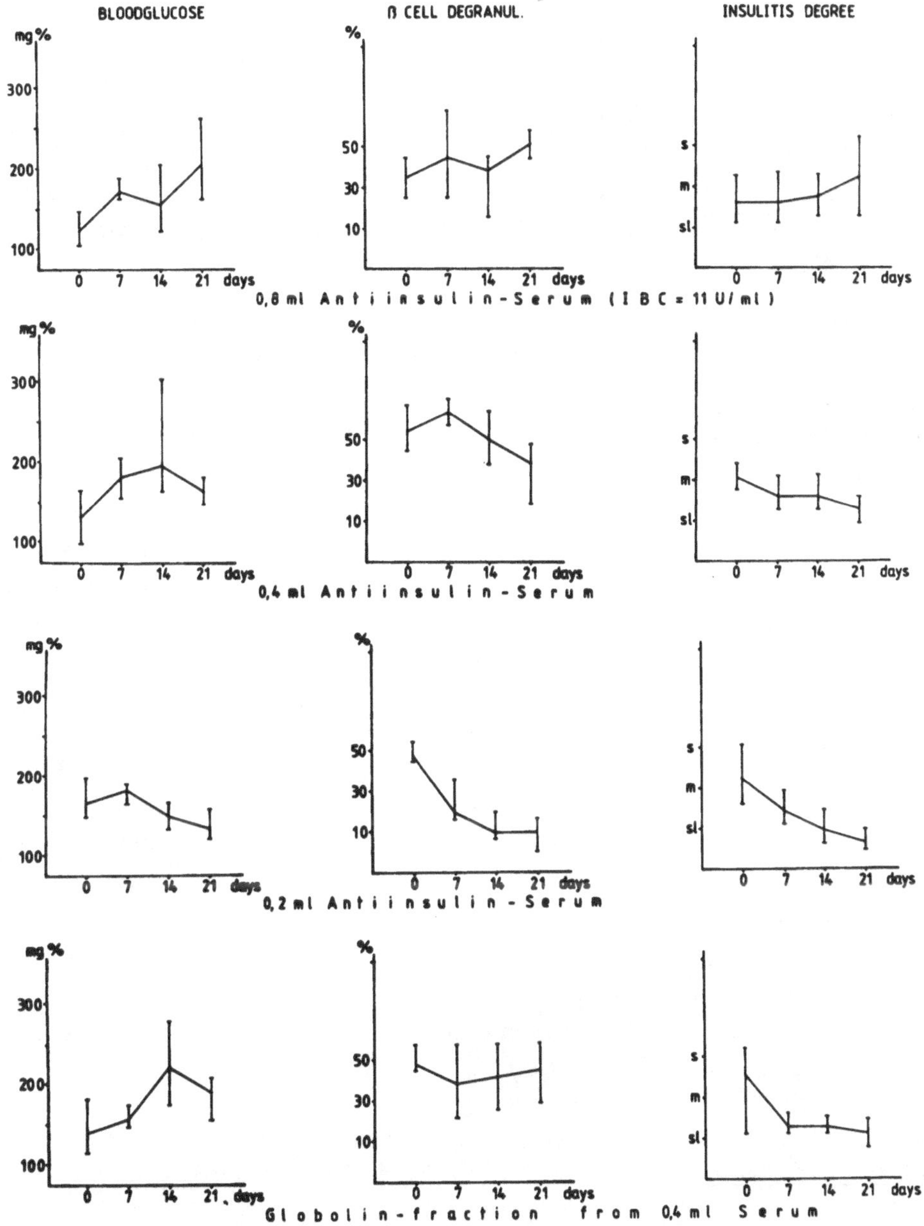

Fig.9: Synopsis of findings in preimmunized NMRI mice after repeated injection of different amounts of guinea pig anti-insulin serum.

Results

Of 15 mice killed immediately after the end of the assay, 13 showed medium to severe "insulitis" with intra- and periinsular infiltration of lymphocytes, monocytes and plasma cells. ß cells were degranulated to between 10 and 50%. At this stage the pathologic changes are very similar to those found in non-preimmunized animals.

The effect of preimmunization is manifested during the following weeks: Symptoms of inflammation in the islets of Langerhans regress like they do in non-preimmunized animals, but insulitis is found to persist (Fig.9). Chronic insulitis was most impressive in the animals treated with 0.8 ml antibovine insulin serum, which all showed florid insulitis 2 weeks after passive immunization with marked degranulation of ß cells and blood sugar levels between 100 and 200 mg/dl. Three weeks after immunization insulitis is still prominent with a 40-50% degranulation of ß cells and blood sugar levels of 150-200 mg/dl.

The enhancing effect of preimmunization is reflected in the fact that severe acute inflammatory immune response is provoked by even minimal doses of anti-insulin serum. The group treated with 0.2 ml antiserum showed moderate to severe inflammatory reactions and strong degranulation of ß cells immediately after the stop of administration, but the lower dose is unable to induce chronic persistent inflammation. One week after passive immunization insulitis is found in merely a few animals, and by this time degranulation of ß cells is again near normal, blood sugar levels around 150 mg/dl.

D. Immunization against in vivo Islet Cell Fragment

Our observation of passive rather than active immunization against insulin leading to severe pathologic changes in mouse islets, suggests that the chronic type of insulitis in NMRI mice must result from a combined action of repeated islet cell damage by antigen-antibody complexes, and a subsequent lymphoproliferative process induced by immunogenic islet cell fragments. NERUP et al.(14) had shown that insulitis can be induced by immunizing mice against lyophilized calf islet tissue in complete Freund's adjuvant. They had observed mononuclear cell infiltration - especially with lymphocytes - 7 days later in most of the islets. This inflammatory infiltration was markedly regressed after a further 10 days. In a similar experimental study with rats (15), destruction of islet tissue with severe fibrosis was recorded 3 months later. In recent studies on the same topic (16, 17) we tried to induce the cellular response against islets by destroying a certain portion of islet cell tissue, thus liberating some immunogenic islet cell fragments.

140 adult male white NMRI mice (group I) were immunized at weekly intervals with 0.5 ml g.p. serum plus 0.5 ml complete Freund's adjuvant injected s.c. into the back skin. One week after the third injection of foreign protein the animals were given one i.v. injection of Alloxan monohydrate into the caudal vein (75 mg/kg in aqu.sol.). These Alloxan injections were immediately followed by another s.c. application of Freund's adjuvant plus g.p. serum. One half of the mice in this group (Ib) were given a second i.v. injection of Alloxan 5 weeks later, again combined with s.c. application of Freund's adjuvant plus g.p. serum. 80 non-preimmunized mice received the same Alloxan injection (group II), of which 10 got also the second Alloxan dose 5 weeks later (group II b). 30 mice preimmunized like those of group I were left without Alloxan administration to serve as controls (group III).

Results

Under the experimental conditions chosen, a dose of 75 mg/kg produced not more than a low toxic effect. Only 60% of the non-immunized mice developed diabetes; preimmunized animals seemed to be more sensitive showing increased blood sugar levels in 80% of cases. On the other hand, the diabetic condition induced by Alloxan returns to normal more rapidly in preimmunized animals than in the non-immunized group II (Fig. 10).

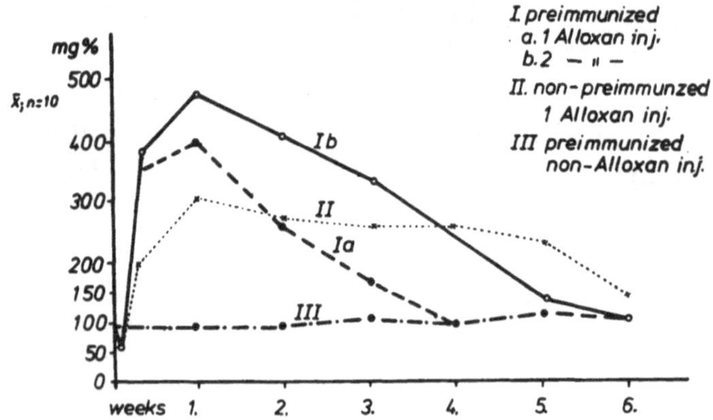

Fig. 10: Blood glucose after Alloxan administration

The second injection of Alloxan provoked rising mean values in the preimmunized mice of group Ib, as compared to animals receiving only one application. Blood glucose levels failed to normalize for as long as 6 weeks in some cases. Maximum values were again found at 600 mg/dl. The non-immunized animals of group II show no essential difference in their blood glucose reactions to the first and second Alloxan application.

48 hrs after Alloxan treatment, islets in non-immunized animals are frequently seen with complete necrosis of ß cells, while α cells are preserved and clearly outlined against the necrotic tissue. ß cell necroses seem to remain non-reactive. In preimmunized mice the islets of Langerhans show different behaviour: 24 hrs after the injection of Alloxan we see a massive, diffuse infiltration of granulocytes (Fig.11a). Another striking contrast to non-immunized animals is the increasing evidence of

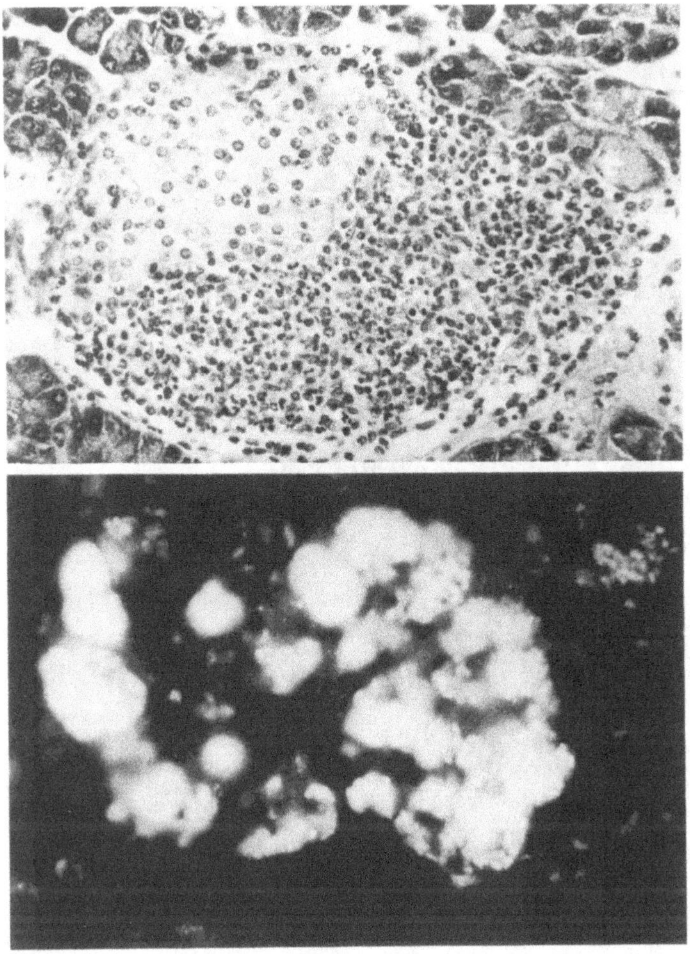

Fig. 11: Pancreas islet of preimmunized NMRI mouse, 48 hrs after Alloxan injection. a) ß cell necrosis and marked leucocytic infiltration (Giemsa, x 300). b) C_3C_4 complement cluster. Immunofluorescene slide coated with antiC_3C_4-globuline (rabbit)

complement factors. Massive accumulation of C_3 and C_4 can be demonstrated in inflamed islets by immunohistochemical methods (Fig. 11b) After the second Alloxan injection the necrotic area is infiltrated not only by granulocytes, but also by numerous monocytes (Fig. 12a). Lymphocytes are seen to immigrate somewhat later while granulocytes disappear.Unlike the pattern observed

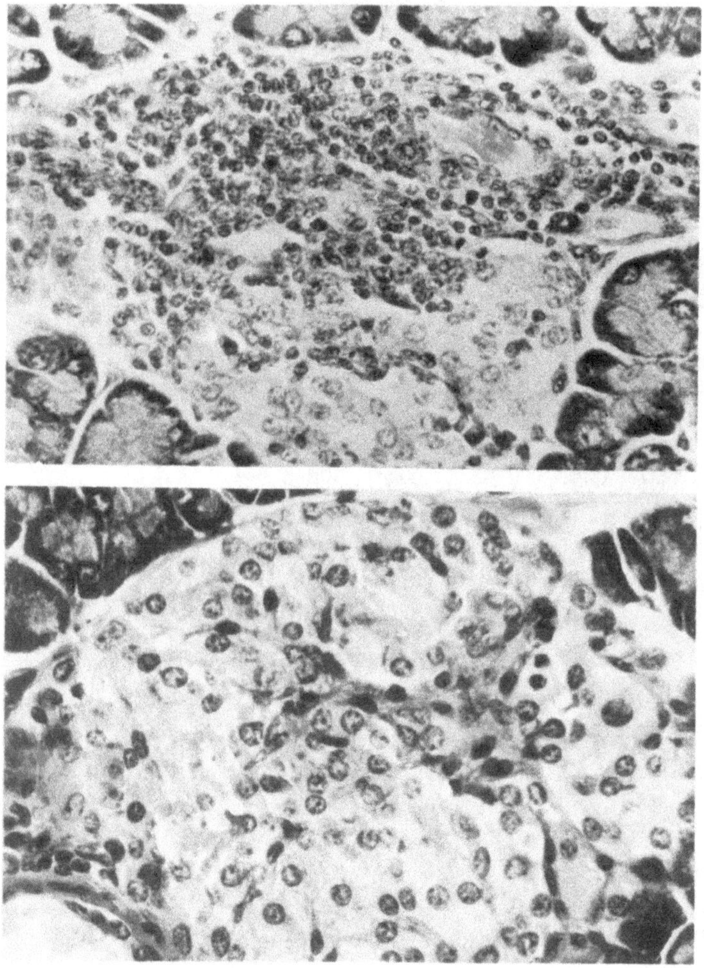

Fig.12: Pancreas islets of preimmunized NMRI mouse 6 weeks after the second Alloxan injection. a) Para- and intrainsular infiltration of round cells (Giemsa, x 300). b) Proliferating sinus endothelial cells (PAS, x 300).

after a single injection, the lympho-monocytic infiltration persists beyond the seventh day and remains visible as late as 2 weeks after the second injection (Fig.12b). Cellular infiltration is paralleled by activation of sinus endothelial cells with proliferation of endothelial cells and nuclear swelling.

At later stages lympho-monocytic cells are predominantly found in the islet periphery and near the vascular pole in parainsular and paraductular arrangement.

The final stage of chronic progressive insulitis following the second Alloxan injection in preimmunized animals, is characterized by fibrosis and hyalinization of islets. Aldehyd fuchsin staining reveals ß cells with either severe degranulation or, occasionally, with hypergranulation and transfixed secretion. Another interesting feature is found 3 weeks after the second injection: insulin antibody-producing plasma cells within the parapancreatic lymph nodes, predominantly in the medullar area.

Summary and Conclusion

Active immunization of experimental animals with heterologous insulin will provoke morphologic changes in the islets of Langerhans reflecting the functional enhancement and eventual exhaustion of ß cell activity. Besides islet hyperplasia, degranulation of ß cells and an altered ratio of α/ß cells are regular findings after long-term immunization of guinea pigs and mice. Chronic progressive and aggressive insulitis cannot be experimentally induced by repeated injection of insulin alone. Transient intrainsular infiltration in white NZ rabbits, or parainsular infiltration in NMRI mice, are only induced by concomitant unspecific activation of the cellular immune response by application of adjuvant. Chronic insulitis is induced in mice by passive transfer of anti-insulin serum which may eventually result in complete destruction of Langerhans' islets. Changes like those observed in the initial phase of human diabetes type I, are reproduced experimentally not by active immunization against insulin, but rather by direct damaging of ß cells with concomitant activation of the cellular immune response. Accordingly, the induction of chronic progressive insulitis is possible by passive transfer of guinea pig insulin antibodies as well as by repeated administration of Alloxan to preimmunized mice. Experimental investigations have shown that chronic progressive insulitis is enhanced and prolonged rather by the effect of an autoimmune process induced by ß cell fragments, than by immunization against molecular insulin. Our review may further illustrate the role of adjuvants or other manipulations of the immune responsiveness in the development of "insulitis", a role which certainly deserves stronger consideration in the evaluation of experimental models.

References

1. Freytag,G.: Experimentelle Immunpathologie des Pankreas nach Einwirkung von Insulin-Antikörpern. Habilitationsschrift Hamburg 1969
2. Renold, A.E., Soeldner,J.S., Steinke,J.: Ciba Found. Coll.Endocrinol. 15, 122-134 (1964)
3. Federlin,K.: Immunopathology of Insulin. Clinical and Experimental Studies. Mongr.Endocrinol.Vol.6. Springer, Berlin-Hedielberg-New York 1971
4. Toreson,W.E., Lee,J.C., Grodsky,G.M.: Amer.J.Pathol. 52, 1099-1115 (1968)
5. v.Meyenburg,H.: Schweiz.med.Wochenschr. 70, 554-557 (1940)
6. Gepts,W.: Diabetes 14, 619-633 (1965)
7. Klöppel,G., Altenähr,E., Freytag,G., Jansen,F.K.: Virchows Arch.A path.Anat. 364, 333-346 (1974)
8. Jansen,F.K., Freytag,G.: Diabetologia 9, 191-196 (1973)
9 Lacy,P.E., Wright,P.H.: Diabetes 14, 634-642 (1965)
10. Cochrane,L.G., Weigle,W.D., Dixon,F.J.: J.exp.Med. 110, 481-494 (1959)
11. Freytag,G., Klöppel,G., Howe,I.: Verh.dtsch.Ges.Path. 53, 423-429 (1969)
12. Wrede,G., Freytag,G., Kiesel,U., Kolb,H.: unpublished results (1979)
13. Lange,R., Freytag,G.: Unpublished results (1976)
14. Nerup,J., Andersen,O.O., Bendixen,G., Egberg,J., Gunnarson, R., Kromann,H., Poulsen,J.E.: Horm.Metab,Res, 6, 173-175 (1974)
15. Heydinger,D.K., Lacy,P.E.: Diabetes 23, 579-582
16. Freytag,G.: Verh.dtsch.Ges.Path. 61, 339+ (1977)
17. Freytag,G., Kiesel,U.: Diabetologia 13, 394+ (1977)

THE ROLE OF AUTOIMMUNE PROCESSES IN THE DEVELOPMENT OF INSULIN-DEPENDENT DIABETES MELLITUS IN MICE TREATED WITH STREPTOZOTOCIN

S. Shin[1], S.-G. Paik[1] and N. Fleischer[2]

Departments of [1]Genetics and [2]Medicine, and Diabetes Research and Training Center, Albert Einstein College of Medicine
Bronx, New York 10461, U.S.A.

Introduction

The acute, juvenile-onset, insulin-dependent (Type I) diabetes mellitus has clinical and epidemiological manifestations that are quite different from those of the maturity-onset (Type II) diabetes, and most certainly represents a genetically distinct disease. Increasing evidence, both clinical and experimental, suggests that the development of the former is mediated by autoimmune processes.

Pancreatic islets of children with newly-diagnosed insulin-dependent diabetes frequently contain infiltrating mononuclear lymphocytes, exhibiting what is commonly referred to as "insulitis" (1). Many juvenile diabetics have circulating antibodies against the islet cells (2), as well as lymphocytes with cytolytic activity against human insulinoma cells in culture (3). Epidemiologic studies in several countries have independently established that a number of alleles of the HLA gene complex, especially of the HLA-D locus, are associated with a significantly elevated risk to Type I diabetes (reviewed in 4). These observations together indicate that some form of immunological mechanisms may play a role in the etiology of the disease.

Experimental evidence in support of this view comes from several laboratories. In a series of experiments, Like and Rossini and their coworkers demonstrated that the induction of insulin-dependent diabetes in mice and rats by the beta-cell toxin, streptozotocin, typically proceeds in two quite different pathways (5). When a single, sublethal, high dose is given

Basic and Clinical Aspects of Immunity to Insulin

to susceptible animals, rapid destruction of the islet beta-cells ensues, followed almost immediately by a profound and permanent hyperglycemia. On the other hand, when the same total dose of streptozotocin is given as five small daily doses, insulitis associated with the induction of type C viruses in the beta-cells develops, followed by a delayed but progressive hyperglycemia (5). Furthermore, both the insulitis and the subsequent development of hyperglycemia are prevented by rabbit antisera directed against mouse lymphocytes (6). Similarly, rabbit antiserum against rat lymphocytes can prevent the development of spontaneous insulin-dependent diabetes which occurs with a high frequency in the non-obese BB/W rats (7).

The involvement of the host immunological mechanisms in the development of insulin-dependent diabetes is supported also by the work of Buschard and Rygaard (8), who reported that the injection of multiple low doses of streptozotocin, which was shown earlier to induce hyperglycemia in immunocompetent mice (5), was without effect in the athymic nude (nu/nu) mouse. In addition, certain viruses known to induce the diabetic syndrome in various inbred strains of mice, such as the M-strain of encephalomyocarditis virus (EMC) (9), could not induce hyperglycemia in BALB/c nude mice as readily as they could in euthymic heterozygous (+/nu) BALB/c mice (10). Most provocative in this regard was their report that human peripheral blood lymphocytes obtained from newly-diagnosed juvenile diabetics were sometimes able to induce hyperglycemia in nude mice (11). Although preliminary in nature, these observations appeared to imply that the induction of experimental diabetes in mice is critically mediated by autoreactive immune lymphocytes that recognize the pancreatic beta-cells in an organ-specific, species-nonspecific manner. Unfortunately, however, subsequent efforts in a number of laboratories failed to confirm the reports of Buschard and his collaborators (12-15).

The possibility that viral infection may be one of the primary causes of juvenile-onset diabetes in humans has been considered widely (16, 17). In a well-known recent report, it was shown that a strain of Coxsackie B virus isolated from the pancreas of an acutely-ill diabetic child can induce insulin-dependent diabetes when injected into mice (18). However, all of the viruses implicated in diabetogenesis are widespread in human populations and only a small fraction of those who become infected with any one of them will actually develop diabetes. In fact, a recent survey concluded that an acute infection with Coxsackie B4 virus does not normally lead to the development of Type I diabetes (19). There is as yet no direct proof that, even in those who have developed diabetes after a known infection by one of the viruses, the virus was indeed the direct cause of the disease.

An attractive hypothesis consistent with the clinical and experimental observations summarized above is the following: Regardless of what the primary initiating event may be (virus infection, subclinical chemical insult, etc.), the immediate etiologic antecedent of insulin-dependent diabetes is the generation of autoreactive lymphocytes directed against the pancreatic beta-cells. Severe insulin deficiency, according to this hypothesis, is a result of the subsequent destruction of the majority of the beta-cells by the activated immunocytes. This notion assumes that the antigenic determinants recognized by the autosensitized immune lymphocytes (most probably T-cells) are localized at the islet beta-cells and shared in different species.

Our studies to be described in this paper were carried out to test this hypothesis. We investigated the experimental parameters needed for the induction of insulin-dependent diabetes in normal and congenitally athymic (nude) BALB/c mice following treatment with streptozotocin. More specifically, we sought to reexamine critically the role of thymus-dependent immunity in the induction process. Some of these results have been reported previously (20, 21).

Results

Induction of Persistent Hyperglycemia with Streptozotocin. Phenotypically normal heterozygous (+/nu) euthymic mice and their homozygous mutant (nu/nu) athymic littermates of BALB/c background were injected with streptozotocin (Sigma; mixed anomers) immediately after dissolving the toxin in sterile citrate buffer, pH 4.5, according to the procedure described by Like and Rossini (5). The development of hyperglycemia was then monitored by following the changes in plasma glucose levels (21). Results are summarized in Table 1.

Table 1. Induction of Hyperglycemia with Streptozotocin in BALB/c Mice

Genotype of mice	Treatment with streptozotocin	Sex	% Incidence of hyperglycemia §		Mean plasma glucose level (mg/100 ml) ψ	
+/nu	None (buffer alone)	M	0	(0/8)	156 ± 14	(n=8)ξ
		F	0	(0/15)	156 ± 23	(n=15)ξ
	Single high dose (200 mg/kg b.w.)	M	100	(13/13)	517 ± 86	(n=12)ϕ
		F	77	(10/13)	474 ± 159	(n=8)ϕ
	Multiple low doses (5 x 40 mg/kg b.w.)	M	100	(18/18)	502 ± 172	(n=17)ϕ
		F	15	(2/13)	(229, 480)θ	
nu/nu	None (buffer alone)	M	0	(0/9)	167 ± 28	(n=9)ξ
		F	0	(0/11)	155 ± 21	(n=11)ξ
	Single high dose (200 mg/kg b.w.)	M	91	(10/11)	554 ± 131	(n=10)ϕ
		F	73	(8/11)	515 ± 194	(n=8)ϕ
	Multiple low doses (5 x 40 mg/kg b.w.)	M	17	(3/18)	(235, 244, 248)θ	
		F	7	(1/14)	(267)θ	

Males (M) and females (F) of heterozygous normal (+/nu) or homozygous mutant nude (nu/nu) mice were injected i.p. with streptozotocin, and the plasma glucose level of each mouse was determined twice weekly thereafter for 4 weeks. Control mice were injected with the diluant only.

§ Cumulative incidence of hyperglycemia, as of 28 days after the last injection of streptozotocin. For the present study, mice with glucose values above 220 mg/100 ml (normal mean + 2 S.D.) were considered to be hyperglycemic. (No. of hyperglycemic mice/No. of treated mice)

ψ Non-fasting plasma glucose level, 21 days after the last injection, mean ± S.D. (n: No. of mice surviving on day 21, from which the glucose values were obtained)

ξ These values represent the normal non-fasting glucose levels of the control groups not treated with streptozotocin.

ϕ Mean glucose value of the hyperglycemic mice surviving on day 21.

θ Glucose values of individual hyperglycemic mice.

The injection of a single high dose of streptozotocin (200 mg/kg body weight) induced severe hyperglycemia in both +/nu and nu/nu mice. Elevated glucose levels were apparent in mice receiving this dose within 2 days after the injection, and persisted until the mice died or until the experiment was terminated 60 days later. Female mice were markedly less susceptible compared to males; whereas 100% of the male mice of either genotype developed hyperglycemia, 23% of +/nu females and 27% of nu/nu females did not develop hyperglycemia at all (see Table 1).

In contrast, the induction of hyperglycemia in mice injected with multiple low doses of streptozotocin (40 mg/kg body weight/day for 5 consecutive days) was strikingly different between the +/nu and nu/nu genotypes, especially in male mice. The majority of +/nu males developed pronounced hyperglycemia by the 7th day after the last injection; eventually, by the 3rd week, 100% of these mice became hyperglycemic. However, very few nu/nu males treated identically developed hyperglycemia; the cumulative incidence of hyperglycemia on 28 days after the last injection was only 17%. Even in those nude males that were classified as hyperglycemic in this group, the plasma glucose levels were only minimally higher than the pretreatment level; almost none reached the extremely high glucose values observed in the +/nu males treated identically (see Table 1). Once again, female mice of either genotype were markedly less susceptible to the diabetogenic effects of streptozotocin. This phenomenon will be discussed later.

Streptozotocin-Induced Hyperglycemia is Insulin-Dependent. The severe hyperglycemia induced in mice by streptozotocin, either with the single high dose or with the multiple low dose schedule, is a result of insulin insufficiency. We demonstrated this first by directly measuring the plasma insulin levels of hyperglycemic mice by radioimmunoassay. The results showed that in both groups of mice, elevated plasma glucose levels were always associated with decreased plasma insulin levels (Fig. 1).

More direct evidence for the insulin dependence was obtained in moribund hyperglycemic nude mice implanted with a hamster insulinoma, which had been shown previously to maintain its insulin-producing capacity through serial transplantations in nude mice (22). Representative results of this experiment are summarized in Fig. 2. One group of the diabetic mice died shortly after the transplantation, before the hamster tumor growth was apparent, presumably due to the severe hyperglycemia. In another group, in which palpable tumor nodules developed and continued to grow in size, the plasma glucose levels gradually decreased and finally returned to the normal range as the insulin-secreting tumors grew; eventually, these once hyperglycemic mice became hypoglycemic. These observations clearly show that the hyperglycemia induced by streptozotocin can be corrected by the heterologous insulin produced by the transplanted hamster islet-cell tumor.

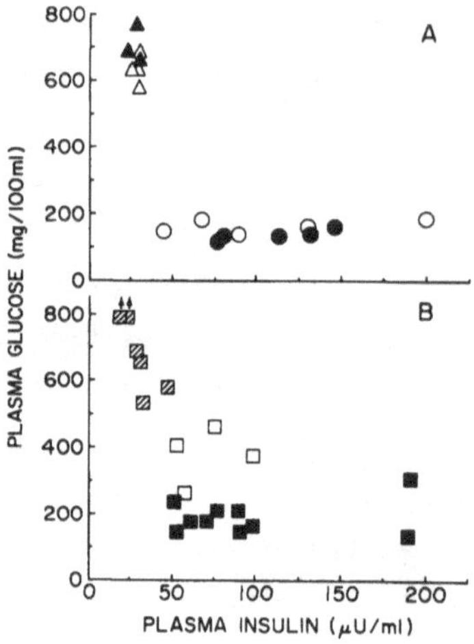

Figure 1. Relationship between plasma glucose and plasma insulin levels in male mice treated with streptozotocin. A: Control mice given a single injection of citrate buffer only (○, +/nu; ●, nu/nu), and severely hyperglycemic mice given a single high dose of streptozotocin 7 days earlier (△, +/nu; ▲, nu/nu). B: Mice given multiple low doses of streptozotocin. ■, normoglycemic nu/nu mice 7 days after the final injection; □, frankly hyperglycemic +/nu mice 7 days after the final injection; ▨, severely hyperglycemic +/nu mice 12 weeks after the injection. The two highest glucose values in this group (arrows) were over 800 mg/100 ml.

Obligatory Role of the Host Thymic Functions in the Induction Process. We now examined directly whether the failure of genetically athymic nude male mice to develop insulin-dependent hyperglycemia after the low dose treatment with streptozotocin was causally related to the absence of thymic functions. Young adult male nu/nu mice were grafted subcutaneously with whole thymuses removed from newborn +/nu mice, and 4 weeks later, the degree of T-cell reconstitution was determined by the titer of hemagglutinating antibodies produced after immunization with sheep red blood cells (SRBC), which are known to be thymus-dependent antigens. Typical responses in 8 adult euthymic (+/nu) mice similarly immunized with SRBC ranged in hemagglutinating titers of from 2^{10} to 2^{12}. Among the 9 nu/nu mice grafted with thymuses, 5 showed no evidence of functional restoration of T-cells since the anti-SRBC titers in these mice were not detectably higher than in sham-operated nu/nu controls ($<2^3$). However, in the remaining

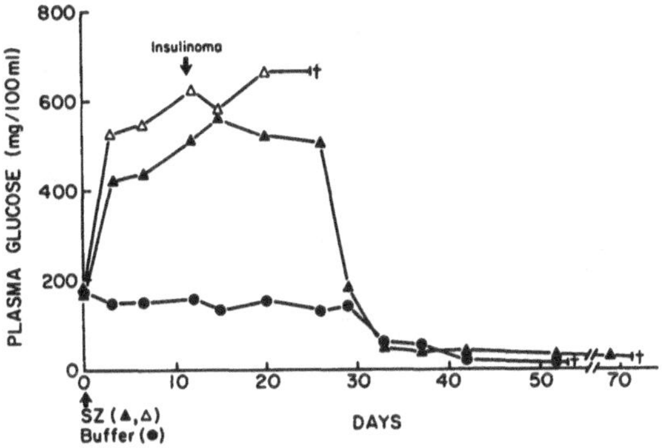

Figure 2. Rescue of moribund diabetic nude mice with a hamster insulinoma implant. On day 0, mice were given either citrate buffer alone (-●-), or a single high dose of streptozotocin of 200 mg/kg body weight (-△-,-▲-). On day 12, each mouse was injected subcutaneously in the flank with 10^7 tumor cells of a Syrian hamster pancreatic islet-cell tumor which had been previously maintained in nude mice by serial heterotransplantation (22). Three of the 7 diabetic mice were rescued in this way; for clarity, results from one such mouse are given here. The time of death of each mouse is indicated by a cross.

---

4 nu/nu mice, the graft was partially successful in restoring T-cell immunity; the anti-SRBC antibody titers in these mice ranged from 2^6 to 2^9.

All of these mice were injected with multiple low doses of streptozotocin. Progressive and permanent hyperglycemia was induced in all of the 4 nude mice in which the thymus graft had resulted in at least partial functional reconstitution, but in none of the 5 nude mice in which the graft failed to restore any T-cell functions (Fig. 3). The severity of hyperglycemia induced in the T-cell-reconstituted nude mice was considerably less than in the fully thymus-competent +/nu mice, indicating that there is an approximate correlation between the degree of hyperglycemia induced by multiple low doses of streptozotocin and the degree of T-cell-dependent functional capacity of the host animal.

Presence of Activated Autoimmune Lymphocytes in Diabetic Mice: Passive Transfer of Glucose Intolerance to Naive Nude Mice. Now we asked whether the +/nu mice, in which severe hyperglycemia has been induced by the multiple low dose injections of streptozotocin, have activated autoimmune

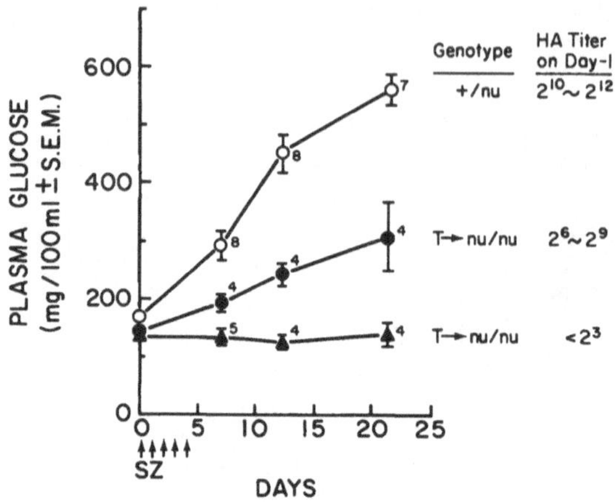

Figure 3. Induction of delayed hyperglycemia in thymus-reconstituted nude mice. Male nude mice were grafted with whole thymus glands from neonatal +/nu mice, and 4 weeks later, tested for thymus-dependent immune functions by immunization with sheep erythrocytes, assayed by hemagglutinating antibodies (HA). The thymus-grafted nude mice (-▲-, -●-) and euthymic control male +/nu mice (-○-) were injected with 40 mg streptozotocin/kg b.w./day for 5 days beginning on day 0, and the rise in plasma glucose levels was followed for 3 weeks. The total number of surviving mice in each group, and the standard error of the mean (vertical bar), are indicated for each data point. (From Paik et al., ref. 21)

lymphocytes that can passively transfer the diabetic syndrome into nude mice not treated with streptozotocin.

Spleen cells were removed from hyperglycemic +/nu mice previously injected with multiple low doses of streptozotocin, and injected into a group of male nude mice via the tail vein. A control group of nude mice was injected with same number of spleen cells removed from nondiabetic (buffer-injected) +/nu mice. The non-fasting plasma glucose levels in both groups of nude mice remained within the normal range. However, the nude mice given the spleen cells from hyperglycemic mice showed significantly abnormal glucose tolerance tests beginning 4 days after the spleen cell transfer. The fraction of recipients showing impaired glucose tolerance reached a peak about 10 days after the transfer, and decreased afterwards so that by the 4th week, most of the nude mice again responded normally to glucose tolerance tests. Data from three such experiments are summarized

Table 2. Passive Induction of Abnormal Glucose Tolerance in Nude Mice by Spleen Cells from Diabetic Mice

Source of spleen cells	Incidence of abnormal glucose tolerance in recipient nude mice Days after spleen cell transfer: 4	7	11	19
None (PBS alone)		0/7	0/7	
Nondiabetic +/nu mice	0/5	0/5	0/5	0/2
Diabetic +/nu mice	1/5	1/4	5/9	2/5

Spleen cells were removed from normal or diabetic male +/nu mice, and 4×10^7 cells were injected into each male nude mouse via the tail vein. On days indicated, each recipient was fasted overnight, and tested for glucose tolerance after injection i.p. of 2 mg glucose/g body weight, using a 20% aqueous solution.

---

in Table 2. The ability of diabetic spleen cells to induce a subclinical diabetic syndrome in naive nude mice was destroyed when the spleen cell preparations were first treated with an anti-Thy 1.2 serum and complement, but not when the spleen cells were depleted of B-cells by passing through a column packed with nylon wool (Fig. 4).

Failure to Identify Beta-Tropic Viruses in Diabetic Mice Induced with Multiple Low Doses of Streptozotocin. We examined the islets of +/nu and nu/nu mice treated with one single high dose or multiple low doses of streptozotocin by electron microscopy in order to determine whether the multiple low dose treatment of +/nu mice resulted in the induction of endogenous type C viruses, as postulated by Like and Rossini (5). Preliminary results indicated that no detectable viral particles were present in the islets of any of these mice (S.-G. Paik, D. M. Phillips and S. Shin, unpublished observations).

Sex Difference in Susceptibility to Low-Dose-Induced Delayed Hyperglycemia. The reasons for the very striking difference between euthymic males and females in the frequency and magnitude of induced hyperglycemia, presented in Table 1, is not yet understood. We found that the critical factor in determining the animal's susceptibility to the diabetogenic effects of multiple low doses of streptozotocin is not the genetic sex of the mouse,

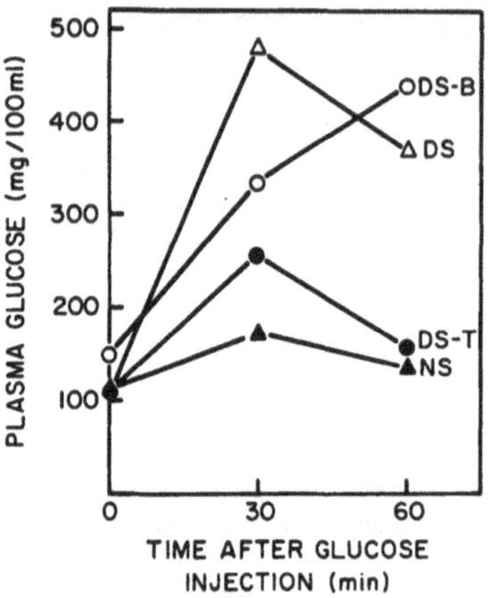

Figure 4. Passive transfer of glucose intolerance by splenic lymphocytes from diabetic mice: Effect of T-cell depletion. Spleen cells from two severely diabetic +/nu males, which had been induced with multiple low doses of streptozotocin 24 days previously, were pooled, and one fraction was depleted of T-cells and another fraction was depleted of B-cells as described in the Text. For control, spleen cells from nondiabetic +/nu males were used without fractionation. Male nu/nu mice were injected with 10^7 spleen cells of each fraction via the tail vein, and tested for glucose tolerance 20 days later. DS (-△-), unfractionated diabetic spleen cells; DS-B (-○-), B-cell-depleted diabetic spleen cells; DS-T (-●-), T-cell-depleted diabetic spleen cells; NS (-▲-), normal spleen cells. (From Paik et al., ref. 21)

but rather it is the balance between estrogens and androgens at the time the animal is injected with the beta-cell toxin.

The implantation of slow-release estrogen capsules (containing 5 mg estradiol in a Silastic tubing) in genetic males renders the mice completely unresponsive to the diabetogenic effects of streptozotocin in low doses, whereas the implantation of androgen capsules in a similar manner renders genetic females as highly susceptible as genetic males (S.-G. Paik, M. A. Michilis, Y. T. Kim and S. Shin, unpublished results). Furthermore, the injection of estradiol into +/nu male mice immediately before each injection of streptozotocin results in a drastically reduced incidence of delayed hyperglycemia. Similarly, injections of testosterone into +/nu females cause the mice to develop delayed hyperglycemia as readily as in genetic males (data not shown).

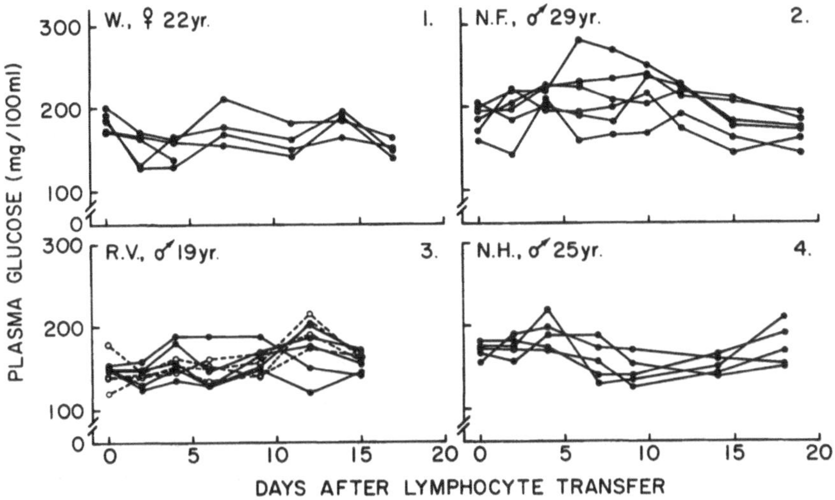

Figure 5. Passive induction of hyperglycemia in nude mice by human blood lymphocytes from Type I diabetics. Peripheral blood lymphocytes were collected from fresh blood of newly-diagnosed, insulin-dependent diabetics, and 10^7 lymphocytes were injected into each nude mouse via the tail vein, as described by Buschard et al. (11). The non-fasting plasma glucose levels of individual recipients were determined periodically thereafter. Glucose values on day 0 represent the control value, immediately before the lymphocyte injection. Unbroken lines connecting filled circles represent the changes in glucose level for individual nude mice. The three broken lines in Experiment 3 represent mice which were injected with lymphocytes enriched for T-cells by passing through a nylon wool column. The sex and age of each patient, from whom the lymphocytes were obtained, are indicated for each experiment.

Passive Induction of Hyperglycemia in Nude Mice by Human Blood Lymphocytes from Insulin-Dependent Diabetes Patients. We carried out a limited series of preliminary experiments to confirm the report of Buschard et al. that the peripheral blood lymphocytes from newly-diagnosed insulin-dependent diabetics are capable of inducing overt hyperglycemia in naive nude mice (10). Our results obtained so far, from the first 4 experiments of this series, are summarized in Fig. 5.

In one of these experiments, in which the blood lymphocytes obtained from a 29-year-old male patient (N.F.) were injected into 6-week-old male nude mice, at least 3 mice (50%) developed transient but significant hyperglycemia (Experiment 2, Fig. 5). None of the nude mice injected with peripheral lymphocytes from the other 3 patients showed comparable evidence of hyperglycemia.

Discussion

These results demonstrate that the induction of insulin-dependent diabetes mellitus by multiple subdiabetogenic doses of streptozotocin requires the participation of host thymic functions. More specifically, the observation that splenic T-lymphocytes from diabetic mice have the capacity to induce a subclinical diabetic syndrome in naive nude mice strongly suggests that this requirement for thymic functions reflects the obligatory role of autoimmune T-cells activated against beta-cell-specific autoantigens, which are presumably generated by the beta-cell toxin.

Our results generally confirm the earlier reports by Like and Rossini and their colleagues (5-7), and by Buschard and his collaborators (8, 10, 11), with certain important differences. Rossini et al. (6) proposed that the induction of insulin-dependent diabetes by low doses of streptozotocin may be due to the induction of endogenous beta-cell-tropic type C viruses by the toxin. As we mentioned earlier, our own studies of thin sections of pancreatic islets by electron microscopy failed to show any evidence of viral particles in mice that developed the delayed hyperglycemic state after the low dose treatment. Our observation that T-cell-depleted splenic lymphocytes from diabetic mice can no longer induce transient glucose intolerance in nude mice also argues against the obligatory role of a newly-induced endogenous virus, since it is difficult to imagine that the selective elimination of T-cells (but not of B-cells) will also result in the removal of virus particles from the spleen cell preparations.

Our results presented in this report differ from the reports of Buschard and Rygaard (8), in that we never observed the induction of severe hyperglycemia in nude mice treated with streptozotocin according to the low dose procedure. In addition, we were unable to confirm their report (10), that the transfer of spleen cells from diabetic +/nu mice to naive nude mice caused frank hyperglycemia in the recipient mice.

Based on these observations then, we may speculate that the diabetogenic viruses and subdiabetogenic doses of streptozotocin are alternative triggering mechanisms, each of which can act independently by inducing the appropriate beta-cell surface modifications that are recognized as neo-antigens by the host immune system. The strain dependence of the susceptibility to diabetogenic viruses (9, 23) or to streptozotocin (24) in mice, and the well-known association between an increased incidence of juvenile-type diabetes and certain specific alleles of the HLA complex in humans (25), may then be seen as reflecting in part the degree of ease with which the relevant autoantigens are generated on the beta-cell surface. The formation of such autoantigens would depend on the existence of the proper surface molecular substrates on the beta-cell (perhaps provided, for example, by the appropriate HLA-A and HLA-B determinants in the case of humans), and their recognition as potential immunogens would in turn require the proper T-cell clonal repertoire (and thus the appropriate HLA-D haplotypes in human cells).

On the other hand, the rapid development of profound and permanent hyperglycemia in mice given the single high dose of streptozotocin would not require the amplification mechanism involving autoimmune host T-cells, since the hyperglycemia in this case would be a direct consequence of the overwhelming physical destruction of the beta-cells by the toxin, as first suggested by Like and Rossini (5). Similarly, an islet-tropic virus may also cause a rapid insulin-dependent diabetes by destroying the majority of beta-cells in an animal. The isolation of a strain of Coxsackie B4 capable of inducing hyperglycemia in mice, from the pancreas of a child with acute diabetic ketoacidosis, (18) may have been an example of this. However, viremia is a very rare event even in fulminant juvenile-type diabetes.

While we have essentially confirmed, and extended, the earlier reports by Buschard and coworkers (8, 10), regarding the insensitivity of nude mice to multiple subdiabetogenic doses of streptozotocin, their subsequent report on the passive transfer of diabetes from humans to mice (11) remains to be confirmed. The very limited data from our own preliminary studies in this direction could be interpreted as evidence that the transient rise in the plasma glucose levels in some of the mice (see Experiment 2, Fig. 5) was caused by the action of activated human lymphocytes which recognize organ-specific, species-nonspecific beta-cell antigens. However, our results also point out the potential difficulty in demonstrating the validity of their hypothesis that the generation of the organ-specific, cross-reacting beta-cell antigens is a critical step in the etiology of insulin-dependent diabetes mellitus (12-15).

The difference between male and female mice in susceptibility to streptozotocin-induced diabetes is especially pronounced in our studies reported here. Similar, though less pronounced, differences have been described by other workers, for both streptozotocin-induced hyperglycemia (26, 27) and virus-induced diabetes (28, 29). Results of our experiments mentioned earlier would appear to suggest that, at least in mice injected with streptozotocin, the sex difference in hyperglycemic incidence may be due in part to the effect of estrogenic steroids on the rate of degradation of the toxin in vivo, or on the rate of its uptake by the beta-cells. However, an influence of estrogens on the host immune reactivity cannot be ruled out at present.

Acknowledgements

We would like to acknowledge the expert technical assistance of Andre L. Brown. This work was supported by a U. S. Public Health Service research grant (AM 26106) and the Genetics Center Grant (GM 19100) to Albert Einstein College of Medicine. S.S. is a recipient of a Faculty Research Award from the American Cancer Society.

References

1. Gepts, W.: Diabetes 14, 619-633 (1965).
2. Lendrum, R., Walker, G., Gamble, D.R.: Lancet i, 880-883 (1975).
3. Huang, S.-W., MacLaren, N.K.: Science 192, 64-66 (1976).
4. Craighead, J.E.: N. Engl. J. Med. 299, 1439-1445 (1978).
5. Like, A.A., Rossini, A. A.: Science 193, 415-417 (1976).
6. Rossini, A.A., Like, A.A., Chick, W.L., Appel, M.C., Cahill, G.F., Jr.: Proc. Nat. Acad. Sci. USA 74, 2485-2489 (1977).

7. Like, A.A., Rossini, A.A., Guberski, D.L., Appel, M.C., Williams, R.M.: Science 206, 1421-1423 (1979).

8. Buschard, K., Rygaard, J.: Acta Pathol. Microbiol. Scand., Sect. C. 86, 23-27 (1978).

9. Notkins, A.L.: Arch. Virol. 54, 1-17 (1977).

10. Buschard, K., Rygaard, J., Lund, E.: Acta Pathol. Microbiol. Scand. Sect. C. 84, 299-303 (1976).

11. Buschard, K., Madsbad, S., Rygaard, J.: Lancet i, 908-910 (1978).

12. Lipsick, J., Beattie, G., Osler, A.G., Kaplan, N.O.: Lancet i, 1290-1291 (1979).

13. Thurneyssen, O., Jansen, F.K., Vialettes, B., Vague, Ph., Selam, J.L., Mirouze, J.: Lancet i, 1291-1292 (1979).

14. Serra, A.S., Farndon, J.R., Shenton, B.K., Johnston, I.D.A.: Lancet i, 1292 (1979).

15. Beattie, G., Lannom, R., Lipsick, J. Kaplan, N.O., Osler, A.G.: Diabetes 29, 146-150 (1980).

16. Gamble, D.R., Taylor, K.W., Cumming, H.: Br. Med. J. 4, 260-262 (1973).

17. Steinke, J., Taylor, K.W.: Diabetes 23, 631-633 (1978).

18. Yoon, J.-W., Austin, M., Onodera, T., Notkins, A.L.: N. Engl. J. Med. 300, 1173-1179 (1979).

19. Riley, W., MacLaren, N., Rand, K., Bejar, R.: Diabetes 29, 53A (1980).

20. Paik, S.-G., Fleischer, N., Shin, S.: Diabetes 29, 52A (1980).

21. Paik, S.-G., Fleischer, N., Shin, S.: Proc. Nat. Acad. Sci. USA 77, (in press) (1980).

22. Shin, S., Baum, S., Fleischer, N., Rosen, O.M.: J. Cell Sci. 18, 199-206 (1975).

23. Yoon, J.-W., Lesniak, M.A., Fussganger, R., Notkins, A.L.: Nature 264, 178-180 (1976).

24. Rossini, A.A., Appel, M.C., Williams, R.M., Like, A.A.: Diabetes 26, 916-920 (1977).

25. Rubinstein, P., Suciu-Foca, N., Nicholson, J.F.: N. Engl. J. Med. 297, 1036-1040 (1977).

26. Rossini, A.A., Williams, R.M., Appel, M.C., Like, A.A.: Endocrinol. 103, 1518-1520 (1978).

27. McLaughlin, J., Taylor, G., MacLaren, N., Krupp, B., Jones, R.: Diabetes 27, 492 (1978).

28. Boucher, D.W., Hayashi, K., Rosenthal, J., Notkins, A.L.: J. Infect. Dis. 131, 462-466 (1975).

29. Morrow, P.L., Freeman, A., Craighead, J.E.: Diabetologia 18, 247-249 (1980).

EFFECT OF INSULIN-BINDING ANTIBODIES ON FREE INSULIN IN PLASMA AND TISSUE AFTER SUBCUTANEOUS INJECTION. A MODEL STUDY.

Viggo Kruse
Novo Research Institute, Novo Allé, DK-2880 Bagsværd, Denmark

Introduction

For more than 20 years it has been known that most insulin-treated diabetics form insulin-binding antibodies as a consequence of the insulin therapy. It is well known that insulin molecules are catabolized more slowly in persons with insulin antibodies than in persons without. Apparent half-lives of plasma insulin as long as 22 hours have been reported in patients with diabetes mellitus (10). This is in sharp contrast to the half-life of about 3 minutes found in persons without insulin antibodies (24). Relatively little is known about the variations in free insulin in the plasma of persons with insulin antibodies, and no attempt appears to have been made to evaluate free insulin in the tissue of such persons.

The concentration of insulin-binding antibodies, as well as the affinity of the antibodies, show large variations between patients. Even in a given patient some antibodies show a low and others a high affinity for insulin, i.e. they are heterogenous with respect to affinity.

Recent work has shown that the affinity of an antibody, usually expressed in terms of the equilibrium constant ($\underline{K}$), is determined almost exclusively by the dissociation rate constant (k_{dis}) of the ligand-antibody complex (4, 18, 25). The asso-

Basic and Clinical Aspects of Immunity to Insulin

ciation rate constant (k_{ass}) varies very little between antibodies of highly different affinity. It should be remembered that K is defined as k_{ass} divided by k_{dis}. The statistical chance for the formation of a ligand–antibody complex is determined by the concentration of the two reactants and the practically invariant association rate constant. As a consequence the rate of formation of ligand–antibody complexes is practically the same for a given concentration of ligand and antibody, regardless of the affinity of the antibody. Although these conclusions were drawn on the basis of studies of several hapten-antibody systems, it is assumed that they also apply to the insulin-antibody system. The stability of the complexes is determined by the dissociation rate constant.

The aim of the present study was to analyse the influence of antibodies on free insulin in plasma and tissue as a function of time during a course of repeated subcutaneous injections of insulin. A computer model was constructed on the basis of known physico-chemical characteristics of the insulin-antibody system and known data on the metabolism of insulin and IgG.

Methods

The insulin model. Figure 1 shows the model used for the simulation of insulin metabolism. The model was developed by Sherwin et al. (24) on the basis of experiments on normal persons made by the glucose-clamp technique. Compartments with insulin are shown as circles and rate constants as arrows. The arrow with asterix indicates where insulin enters the model. The figures by the arrows show the rate constants estimated by Sherwin et al. (24). For example, the rate constant for transport of insulin from compartment 1 to compartment 2 indicates that the fraction 0.142 of the content of comp. 1 is transferred to comp. 2 per minute. The unit for rate constants

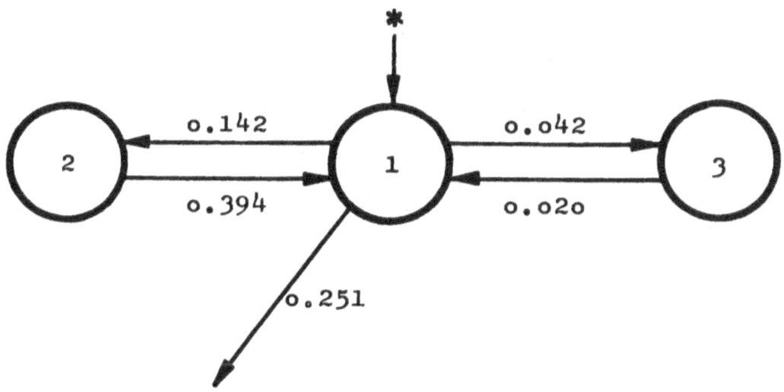

Fig. 1 Compartmental model of insulin kinetics in man. Model and parameters from Sherwin et al. (24)

is per minute (min^{-1}). The constant 0.693 divided by the rate constant gives the time it takes for half of the content to leave the compartment, if it is the only rate constant operating. It is called the half-time or half-life, and has the unit min. The catabolism of insulin was modelled as the irreversible loss of 0.251 of the intravascular pool (comp. 1) per minute (24). The size of compartment 1 is 4.5% of the bodyweight and represents the plasma space. The bodyweight is assumed to be 70 kg and the volume of compartment 1 (=plasma volume=intravascular space) is thus 3.150 l. Compartment 2 is a small rapidly equilibrating extravascular pool with a mean residence time for an insulin molecule of about 3 min. Compartment 3 is a large, slowly equilibrating extravascular pool of insulin with a mean insulin residence time of about 50 min. It is assumed (24) that compartment 2 represents tissues with a high perfusion efficiency, such as liver, kidney, heart and gut, and that compartment 3 represents those tissues that are relatively poorly perfused, such as muscle, adipose tissue and skin. The rate of glucose utilization was found by Sherwin et al. (24) to be closely correlated with the amount of insulin in compartment 3. Glucose utilization was not correlated with insulin in plasma or in the fast equilibrating compartment 2.

Expanded model with insulin antibodies and a subcutaneous insulin depot. The model shown in Fig. 1 was changed so insulin enters the plasma (compartment 1; Fig. 2) from a s.c. insulin depot (compartment 4) by a simple first-order process. The absorption kinetics of most insulins, including the soluble, rapidly absorbed types of insulin, are somewhat more complex than modelled here (8). However, the model is considered adequate for its purpose.

The model was further expanded to have insulin-binding antibodies in the intravascular space (Q_{iv}) as well as in the extravascular space (Q_{ev}). This is modelled as compartment 7 and 13, respectively (Fig. 2). The amount of insulin antibodies (Q) in the extravascular space (compartment 13) is set equal to the amount in the intravascular space (compartment 7) (ref. 2). The exchange of antibodies between the two pools is very slow, the rate constant being set equal to 2 day^{-1} in both directions. Insulin (P) and antibodies (Q) may form insulin–antibody complexes in the intravascular space (PQ_{iv}; compartment 8) as well as in the extravascular space (PQ_{ev}; compartment 14). Since insulin in compartment 2 equilibrates rapidly with plasma insulin in compartment 1, it was considered sufficient in this study to let only the insulin in compartment 3 react directly with antibodies. The rate of formation of intravascular complexes (PQ_{iv}) is $P_{iv}Q_{iv}k_{ass}$, where k_{ass} is the association rate constant. The rate of formation of extravascular complexes (PQ_{ev}) is taken as $P_{ev}Q_{ev}k_{ass}$ multiplied by the factor 0.1, because the concentration of Q in the interstitial fluid is about 1/3 of the concentration of Q in plasma (22, 23) and because a similar, although probably smaller, concentration difference exists for insulin. No reliable estimate of k_{ass} appears to have been made for the insulin-antibody system, so the value of 10^7 l mol^{-1} sec^{-1} was taken from studies on hapten-antibody systems (4, 18, 25). The value for the dissociation rate constant is given later together with the results.

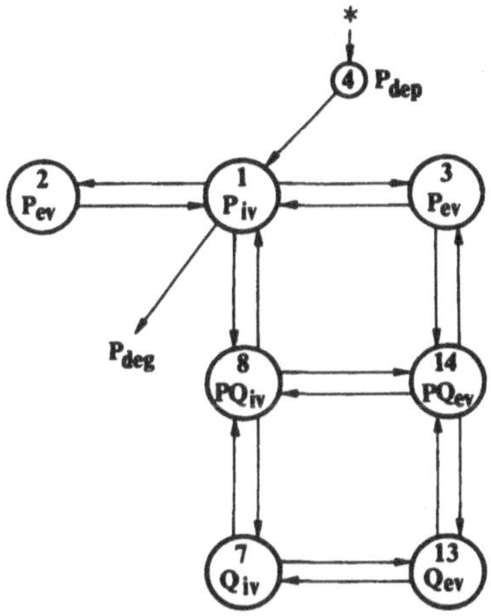

Fig. 2 Model of insulin kinetics in diabetic persons with insulin-binding antibodies. P=insulin; Q=antibody; PQ=insulin–antibody complexes; dep=depot of injected insulin; iv=intravascular; ev=extravascular; deg= degraded

All antibodies have the same k_{ass} and the same k_{dis} in a given simulation run; in other words, the antibodies are completely homogenous with respect to affinity. It is extremely unlikely to find this in real life, but for the present purpose it is useful to study the kinetics of a simplified insulin-antibody system.

The exchange of PQ complexes between compartment 8 and 14 is simulated with the same rate constants as for Q_{iv} and Q_{ev}, although it is realised that complexes of considerably larger size than PQ may be formed under certain circumstances. Each antibody combining site is treated as a single independent site in the model. No synthesis or degradation of antibody was included in the model, since it is the steady-state situation with respect to Q we want to study here. Also the model does not include catabolism of PQ_{iv} and PQ_{ev} - nor does it allow for the formation of large insulin–antibody complexes of the type $PQ_1PQ_2PQ_1PQ_2$ ..., where Q_1 and Q_2 symbolize antibodies which may bind to different parts of the insulin molecule at the same time.

The SAAM27 programme developed by Berman & Weiss (6) was used for the simulations. Testing of the model for errors and consistency was done by introducing known quantities into one or two of the compartments at a time and checking for conservation of mass.

Results

The insulin metabolism in diabetics was studied by injecting 20 U of insulin into compartment 4 at t = 0, and by repeating the injection of 20 U every 12 h for two or four days. The rate constant for absorption from the injection site was 0.006 min^{-1} which is equivalent to a half-life of 2 h for the insulin in compartment 4. This is of the same order of magnitude as observed for Actrapid (8). The time course of free insulin in plasma (compartment 1) and tissue (compartment 3) was studied in simulations with 0.1 U, 1 U or 10 U of antibody binding sites per litre plasma (compartment 7) and with an amount of binding sites in the extravascular space (compartment 13) corresponding to this, i.e. 0.1 U/l, 1 U/l and 10 U/l, respectively, multiplied by the plasma volume (3.150 l).

High-affinity antibodies. Simulations were first carried out with antibodies of very high affinity. The dissociation rate constant for insulin—antibody complexes was thus 0.0001 min^{-1}, which is equal to a dissociation half-life of 5 days.

Figure 3 shows that with a low concentration of antibody binding sites in plasma (0.1 U/l) the plasma free insulin reaches a peak concentration shortly after the injection, and that a steady state is reached after the second injection with peak

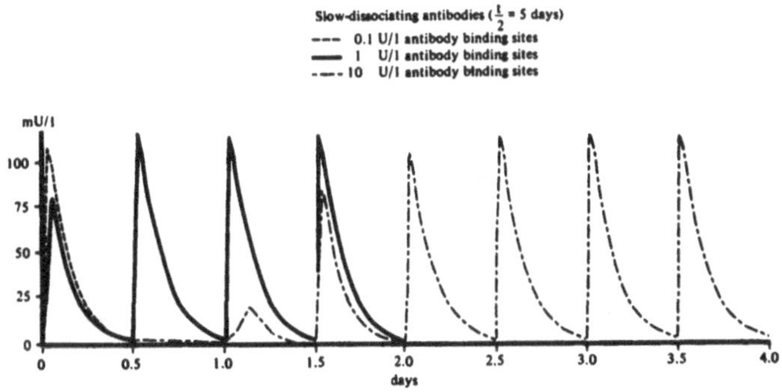

Fig. 3 Plasma free insulin simulated in diabetics with low (0.1 U/l), medium (1 U/l) and high (10 U/l) concentrations of insulin binding antibodies. The curves were generated with high-affinity (slow-dissociating) antibodies; the insulin–antibody complexes had a half-life of 5 days. A dose of 20 U of soluble insulin was given every 12 h. Simulations with 10 U/l binding sites were done for a period of 4 days, the rest for 2 days only.

values of about 120 mU/l (curve masked by the 1 U/l curve). A minimum value of about 3 mU/l is reached just before the next injection.

Tissue free insulin as a function of time is shown in Fig. 4. A delay in peak values relative to free insulin in plasma is observed. This is caused by the relatively low rate constant for transfer of insulin from compartment 1 to compartment 3 (Fig. 1 & 2). The total amount of binding sites in the model, free and bound, intravascular as well as extravascular ($Q_{iv} + PQ_{iv} + Q_{ev} + PQ_{ev}$), in relation to the dose of insulin given with each injection is 0.63 U of binding sites per 20 U of insulin (3.15 per 100). Such a relatively low binding capacity has only a small influence on the time course of free insulin in plasma and tissue. The time course for insulin in a model without any antibodies (not shown) is practically identical to the curves shown after the second injection in the model with 0.1 U/l antibodies (Fig. 3 & 4). Fig. 3 & 4 also show the

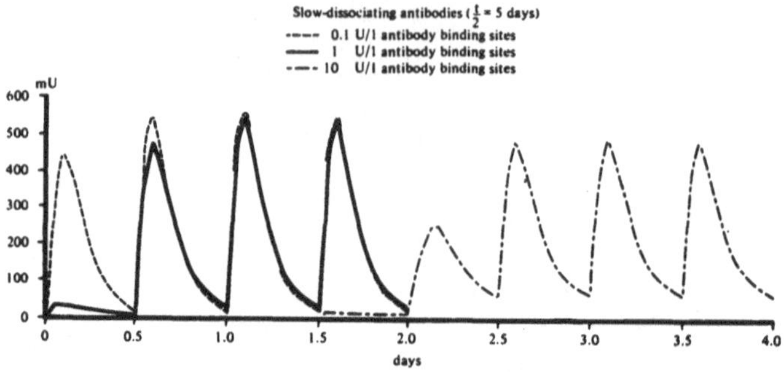

Fig. 4 Free insulin in tissue, obtained from the same simulation as in Fig. 3.

time course for free insulin in plasma and tissue when the antibody concentration is increased by a factor 10 from 0.1 to 1 U/l. The total amount of binding sites in the model is then 6.3 U, which may be compared to the 20 U of insulin given per injection (31.5/100). Steady state is reached after the third injection (Fig. 4). The maximum values for free insulin in plasma and tissue at steady state are only slightly lower than with 0.1 U/l binding sites.

When the antibody concentration is 10 U/l, the total amount of binding sites is 63 U in relation to the insulin dose of 20 U (315/100). In this situation a steady state is not reached until after 6 injections have been given. It is most important to note that free insulin in both plasma and tissue is extremely low - even after 3-4 injections because practically all insulin becomes bound to the antibodies. It takes five injections before a considerable amount of free insulin appears in the tissue (Fig. 4). Free insulin in plasma reaches almost the same peak value in the steady-state situation as when only a low concentration of antibodies is present. However, the peak value for tissue insulin is not quite as high as when less antibodies are present (Fig. 4). This is because enough free binding sites are available in the tissue to blunt the increase in tissue free insulin. It should be noticed that the minimum value for tissue free insulin, which is reached just before a new injection is given, increases with increasing concentration of binding sites.

The situations considered so far are quite realistic as far as the range of antibody concentrations is concerned. However, the dissociation rate constant used in the model is extremely low. A dissociation rate constant of 0.0001 min^{-1} may be found for some of the antibodies in serum from hyperimmunized animals (16), but rarely or never in diabetics, and certainly not in homogenous form without any rapidly dissociating antibodies.

Dissociation studies carried out in vitro at 37°C have shown mean values for slowly dissociating antibodies of 0.0031 min^{-1} ($\frac{t}{2}$ = 0.15 days) (ref. 26) and 0.0049 min^{-1} ($\frac{t}{2}$ = 0.10 days) (ref. 17); and minimum values have been reported to be 0.0009 min^{-1} ($\frac{t}{2}$ = 0.53 days) (ref. 12) and 0.0004 min^{-1} ($\frac{t}{2}$ = 1.2 days) (ref. 7).

In vivo studies have shown that the apparent disappearance rate constant for ^{125}I-insulin given intravenously can be as low as 0.00053 min^{-1} ($\frac{t}{2}$ = 0.9 days) (ref. 10).

Low-affinity antibodies. To evaluate the insulin kinetics when the dissociation rate constant is 1000 times higher, the simulations were repeated with a dissociation rate constant of 0.1 min^{-1} ($\frac{t}{2}$ = 7 min). All other parameters remained unchanged. Dissociation rate constants for rapidly dissociating antibodies have been reported to have a mean of 0.06 min^{-1} ($\frac{t}{2}$ = 12 min) (ref. 26) and 0.148 min^{-1} ($\frac{t}{2}$ = 5 min) (ref. 17). The highest reported single value is 0.35 min^{-1} ($\frac{t}{2}$ = 2 min) (ref. 7).

With only 0.1 U/l antibody binding sites the plasma and tissue curves for free insulin were very similar to the curves found with 0.1 U/l of slowly dissociating antibodies (Fig. 5 & 6 ver-

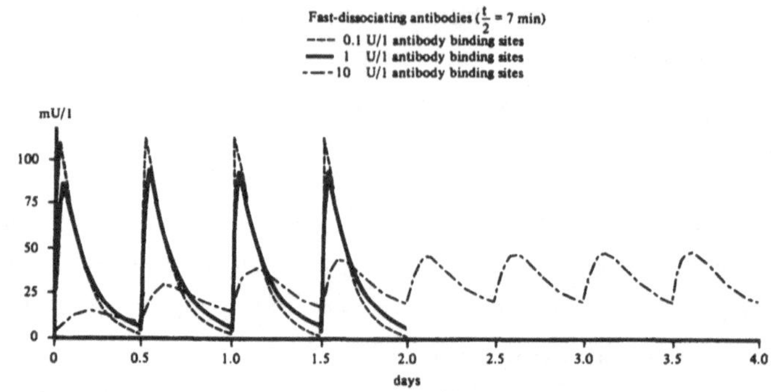

Fig. 5 Plasma free insulin in diabetics with low-affinity (fast-dissociating) antibodies. A half-life of 7 min for the insulin-antibody complexes was used in the simulations. All other parameters were as in Fig. 3.

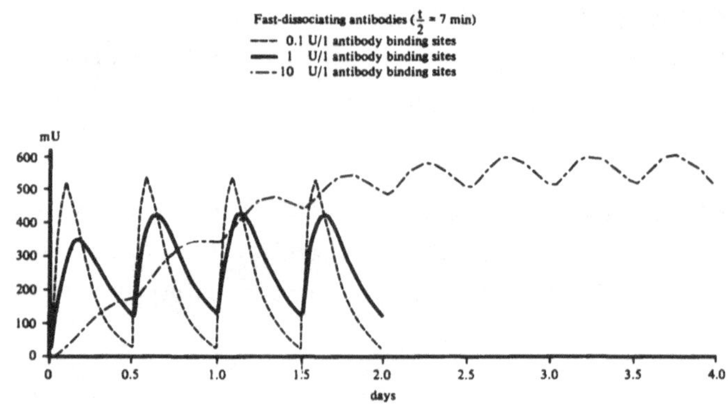

Fig. 6 Free insulin in tissue, obtained from the simulations in Fig. 5.

sus Fig. 3 & 4). However, with 1 U/l and especially with 10 U/l of rapidly dissociating antibodies the peaks of free insulin in plasma become lower and the maxima occur later. Dramatic effects are seen for free insulin in tissue (Fig. 6). With increasing antibody concentrations the minimum values for tissue insulin, observed just before a new injection is given, increase drastically and the peaks become less prominent and are delayed.

Occupancy of binding sites. Figure 7 shows to what degree the binding sites in plasma are occupied in the period between two insulin injections after steady state has been reached. When antibodies have a low dissociation rate constant of 0.0001 min^{-1} and the binding site concentration is 10 U/l, the antibodies are almost totally saturated at all times, whereas when the antibodies have a high dissociation rate constant of 0.1 min^{-1}, there is a net uptake of insulin by the antibodies during the first 2 1/4 h after the injection, and a net release from that time until the next injection is given. The binding capacity of 10 U/l plasma corresponds to a large amount of total binding sites - 63 U for each 20 U of insulin injected (315/100) - half of them in the plasma (32 U) and half of them in the tissue. A change in occupancy of binding sites of about 20% during the interval between two insulin injections (Fig. 7) corresponds to an uptake and release of 20% of 32 U, which is equal to 6.3 U of insulin of each 20 U injected. Something similar occurs in the tissue.

Fig. 7 Variation in saturation of insulin-binding antibodies in the period between two insulin injections. The injections (20 U) were given on day 3.5 and 4.0 after steady state had been reached. The upper curve (- - - -) was simulated with a high concentration (10 U/l) of high-affinity antibodies, and the lower curve (——) with low-affinity antibodies of the same concentration.

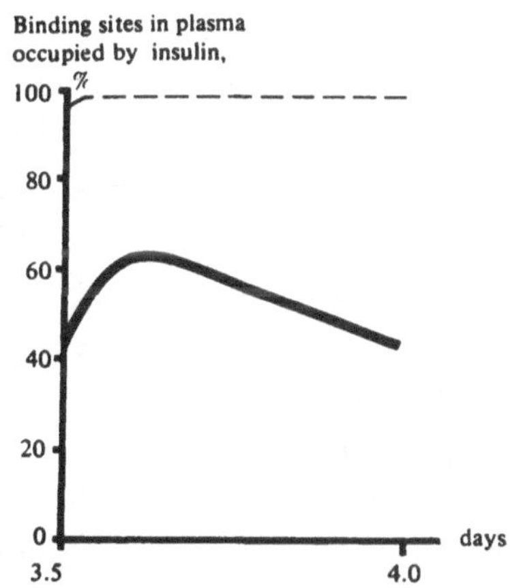

Discussion

A simulation model for the analysis of plasma and tissue free insulin in insulin-treated diabetics with circulating insulin antibodies has been presented. A number of simplifications have been made in order to make the model workable; nevertheless, several essential features are included in the model. The simulations were thus carried out with a wide range of antibody concentrations and with widely different dissociation rate constants. Furthermore, the model contains a delay in the exchange of insulin between plasma and tissue. This appears to be essential for the simulation of realistic tissue values (24). Antibodies in the interstitial fluid (the extravascular space) are also considered in the model. It is likely that some degradation of insulin occurs in connection with compartment 3, but no estimate of this degradation is available. Another approximation concerns the association rate constant. Here it is assumed to be as for haptens. In spite of the simplifications and approximations the model is considered suitable for its purpose.

On the basis of the simulated results, it is to be expected that patients with a high concentration of rapidly dissociating antibodies will show a pronounced hyperglycemia after the main meals due to quite inadequate peaks of free insulin in plasma and tissue. This will happen regardless of what time insulin is given in relation to the meal and regardless of whether rapidly or slowly absorbed insulin is given. It may further be expected that hypoglycemia will occur when the rate of absorption of glucose from gut to blood goes down 2-4 h after the meal, due to the high level of free insulin in plasma and, especially, in tissue. A general pattern like this is often observed in patients with what is called unstable or brittle diabetes (see e.g. 19). Thus it seems likely that brittle diabetes in many cases is caused or precipitated by high concentrations of rapidly dissociating insulin antibodies. The use of insulin preparations with a low absorption rate constant (medium or long-acting insulins) would clearly be contra-indicated for the treatment of such patients. This conclusion was also reached several years ago by Molnar et al. (19), but does not seem to have been generally accepted.

In patients with a high concentration of rapidly dissociating antibodies the diabetic control is likely to improve if the mean affinity increases or the concentration of antibody goes down. A change from conventional to pure insulin has been shown to lower the concentration of antibodies (9).

Several observations reported in the literature support the conclusions about the influence of antibodies on insulin kinetics. Nabarro et al. (20) have shown that the increase in free insulin in plasma after subcutaneous injection of soluble insulin is delayed when antibodies are present. The return of free plasma insulin to the preinjection level is also delayed in comparison to what is found when no antibodies are present. This is in agreement with the results reported here.

Harwood (13) has described a case where a diabetic patient intermittently needed high doses of insulin or no insulin at all. The patient, a diabetic woman, was on 140-180 U/day of protamine zinc insulin. About once a month she went through a period of 5-6 days during which she did not need and did not take any insulin. The period began with hypoglycemic attacks whose control required the repeated ingestion of large amounts of sugar. After 5-6 days the insulin-free period came to an end and she resumed her insulin injections. In Berson & Yalow's laboratory her serum was found to contain 106 U/l antibodies. This is more than ten times higher than the highest antibody concentration used in any of the simulations. The explanation offered was that antibodies were able to "store" sufficient insulin for about 5 days' requirements for insulin, and that the insulin-antibody complexes released considerable amounts of insulin over several days after the last injection of insulin. On the basis of the results presented here (Fig. 5 & 6) this explanation seems quite reasonable.

A case has been reported where a new-born baby with a high titer of insulin antibodies presented with frequent attacks of hypoglycemia with tremors during the first few months of life (21). These symptoms could be alleviated by artificial feeding. The mother also had a high titer of antibodies. It was assumed that the antibodies had been transferred from mother to baby via the placenta.

Goldman et al. (12) have described five patients who had circulating autoantibodies against insulin and an apparently normal B-cell response to glucose stimulation. The patients often had severe fasting hypoglycemia and postprandial hypoglycemia. Intravenous glucose infusion was used to relieve the patients' hypoglycemia. In one patient hypoglycemia reoccurred 90 min after the glucose infusion was stopped. Brain damage was observed in one of the other patients after unattended hypoglycemia. The measured antibody concentrations (4-14 U/l estimated from Scatchard plots) and dissociation rate constants make it likely that insulin which dissociated from the antibody complexes caused the hypoglycemia. Følling & Norman (11) and Ichihara et al. (15) have each published observations on a patient with a similar syndrome. Følling & Norman (11) found a pronounced hyperglycemia 1-2 h after an oral glucose load (1 g/kg body weight). This was followed by severe hypoglycemia 2-5 h after the glucose load. The patient had "several" U/l of insulin antibodies in the serum. The increase in total insulin in response to the glucose load was "very large" and the elevated concentration of total insulin persisted into the period with hypoglycemia. A similar syndrome has recently been produced experimentally in an adult mini-pig (14).

The mechanism suggested to be responsible for this syndrome was (12, 15) that insulin is secreted in large amounts by the pancreas in response to a high influx of glucose from gut to blood, and many insulin—antibody complexes are formed. When the influx of glucose from gut to blood is low, as it is during the postabsorptive period, insulin will dissociate from the complexes in amounts large enough to cause severe hypoglycemia, if the pool of complexes is large and the dissociation rate constant is high. This release of insulin is not under feed-back control, in contrast to the release of insulin from the B-cells, as discussed by Ichihara et al. (15) and Goldman et al. (12).

Concluding Remarks

There can be little doubt that antibodies can exert an influence on the level of free insulin in plasma and tissue in special cases. This has been particularly well demonstrated in patients who do not have diabetes mellitus, but who have high concentrations of circulating insulin autoantibodies (11, 12, 15, 21). The results presented here indicate that in certain situations antibodies have a considerable influence in diabetics as well. It has, however, been difficult experimentally to demonstrate such an effect in diabetics (1, 3, 5). This may be due to the use of inadequate methods for the determination of antibody characteristics (concentration, dissociation rate constants, etc.) and shortcomings of the chosen experimental technique.

References

1. Andersen, O.O.: Acta Endocrinol. 83, Suppl. 205, 231-238 (1976).
2. Andersen, S.B.: Metabolism of human gamma globulin (γ_{SS}-globulin). 139 pp. Blackwell Scientific Publications, Oxford, 1964.
3. Asplin, C.M., Hartog, M., Goldie, D.J.: Acta Endocrinol. 87, 330-338 (1978).
4. Barisas, B.G., Singer, S.J., Sturtevant, J.M.: Immunochemistry 12, 411-421 (1975).
5. Baxter, R.C., Yue, D.K., Turtle, J.R.: Clin. Chem. 22, 1089-1094 (1976).
6. Berman, M., Weiss, M.F.: SAAM Manual. U.S. DHEW publication no. NIH 76-730, U.S. Government Printing Office, Washington DC, 1976.
7. Berson, S.A., Yalow, R.S.: J. Clin. Invest. 38, 1996-2016 (1959).
8. Binder, C.: Absorption of injected insulin. 87 pp. Munksgaard, Copenhagen, 1969.

9. Bruni, B., D'Alberto, M., Osenda, M., Ricci, C., Turco, G. L.: Diabetologia 9, 492-498 (1973).

10. Davidson, J.K., DeBra, D.W.: Diabetes 27, 307-318 (1978).

11. Følling, I., Norman, N.: Diabetes 21, 814-826 (1972).

12. Goldman, J., Baldwin, D., Rubenstein, A.H., Klink, D.D., Blackard, W.G., Fisher, L.K., Roe, T.F., Schnure, J.J.: J. Clin. Invest. 63, 1050-1059 (1979).

13. Harwood, R.: N. Engl. J. Med. 262, 978-979 (1960).

14. Heding, L.G.: Diabetologia 19, 282 (1980).

15. Ichihara, K., Shima, K., Saito, Y., Nonaka, K., Tarui, S., Nishikawa, M.: Diabetes 26, 500-506 (1977).

16. Kruse, V.: Scand. J. Clin. Lab. Invest. 39, 215-221 (1979).

17. Kurtz, A.B., Matthews, J.A., Nabarro, J.D.N.: Diabetologia 15, 19-22 (1978).

18. Levison, S.A., Hicks, A.N., Portmann, A.J., Dandliker, W. B.: Biochemistry 14, 3778-3786 (1975).

19. Molnar, G.D., Taylor, W.F., Langworthy, A.L.: Mayo Clin. Proc. 47, 709-719 (1972).

20. Nabarro, J.D.N., Mustaffa, B.E., Morris, D.V., Walport, M.J., Kurtz, A.B.: Diabetologia 16, 5-12 (1979).

21. Nakagawa, S., Suda, N., Kudo, M., Kawasaki, M.: Diabetologia 9, 367-375 (1973).

22. Olszewski, W.L., Engeset, A.: Lymphology 11, 156-164 (1978).

23. Poulsen, H.L.: Scand. J. clin. Lab. Invest. 34, 119-122 (1974).

24. Sherwin, R.S., Kramer, K.J., Tobin, J.D., Insel, P.A., Liljenquist, J.E., Berman, M., Andres, R.: J. Clin. Invest. 53, 1481-1492 (1974).

25. Smith, T.W., Skubitz, K.M.: Biochemistry 14, 1496-1502 (1975).

26. Yue, D.K., Baxter, R.B., Turtle, J.R.: Biochim. Biophys. Acta 444, 231-239 (1976).

IMMUNOGENICITY OF INSULIN IN RELATION TO ITS PHYSICO-CHEMICAL PROPERTIES

B. Hansen, J. Høiriis Nielsen and B. Welinder
Hagedorn Research Laboratory
DK-2820 Gentofte, Denmark

Introduction

The immunogenicity of insulin preparations is dependent on the presentation of immunogenes to the recipient and on factors in the recipient being either experimental animals or the diabetic patient. The antigenicity of insulin has been thoroughly studied since Berson and co-workers in 1956 (1) reported the presence of circulating insulin-binding immunoglobulins in sera of diabetic patients treated with insulin. Berson and Yalow (2) demonstrated a lower antigenicity of conventional porc insulin as opposed to beef insulin, and this difference has been confirmed by several investigators.

It is also well-established that purification of conventional porcine insulin can reduce the immunogenicity (3,4,5,6,7,8,9). Already in 1964 Deckert (3) observed in rabbits that amorphous porcine insulin isolated early in the isolation and purification procedure was more immunogenic than the final recrystallized porcine insulin, and it was suggested that the impurities might act as an adjuvant enhancing the formation of insulin antibodies.

Although this conclusion still is valid for conventional insulin it cannot alone explain the immunogenic behaviour of highly purified insulin preparations.

It has been noticed that bovine insulin impurities were highly

Basic and Clinical Aspects of Immunity to Insulin

immunogenic in rabbits (8). In spite of this recognition investigations have shown that increased purity of the bovine insulin not necessarily was associated with decreased insulin antibody formation (7). It was proposed, therefore, that species difference, in this case, is more important than the purity of insulin. Furthermore, homologous insulin preparations have shown antibody production in cattle, sheep and goat (10). A possible explanation would be that the antigenic stimulus was created during or after the extraction and isolation of the insulin from the pancreas. The antigenic determinant could be defined chemical modifications, changes in structure or formation of aggregates of the insulin molecule itself.

Composition of insulin preparations

A number of contaminants have been identified, even in recrystallized insulin, e.g. naturally occurring insulin related compounds like proinsulin, intermediate split-products and arginine insulin. During the isolation, purification and storage process derivatives like ethylesterinsulin, desamidoinsulin, non-convertible dimers and maybe higher polymers of unknown structure are formed.

When recrystallized insulin is fractionated according to molecular weight on Sephadex G-50 in 1 M acetic acid the so-called a-, b- and c-fraction can be obtained (12,13,14). Recrystallized insulin purified by gel-chromatography gives a compound for which the term single peak has been used. This single peak insulin is made up of 99% of insulin containing 5-10% desamidoinsulin.

Further purification, e.g. using ion exchange chromatography in dissociating media, a technique that will separate according to net charge yields highly purified insulin also called "single component" insulin or "monocomponent" insulin. Highly purified insulin is composed of more than 99% of insulin.

Besides the above mentioned compounds insulin preparations may contain other pancreatic peptides, e.g. glucagon, pancreatic polypeptide, somatostatin and vaso-active intestinal peptide towards which antibodies have been detected in diabetic patients treated with conventional insulin (11).

Self-association of insulin

The molecular weight of insulin as estimated by gel-chromatography is dependent on several factors, the most important being pH and composition of the solvents, the insulin concentration and the metal ion content.

If pH and/or the buffer substance leads to denaturation and/or dissociation, the molecular weight of the monomer 6000 daltons will be found, e.g. by gel-chromatography in 1 M acetic acid where substances like proinsulin, intermediate forms, non-convertible dimer and higher polymers can be detected.

It is well-known that in neutral or slightly alkaline media insulin has a marked tendency to form reversible aggregates, especially in the presence of zinc ions (for a review see (15)).

In the crystalline form the stable unit is the hexamer consisting of 3 dimers complex bound to two zinc atoms (16) or in the presence of high salt concentrations hexamers with 4 zinc atoms (17). Such zinc insulin complexes are also found in neutral or slightly alkaline aqueous solutions as demonstrated by ultracentrifugation (18, 19) and paper electrophoreses (20).

We have studied the aggregation of insulin with or without zinc by gel-chromatography in weakly alkaline solutions. When crystalline porcine insulin containing 0.5% zinc labelled with ^{65}Zn was subjected to chromatography on Sephadex G-75 at pH 8.8, an elution profile appeared indicating the presence of three separate fractions (fig. 1, upper panel). The distribution of

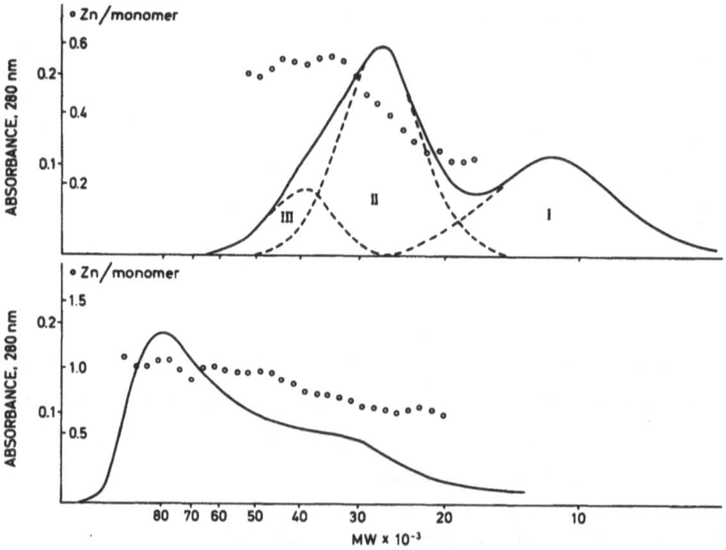

Fig. 1

Gel-chromatography on Sephadex G-75 (50 x 1.5 cm) in barbital buffer (0.01M), 0.05M NaCl, pH 8.8, of 20 mg crystalline porcine insulin containing 0.5% zinc (upper panel) or 27 mg insulin containing 1% zinc (lower panel).

The insulin was dissolved in 1 ml buffer and allowed to equilibrate for 1 hour with 50 µl carrier-free $^{65}ZnCl_2$. The absorbance at 280 nm and radioactivity of the effluent was monitored continously, and the number of Zn-atoms per monomer insulin was calculated from the total amount of insulin and zinc present. The molecular weight scale was constructed on the basis of the localization of a number of proteins with known molecular weights.

radioactivity showed that only fraction II and III contained zinc, while fraction I with an apparent molecular weight about 12,000 daltons was without zinc. By calculating the zinc content of fraction III with an apparent molecular weight about 40,000 daltons, 0.5-0.6 zinc atoms per insulin monomer was found. The zinc content decreased within peak II with the apparant molecular weight 24,000 daltons to 0.2-0.3 atoms per monomer.

If the zinc content was increased to 1% a displacement towards higher molecular weights was found (fig. 1, lower panel). Soluble aggregates with apparent molecular weight about 70,000-80,000 daltons and a zinc content about 1 atom per insulin monomer were present. Under this condition no zinc-free insulin corresponding to fraction I was seen.

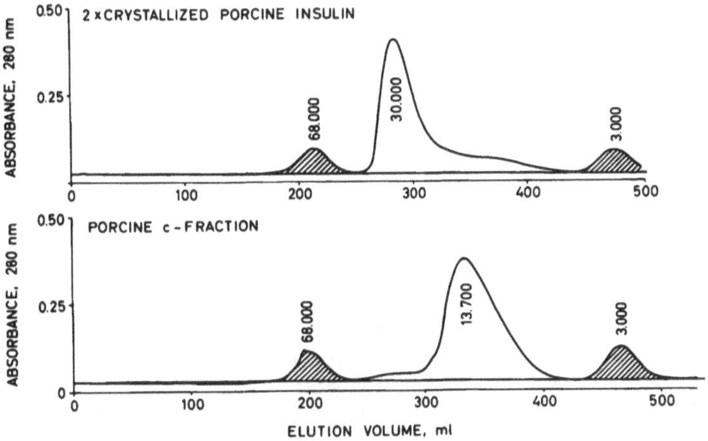

Fig. 2

Gel-chromatography of 2 x crystallized porcine insulin containing 0.5% zinc (upper panel) and zinc-free c-fraction of the same insulin (lower panel) on a 97 x 2.5 cm Sephadex G-75 column eluted at 21.0 ml/h with 0.9% NH_4HCO_3 adjusted to pH 7.30 with glacial acetic acid. The hatched peaks are co-chromatographed molecular weight standards, bovine serum albumin (68.000) and acetone as marker for the lower separation cut-off (MW=3.000). Insulin load was 40 mg in both cases.

If the pH during gel-chromatography was lowered to near physiological values, i.e. 7.3, and insulin with a zinc content of 0.5% was applied most of the insulin appeared as hexamers (fig. 2, upper panel), although some tailing corresponding to both higher and lower molecular weight was seen.

Using the same conditions, Zn-free insulin (c-fraction) eluted mainly as dimer (fig. 2, lower panel).

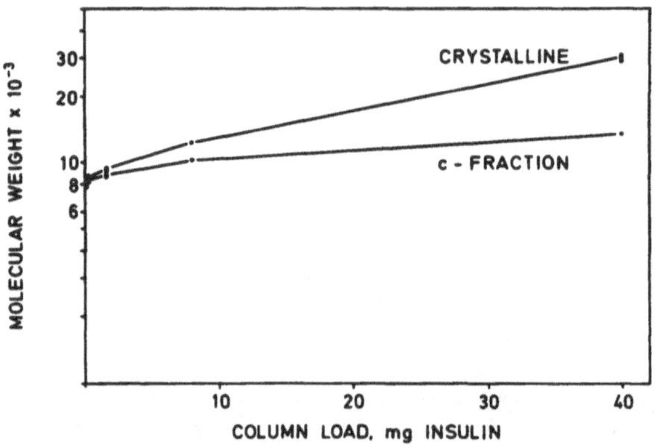

Fig. 3

The apparent molecular weight of insulin in relation to column load. Experimental conditions as in fig. 2. Upper curve: 2 x crystallized porcine insulin, 0.5% zinc. Lower curve: Zinc-free c-fraction of the same insulin.

If the insulin concentration was increased the apparent molecular weight also increased (fig. 3). The upper curve shows the molecular weight of insulin containing 0.5% zinc, while the lower curve shows the molecular weight of zinc-free insulin. At low concentrations both compounds approximate the monomer.

If the buffer was changed to one commonly used in injection-solutions of insulin, a somewhat different elution profile was found (fig. 4). The upper panel shows the elution profile of 2 x crystallized porcine insulin containing 0.5% zinc. The solid line represents a column load of 8 mg (200 IU/ml) the dashed line 0.4 mg (10 IU/ml). A major peak is seen around 30,000 daltons and a minor peak about 43,000 daltons. The middle panel shows the same experiment performed with highly purified crystalline porcine insulin with the same zinc content and column loads. Only one fraction with an apparent molecular weight about 30,000 daltons was found at both insulin concentrations, and the minor peak representing higher molecular weight substances disappeared.

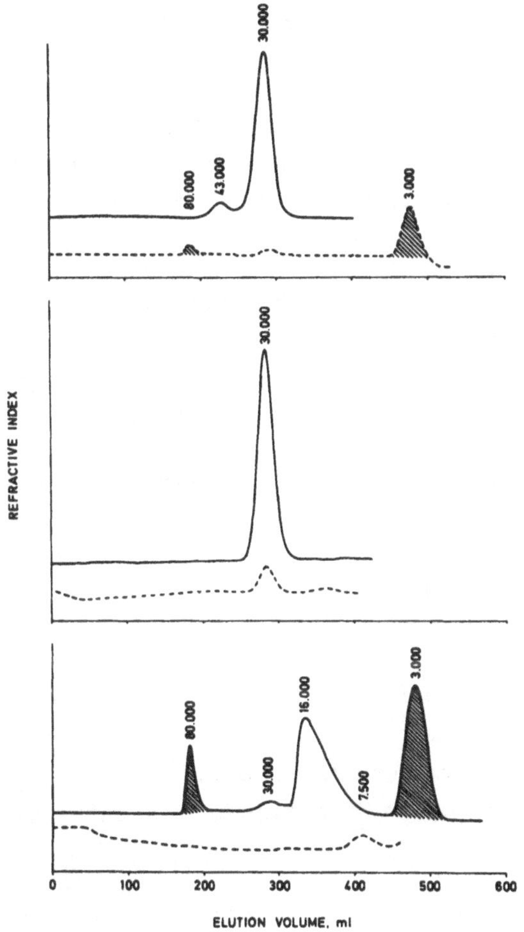

Fig. 4

Gel-chromatography of 3 different insulins on a 94 x 2.5 cm Sephadex G-75 column eluted at 24.0 ml/h with 1/75M phosphate buffer, pH 7.30, containing 0.7% NaCl, 0.07% phenol and 0.15% m-cresol. The solid lines represent a column load of 8.0 mg, the dashed lines 0.4 mg. The hatched areas indicate the upper (Dextran-blue) and lower (acetone) fractionation limits of the column.

The upper panel represents 2 x crystallized porcine insulin containing 0.5% zinc, the middle panel is the elution pattern of highly purified porcine insulin with 0.5% zinc, and the lower panel shows highly purified insulin treated with surplus of EDTA, i.e. highly purified zinc-free insulin.

The lower panel shows the same experiment performed with highly purified crystalline porcine insulin treated with a surplus of EDTA in order to remove the zinc ions. At the high insulin concentration a displacement towards low molecular weight around 16,000 daltons was seen, although there still remained some of the 30,000-dalton compound. At the low insulin concentration only molecules around 7,500 daltons were detected.

Thus, the insulin hexamer seems to be a relatively stable unit which is not readily dissociated by simple dilution. When zinc is removed the hexamer breaks up and zinc-free tetramers, dimers and monomers are formed in an equilibrium dependent on the insulin concentration.

These results indicate that zinc-containing aggregates of variable sizes and zinc contents will be present in insulin solutions depending on pH, buffer constituents, insulin concentration, zinc concentration and purity of the insulin.

In addition to these more or less reversible aggregates insulin seems also to form polymers where insulin molecules are covalently linked together in a sofar unknown manner. As mentioned above a non-convertible dimer has been demonstrated by gel-chromatography in acetic acid.

This and other polymers are supposed to be formed during the preparation and storage of the insulin. It seems conceivable that the probability for such compounds to occur increases if self-association of the above mentioned zinc-dependent type is allowed to take place.

Therefore, we may conclude from these observations that in order to avoid formation of possible highly antigenic polymers highly purified insulin preparations in low concentrations and in the absence of metal ions should be attempted.

This concept is supported by recent work of Arquilla et al. (21,22) who studied the effect of zinc ions on the conformation of antigenic determinants of bovine insulin. When comparing zinc insulin with zinc-free insulin they were able to demonstrate differences in circular dichroism spectra, and they proposed that these differences were due to either aggregation or changes in the structure of the insulin monomers within the aggregated insulin. Furthermore, they were able to demonstrate that immunoresponse was dependent on the type of insulin employed.

Association between insulin and protamine

With the aim of retarding the action of insulin two principles have been used. One is the incorporation of a surplus of zinc into the zinc-insulin crystals and hereby change the solubility and the other is to form a complex where insulin is bound to protamine resulting in a compound which is heavily soluble at neutral pH.

Protamine isolated from the rainbow trout is a mixture of 6 major and some minor compounds of very similar structure. The overall amino acid composition of purified protamine from rainbow trout is found to be: $Arg_{22.1}$ $Ser_{3.5}$ $Pro_{2.7}$ $Gly_{2.2}$ $Ala_{0.5}$ $Val_{1.8}$ $Ile_{0.2}$ giving an average molecular weight for the free protamine base of appr. 4.400 (23,24,25).

When forming the complex a certain amount of protamine (appr. 10% of the amount of insulin by weight) is added, which at neutral pH will bind all the insulin (the isophane proportion) and consequently neither protamine nor insulin will be in solution.

The precipitation takes first place as amorphous particles consisting of both heavily soluble and readily soluble compounds, but by time the soluble compounds are transformed into the heavily soluble and the characteristic NPH-insulin crystals can be formed (26).

In this state the arginine residues in protamine are supposed to be bound to the A21 asparagine in the insulin molecules in the proportion 6 molecules of insulin to 1 molecule of protamine. The binding is of a character not allowing exchange with added free insulin. Although X-ray crystallography has not yet been carried out on the protamine insulin crystal it is conceivable that the configuration differs fundamentally from that of the above mentioned Zn-insulin crystals and soluble aggregates.

In the tissue protamine is degraded by plasmin to smaller peptides being sensitive to carboxypeptidase cleavage resulting in release of insulin.

Precipitation of insulin with protamine is not a selective process and protamine will probably also bind proinsulin, dimers of insulin as well as aggregated forms of insulin, which means that the molecular state of the insulin moiety of the NPH-insulin crystal will, to a certain extent, reflect the molecular form present in the insülin solution to which protamine is added.

Immune response in rabbits

In order to evaluate the impact of the concept discussed in the preceeding sections we have tested the immunogenicity of various highly purified porcine and bovine insulin preparations (proinsulin-like immunoreactivity < 5 ppm) which may primary vary in the physico-chemical state of the insulin molecules.

Immunization and antibody determination

Preliminary studies indicated that insulin antibodies were not formed in rabbits given highly purified insulin without adjuvant. In order to enhance the response all insulin preparations were, therefore, emulsified in a standardized way with Freund's complete (FCA) or incomplete (FIA) adjuvant.

Rabbits (outbred white or WIGA chinchilla, female/male, 2-4 kg) were injected subcutaneously every 10th day with 20 IU of insulin. In each experiment 10 rabbits were immunized.

The soluble forms of porcine and bovine insulin and the NPH-porcine insulin were administered in FCA at the first injection and in FIA in subsequent injections. The NPH-bovine insulin was throughout administered in FIA.

The presence of antibodies was either analyzed by the double antibody technique described by Ortved Andersen (27) or the more sensitive PEG-precipitation technique (28,29,30).

All samples were analyzed by final serum dilution of 1:10. 100 µl rabbit serum, 100 µl ^{125}I-insulin (about 2 µU/ml), 800 µl 0.04 M phosphate buffer, pH 7.4 with 0.15 M natrium chloride and 0.5% human albumine were incubated for 48 h at 4°C. 500 µl PEG 6000 (360 g/l) was added, mixed on Rotamixer and the sample was left to stand for 1 h at 20°C.

After centrifugation for 10 min at 3000 rpm the supernatant was decanted off and scraped, ^{125}I-insulin in precipitate was counted (T). In each test was included a sample with an excess guinea-pig anti insulin (Max binding, T_M) and a sample with rabbit serum from non-immunized rabbits (Zero sample, T_0). The results were calculated as follows:

$\%B = (T-T_0)/(T_M-T_0) \cdot 100.$

Immune response to crystalline insulin

The development of insulin antibodies after immunizing rabbits with a neutral solution of the highly purified crystalline porcine insulin is shown in fig. 5. ^{125}I-insulin-binding activity above the detection limit was observed in all animals tested. When rabbits were immunized with a neutral solution of the same highly purified insulin having the same Zn-content, but where crystallization with zinc prior to the preparation of the injection solution was avoided, a decrease in antibody formation both in terms of frequency among animals and in the level of ^{125}I-insulin binding was shown (fig. 6). The composition of the preparations was exactly the same and yet a decrease in insulin antibody formation was demonstrated.

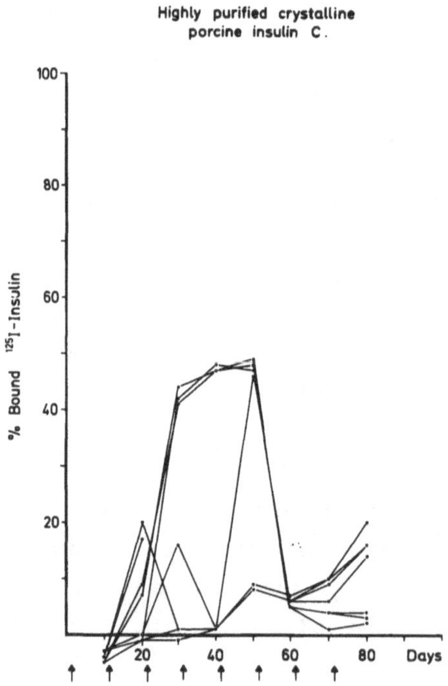

Fig. 5

Immunogenicity of highly purified crystalline porcine insulin. The highly purified porcine insulin was crystallized with zinc. The test was performed on a solution (40 IU/ml) of the compound.

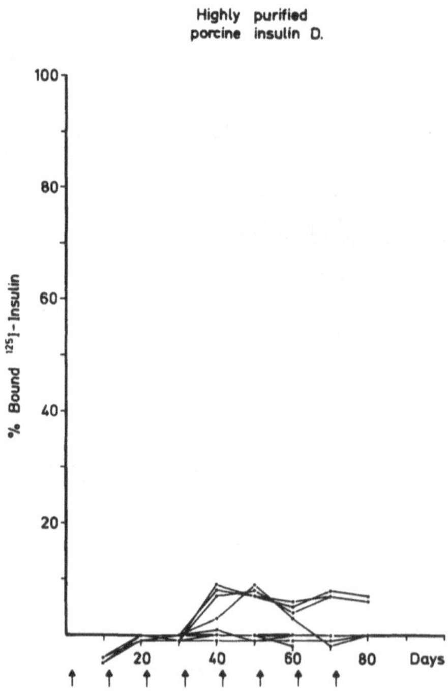

Fig. 6

Immunogenicity of highly purified porcine insulin. The highly purified porcine insulin was the same as described in fig. 5, but crystallization with zinc was omitted. The test was performed on a solution (40 IU/ml) of the compound having exactly the same composition (i.e. containing the same amount of zinc) as the one used in fig. 5.

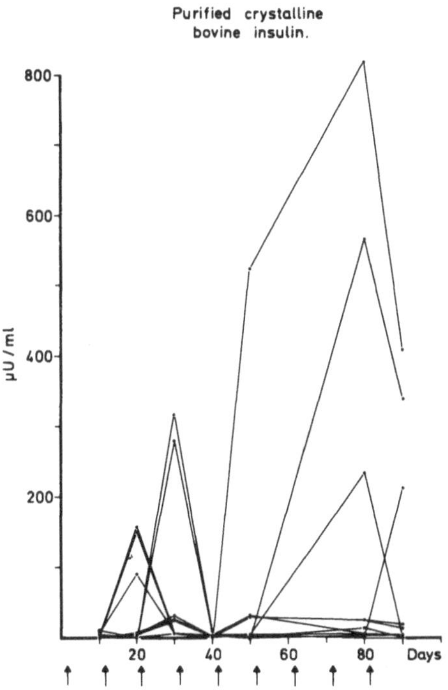

Fig. 7

Immunogenicity of highly purified crystalline bovine insulin isolated by crystallization with zinc. The test was performed on a solution (40 IU/ml) of the compound.

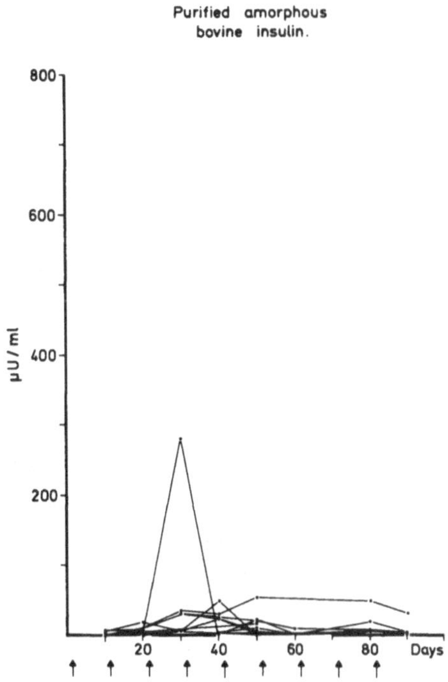

Fig. 8

Immunogenicity of highly purified bovine insulin isolated in amorphous form. The test was performed on a solution (40 IU/ml) of the compound.

Immunization experiments with soluble bovine insulin are shown in figs. 7 and 8, employing the double antibody technique for determination of insulin antibodies. The immune response to highly purified crystalline bovine insulin was positive in all animals (fig. 7). In contrast, the immunogenicity of highly purified bovine insulin isolated in amorphous form only showed a low response, even though positive in 7 out of 9 animals (fig. 8). It should be mentioned that using the PEG-precipita-technique for determining the antibody response a much higher level of insulin antibodies was found in both cases as compared to porcine insulin.

The experiments indicate that a decrease in antibody formation is not related to the purity of the insulin but might well be related to structural differences within crystallized and non-crystallized insulin preparations.

Immune response to protamine insulin

When highly purified NPH-porcine insulin was employed for immunization it was not possible to detect any insulin antibody formation throughout the test (fig. 9), even though the NPH-porcine insulin was prepared in conventional manner from highly purified crystalline porcine insulin. Apparently protamine will bind the porcine insulin in a way preventing the formation of antigenic aggregates or polymers.

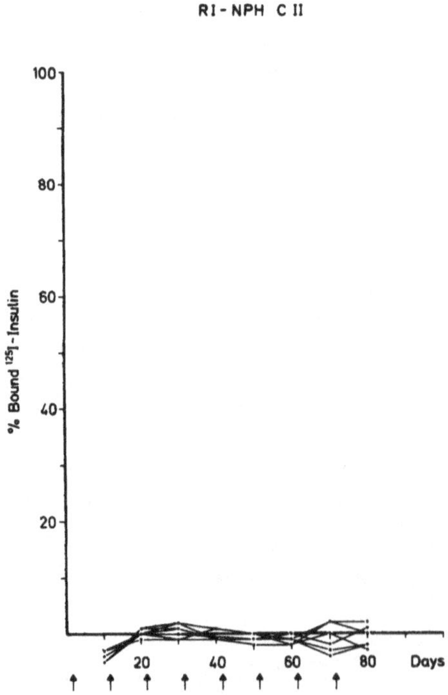

Fig. 9

Immunogenicity of NPH-porcine insulin prepared in conventional manner from highly purified crystalline porcine insulin.

The highly purified porcine insulin used for the preparation of the NPH-insulin was the same as described in fig. 5. The test was performed on a suspension (40 IU/ml) of the compound.

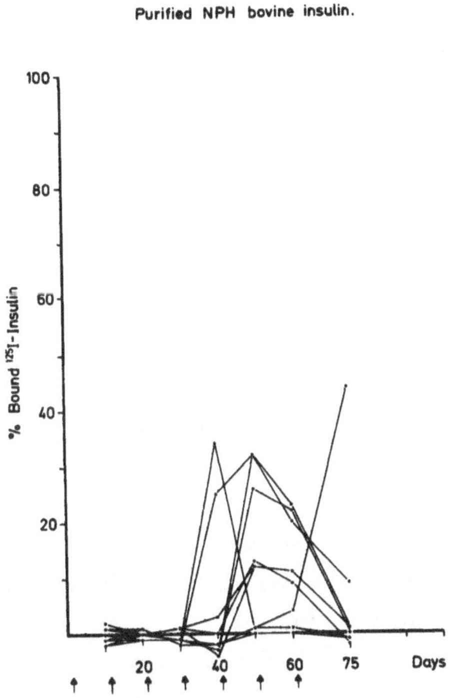

Fig. 10

Immunogenicity of NPH-bovine insulin prepared in conventional manner from highly purified crystalline bovine insulin.

The test was performed on a suspension (40 IU/ml) of the compound.

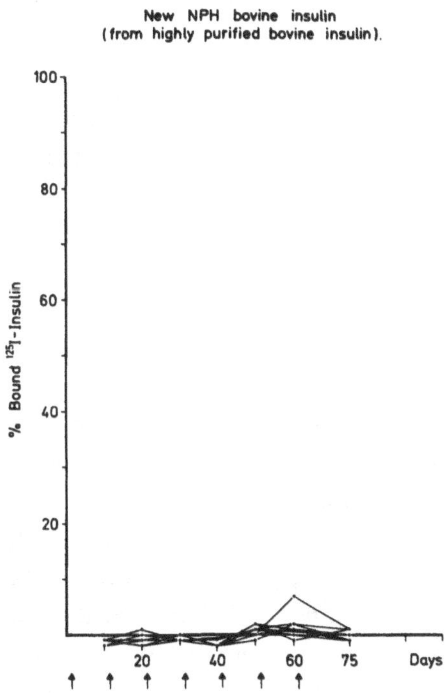

Fig. 11

Immunogenicity of New NPH-bovine insulin isolated directly from dissociating medium after reaction of the highly purified bovine insulin with protamine.

The test was performed on a suspension (40 IU/ml) of the compound.

When highly purified NPH-bovine insulin was employed it was contrary to the experiments using porcine insulin possible to demonstrate immunogenicity as shown in fig. 10. Even though the NPH-bovine insulin is prepared from highly purified crystalline bovine insulin in the same way as the porcine preparation, the binding to protamine was apparently not sufficient to prevent the formation of antigenic forms of the bovine insulin. It might also be that the antigenic compounds already formed during isolation and crystallization of the bovine insulin are bound to protamine as discussed above. Therefore, the highly purified bovine insulin was isolated directly from dissociating medium by reaction with protamine to secure that a monomeric bovine insulin will be bound. Experiments with this preparation showed that insulin antibodies could not be detected (fig. 11).

Conclusion

From these studies of the physico-chemical behaviour of insulin under various conditions and the immunogenicity of the different insulin preparations we may postulate the hypothesis that the immunogenicity of insulin is dependent on the molecular state of the molecule. If the insulin molecule is treated in a manner avoiding contemporary high concentration and avoiding the introduction of the crystallization procedure with zinc, or when the insulin in the isolation phase in a monomeric state is bound to protamine it is possible to diminish or even eliminate the immune response, at least in rabbits. Thus, we may conclude that immunogenic determinants of insulin may be expressed during the isolation procedure and that the native insulin monomer by itself may be only a weak immunogene.

References

1. Berson, S.A., Yalow, R.S., Baumann, A., Rotschild, M.A. and Newerly, K.: J. clin. Invest. 35, 170-190 (1956).
2. Berson, S.A. and Yalow, R.S.: Am. J. Med. 40, 676-690 (1966).
3. Deckert, T.: Thesis. Munksgaard, Copenhagen (1964).
4. Deckert, T., Andersen, O.O. and Poulsen, J.E.: Diabetologia 10, 703-708 (1974).

5. Deckert, T.: In: Nordisk Symposium on Childhood Diabetes, Oslo Norway (1976), pp. 197-208. Published by Nordisk Insulinlaboratorium.

6. Fankhauser, S.: Schweiz. Med. Zeitschrift 106, 1218-1225 (1976).

7. Chance, R.E., Root, M.A. and Galloway, J.A.: Acta Endocrinol. 205, 185-196 (1975).

8. Schlichtkrull, J.: 5th E.F.F. Copp Lecture. University of Southern California Medical Center, March 16 (1973).

9. Schlichtkrull, J.: Horm. Metab. Res. 5 (suppl.) 134-143 (1974).

10. Neubauer, H.P. and Schöne, H.H.: Diabetes 27, 8-15 (1978).

11. Bloom, S.R.: Hormonal Contaminants of Insulin. In: Gut Hormones. Churchill Livingstone, Edinburgh, London and New York (1979), p. 318.

12. Steiner, D.F. and Oyer, P.E.: Proc. Nat. Acad. Sci., USA, 57, 473-480 (1967).

13. Steiner, D.F., Hallund, O., Rubenstein, A., Sooja, C. and Bayliss, C.: Diabetes 17, 725-736 (1968).

14. Steiner, D.F., Kemmler, W., Clark, J.L. Oyer, P.E. and Rubenstein, A.H.: The biosynthesis of insulin. In: Handbook of Physiology, sect. 7, Endocrinology I. Am. Physiol. Soc., Washington D.C. (1972), pp. 175-198.

15. Klostermeyer, H. and Humbel, R.E.: Angew. Chem., Int. Ed. (Engl.) 5, 807-811 (1966).

16. Adams, M.J., Blundell, T.L.,Dodson, E.J., Dodson, G.G., Vijayan, M., Baker, E.N., Harding, M.M., Hodgkin, D.C., Rimmer, B. and Sheat, S.: Nature 224, 291-495 (1969).

17. Schlichtkrull, J.: Dissertation. Munksgaard, Copenhagen (1958).

18. Jeffrey, P.D.: Biochemistry 13, 4441-4447 (1974).

19. Cunningham, L.W., Fisher, R.L. and Vestling, C.S.: J. Am. Chem. Soc. 77, 5703-5707 (1955).

20. Brunfeldt, K., Hansen, B. and Nielsen, J.H.: Acta Endocrinol. 61 (no. 3), 561-576 (1969).

21. Arquilla, E.R., Thiene, P., Brugman, T., Ruess, W. and Sugiyama, R.: Biol. J. 175, 289-297 (1978).

22. Valdes, I., Michalski, R.E., Thompson, R. and Arquilla, E.R.: Diabetes 29 (suppl. 2), 36a. Abstract no. 142.

23. Ando, T. and Watanabe, S.: Int. J. Protein Res. 1, 221-224 (1969).

24. Dixon, G.H. and Smith, M.: Progr. Nucl. Acid Res. 8, 9-34 (1968).

25. Ling, V., Jugil, B. and Dixon, G.H.: J. Biol. Chem. 246, 1168-1176 (1971).

26. Krayenbühl, C. and Rosenberg, Th.: Crystalline protamine Insulin. Report: Steno Memorial Hospital, Copenhagen (1946), pp. 60-73.

27. Andersen, O.O., Brunsfeldt, K. and Abildgaard, F.: Acta Endocrinol. 69, 195-208 (1972).

28. Desbuquois, B. and Aurbach, G.D.: J.Clin.Endocrinol. 33, 732-738 (1971).

29. Unpublished method, developed by J. Vikelsøe.

30. Vini, A.I., Joffe, B.I. and Seftel, H.C.: South African Med. 1976, p. 587.

POTENTIATION OF INSULIN IMMUNOGENICITY BY DIFFERENT TYPES OF ADJUVANT

H. P. Neubauer and H. H. Schöne
Hoechst Aktiengesellschaft
D-6000 Frankfurt 80, Federal Republic of Germany

In an effort to elucidate the immunogenic properties of insulin we have hyperimmunized hundreds of animals belonging to nine different species within the last 6 or 7 years. All kinds of insulin preparations were subjected to our investigations and part of the results have been published elsewhere.

However, the variability of problems to be tackled on one hand, and the abundance of immunological data obtained on the other, provide an excellent opportunity to study other phenomena and parameters connected with antibody development in receptor animals. It is generally accepted that the insulin molecule in itself with its 51 amino acids constitutes a rather weak immunogen. Therefore, in endeavouring to imitate the immunological processes observed in diabetic patients while under insulin therapy, it becomes mandatory to administer in most animal studies insulin preparations in combination with an immune-stimulatory drug.

Besides the complete adjuvant of Freund (CFA) the incomplete adjuvant of Freund and polyacrylic acid in combination with insulin have been tested with the purpose to achieve an increase of immunological response. Based upon the fact that an even more pronounced stimulation of the immune-system will result, if the rather small insulin molecule is being plugged upon a larger protein molecule as a sort of haptene, we asked for the cooperation of our synthesis department to conjugate

Basic and Clinical Aspects of Immunity to Insulin

bovine insulin with BSA.* This conjugate was mixed with complete adjuvant of Freund and administered to a collective of six sheep and six goats.

In order to achieve a certain degree of standardization which would allow comparison of results obtained, a rather rigid <u>experimental design</u> (Fig. 1) was adopted for the performance of most of these investigations. As a rule the insulin treatment was initiated with 1 IU/kg bodyweight, followed by booster doses at weekly intervals. To avoid a suppression of incipient antibodies, it was deemed necessary to reduce the weekly insulin doses logarithmically up to the fifth injection. From here on the uniform amount of 0.2 IU/kg bodyweight was administered till the end of the trials which generally lasted over a period of 12 weeks. Only the first five insulin doses within each series were mixed with an equal volume of the respective adjuvant immediately prior to injection; between the 6th and 12th week no adjuvant was added. The insulin injections were given by the subcuta-

Time of Injection	Insulin Doses	Mode of Application
1. Day	1 IU/Kg	• Complete Freunds Adjuvant
8. "	0,5 "	• "
15. "	0,25 "	• "
22. "	0,125 "	• "
29. "	0,0625 "	• "
From then on 0,2 IU/Kg once every week for at least 12 weeks		
Antibody determination by Radioimmuno-Assay according to Meade and Klitgaard		

Fig. 1

Immunization Schedule

*The authors would like to take the occasion and at this point thank Drs. Geiger and Wissmann for their excellent assistance in this matter.

neous or intradermal route. Prior to the administration, a blood sample was withdrawn and the plasma content of specific antibodies was determined by means of radioimmunoassay.

In the case of the conjugated insulin preparations only, the customary method was abandoned in favour of a procedure described in literature. According to this, rather small doses of conjugated hormone were mixed with adjuvant and the combination was administered at intervals of 10 days, whereby half of the individual dose was given intradermally or subcutaneously and the other half intramuscularly. The initial insulin bolus contained 1 mg of the hormone per goat or sheep and all the following booster doses contained 0.5 mg insulin per animal. In general, one initial and two booster doses sufficed to yield high antibody titers in most cases.

The results obtained give unmistakable proof that insulin alone is not sufficient to stimulate antibody production in the species used in the present investigations, i.e. when administered over a relatively short period of 12 weeks. Neither dogs (Fig. 2), nor swine (Fig. 4) and sheep (Fig. 3) responded with antibody development following the systematic inoculation of the otherwise highly immunogenic bovine hormone within this fixed period.

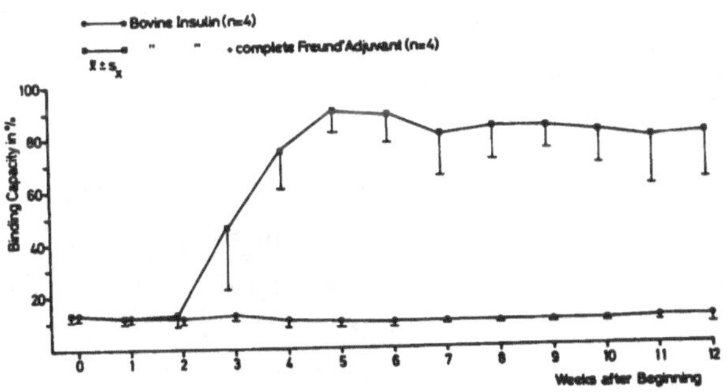

Fig. 2

Influence of Adjuvant on the Development of Antibodies against Heterologous Insulin in Dogs

Therefore, we decided to prolong the immunization procedure for this collective of sheep to six month

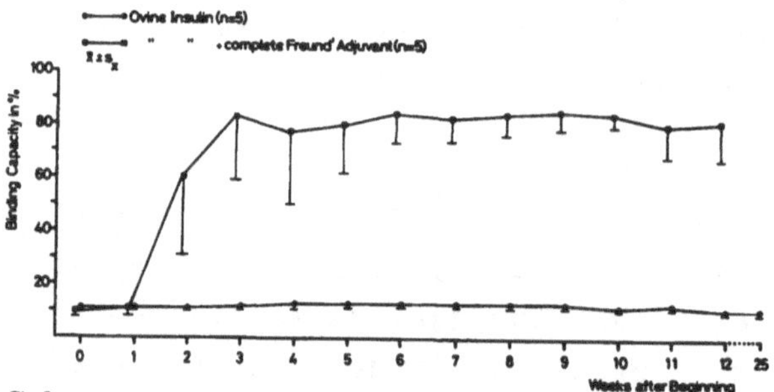

Fig. 3

Influence of Adjuvant on the Development of Antibodies against Insulin in Sheep

but as also demonstrated in Fig. 3 to no avail.

However, in all three species mentioned the addition of complete Freund adjuvant resulted in an acute rise in antibody production within 3 or 4 weeks after the initial dose (Fig. 2 - 4).

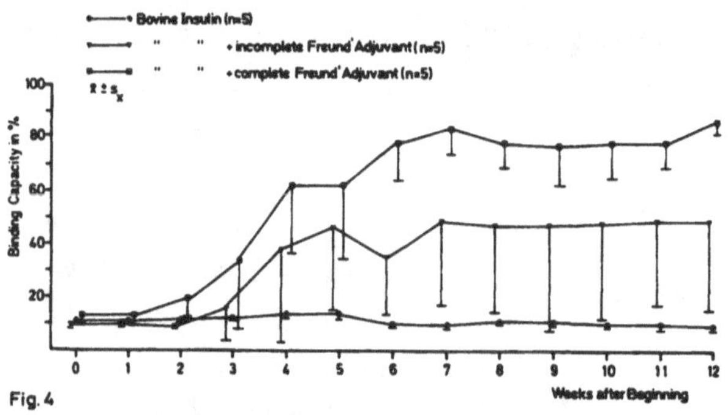

Fig. 4

Influence of Adjuvant on the Development of Antibodies against Heterologous Insulin in Pigs

In another series of experiments we made an attempt to compare the immune stimulating effects between complete and incomplete Freund adjuvant in pigs. The absence of Mycobacteria from the adjuvant seems to exert a distinct influence upon antibody production if compared to CFA. As demonstrated in Fig. 4, there is a significant difference in tracer binding between the two groups. Again, as already mentioned, no stimulation of antibody development without adjuvant could be observed.

Earlier investigations had revealed that polyacrylic acid derivatives are causing a distinct activation of T-Lymphocytes. Suggestion was made that this group of chemical substances might also stimulate immune response against weak immunogens in receptor animals. Because of its well-defined chemical structure and the excellent methods of assays available for detection, insulin was figured to be a suitable immunogen for investigations in this field of endeavour. The results of this study showed that polyacrylic acid stimulates antibody development in dogs, though to a much lesser degree (Fig. 5). Out of five dogs, only two responded to the insulin injections with antibody formation, but the tracer binding capacity was much lower in comparison to the effect of CFA and the period of immunological latency was extented. In other words polyacrylic acid proved to be a rather weak adjuvant and, therefore, unfit for promoting immune response at least during the 12 week observation period.

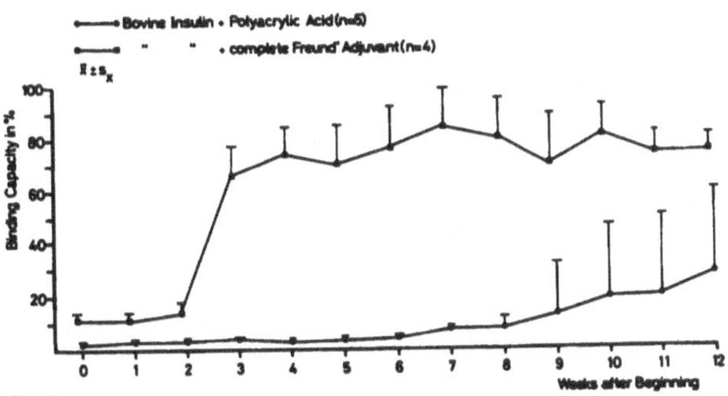

Fig. 5

Influence of Polyacrylic Acid on the Development of Antibodies against Heterologous Insulin in Dogs

The BSA conjugated insulin in combination with complete Freund's adjuvant proved also to be highly immunogenic . In response to the administration of the preparation, an acute rise in insulin antibody development occured. In antibody dilution tests a much higher titer could be determined in comparison to sera from earlier experiments using unconjugated insulins, but they did not reach our expectations.

Therefore, it was surprising that another hormone, in both structure and molecular weight quite similar to insulin, did yield different results when used in the same experimental design. Hyperimmunization of two sheep with Relaxin resulted in a rapid rise in antibody production and even dilutions of 1 : 1 Mill. were left with enough avidity to allow approximately 95 % tracer binding (Fig. 6).

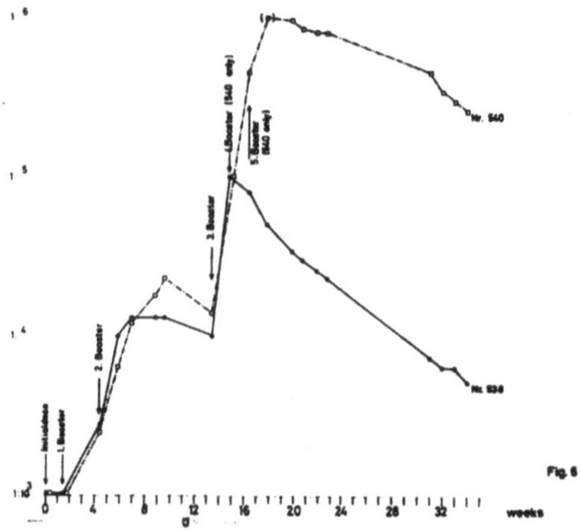

Development of Antibodies against Relaxin in Sheep

It should be noted, that the Relaxin was isolated from ovaries of pregnant sows by Dr. Schwabe, Charleston, South Carolina, and the conjugation with BSA was performed by Drs. Geiger and Wissmann.

The fact that the chemical structure of Relaxin has a distinct similarity to that of the insulin molecule permits the assumption that it will receive more attention in the field of immunology also.

In summarizing the results obtained one can conclude that:

1.) The insulin molecule is a weak immunogen. In dogs, sheep and pigs no immune response could be observed within the 12-week study period, i.e. when used without an adjuvant.

2.) From all adjuvants tested, the complete adjuvant of Freund (CFA) best potentiated the immunogenicity of insulin.

3.) The incomplete adjuvant showed a distinctly lower immune stimulatory effect in comparison to the complete form.

4.) Polyacrylic acid is not satisfactory when used as an adjuvant.

5.) Hyperimmunizations with BSA-conjugated Relaxin in combination with CFA yield anti-Relaxin antibodies with an extremely high titer of dilution.

USE OF MODIFIED INSULINS FOR THE SEPARATION OF INSULIN ANTIBODIES BY AFFINITY CHROMATOGRAPHY

K.-G. Petersen, K. Schlüter, A. Schüttler[δ] and D. Brandenburg[δ]
Medizinische Universitätsklinik, 78oo Freiburg,
δDeutsches Wollforschungsinstitut, D-51oo Aachen,
Federal Republic of Germany

Introduction

Affinity immunoadsorbent fractionation has been widely used to purify antibodies and antigens and to characterize binding sites (1, 5). With regard to insulin such studies have not been reported.

We have now studied the commercially available epoxy-activated sepharose 6 B as matrix for affinity chromatography of guinea pig anti-bovine insulin antibodies. Bovine insulin, des B1-3, 4 pyr bovine insulin, des A1-B1 bovine insulin, des octa-peptide porcine insulin and the bovine B1-B1' and B29-B29' insulin dimers were used as ligands.

Methods

5 g of epoxy-activated sepharose (pharmacia) were swollen for two hours with distilled water and washed by six fold sedimentation. 2 mg of each insulin preparation were dissolved in 5 ml 0.1 M $NaHCO_3$ buffer (0.1 M, pH: 9.5) containing NaCl (0.5 M) and added to the gel. Coupling was done at 37° C for 16 hours in a water bath shaker. Excess groups were blocked by adding ethanolamin (1 M final concentration) for 2 hours. The product was packed into columns (0.7 x 200 mm)

Basic and Clinical Aspects of Immunity to Insulin

and washed six times alternating with 50 ml of 0.03 M tris, pH 9.5 and 0.1 M acetic acid pH 4.5. When using gradients denaturation of antibodies by low pH was minimized by elution into saturated tris solution pH: 10.5. Insulin antibodies were measured by the cellulose adsorption method as described (3). Binding curves were evaluated by a modified Scatchard plot (4) with a computer program.

Results

0.1 ml of pooled anti-bovine insulin antibody serum from guinea pig ($K_1 = 2.5 \times 10^{11}$ l/M) was applied to an insulin epoxy-activated sepharose column under optimal binding conditions (pH: 8.5). The column was then eluted for 3 hours with starting buffer (0.03 M tris, pH: 8.5) followed by a stepwise pH gradient (0.1 M acetate, pH: 4.5; 0.1 glycine, pH 3.5 and 2.5 each containing 0.1 M NaCl). 2 ml fractions were collected. Serum proteins were almost quantitatively recovered in the eluates, indicating that binding by unblocked activated groups did not occur. The antibodies remained bound to the immunoadsorbent despite an environment of pH 2.5.

Identically negative results were obtained with alternative eluents: one step acetic acid pH 2.5, one step propionic acid pH 2.5, use of a chaotropic salt: sodium thio-cyanate 3 M or reduction of polarity by addition of dioxane 10 %. The antibodies remained also bound to the immunoadsorbent under these conditions when CN-Br activated sepharose 4B was used as a matrix. A small amount of antibody was eluted in the void volume after application of the serum to the column at pH 4.5 where antibody binding is partly inhibited. These negative results induced us to study the properties of modified insulins bound to the hydrophobic arm of epoxy-activated sepharose 6B.

The binding constants of the modifications are 2 to 3 decades lower compared to insulin.

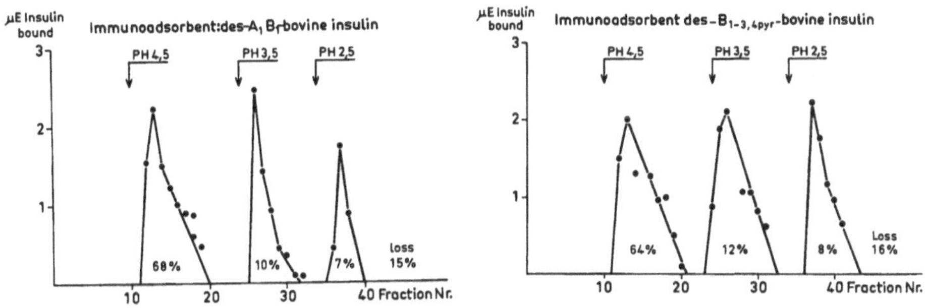

Fig. 1A and B: Separation of guinea pig anti insulin antibodies by pH gradient on immunoadsorbents with modified insulins. A = des B1-3, 4 pyr bovine insulin, B = des A1-B1 bovine insulin. Affinity constants of the eluates from A: pH 4.5, K = 5.1×10^{10} 1/M; pH 3.5, K = 0.6×10^{11} 1/M; pH 2.5, K = 1.4×10^{11} 1/M and B: pH 4.5, K = 4.2×10^{10} 1/M; pH 3.5, K = 0.8×10^{11}; pH 2.5, K = 1.1×10^{11}.

B1-3, 4 pyr bovine insulin as shown in fig. 1A retaines the antibodies completely on the column at pH 8.5. Prolonged washing did not remove any binding activity. The pH gradient removed 64% of binding activity at pH 4.5, 12 % at pH 3.5 and 8 % at pH 2.5. 16 % of the binding activity was lost. As indicated in the legend of Fig. 1 the affinity of the eluate fractions increased from 5.1×10^{10} to 1.4×10^{11} 1/M with decreasing pH.

In comparison des A1-B1' bovine insulin (figure 1B) which is biologically inactive showed nearly the same elution pattern indicating that the A1-position is more critical for metabolic effects, than for the binding of antibodies. Again the antibodies were retained completely at pH 8.5. The affinity increased like-wise slightly with decreasing pH.

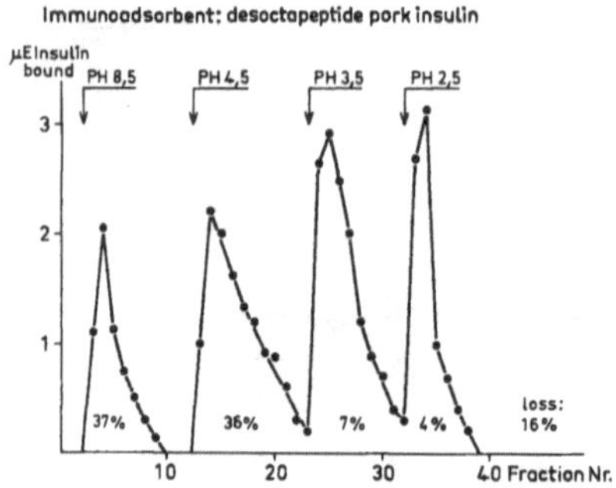

Fig. 2: Elution pattern of antibodies bound to immobilized desoctapeptide insulin. Affinity pH 8.5, K = 8.2 x 10^9 1/M; pH 4.5, K = 2.3 x 10^{10} 1/M; pH 3.5, K = 2.4 x 10^{10} 1/M; pH 2.5, K = 2.8 x 10^{11} 1/M.

Porcine desocta-peptide B23-30 insulin, has no measurable biological acitivity. Used as immunoadsorbent (figure 2) it did not completely retain the antibodies. 37% of binding activity were eluted at pH 8.5. As indicated in the legend of Fig. 2 the void volume fraction eluting at pH 8.5 has an insulin binding affinity of 8.2 x 10^9 1/M which increased with decreasing pH to 2.8 x 10^{11} 1/M.

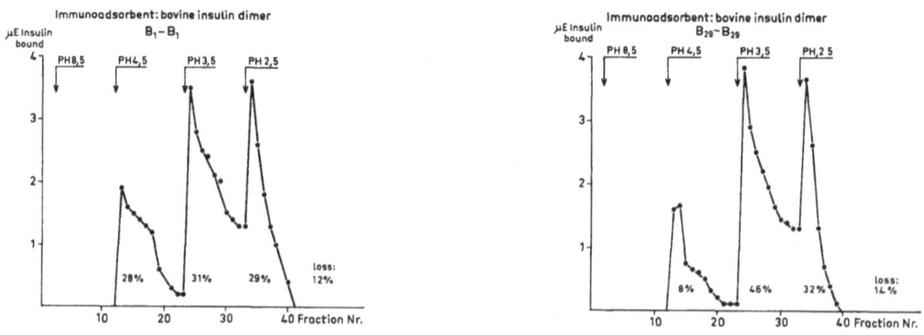

Fig. 3A and B: Separation of guinea pig anti insulin antibodies bound to B1-B1'(A) and B29-B29'(B) sepharose by a pH gradient. Affinity of the eluates to insulin, B1-B1': pH 4.5, K = 3.4 x 10^{11} 1/M; pH 3.5, K = 3.1 x 10^{10} 1/M; pH 2.5, K = 1.9 x 10^9 1/M; B29-B29': pH 4.5, K = 4.1 x 10^{10} 1/M; pH 3.5, K = 3.2 x 10^{10} 1/M; pH 2.5, K = 2.7 x 10^{10} 1/M.

The bovine insulin dimers B1-suberoyl-B1 and B29-suberoyl-B29 were also tested (Fig. 3 A, B). The antibodies were completely retained on both columns at pH 8.5. As can be seen in figures 4 and 5 the elution profiles were different. The B1-B1' bovine insulin immunoadsorbent released 28% of the antibodies at pH 4.5, while B29-B29' releases only 8% and retains the antibodies down to lower pH values. B1-B1' dimer revealed decreasing affinities with decreasing pH, while the affinities of the eluates from the B29-B29' immunoadsorbent were almost constant with decreasing pH.

Discussion

Purified antibodies are essential for the immunological characterization of insulin bound to receptors in order to reduce background activity. Purification was achieved by the use of modified insulins. Bovine insulin immunoadsorbent did not allow the purification and separation of insulin antibodies. Scatchard plots of insulin binding curves of the guinea pig antiserum pool used in the immunoadsorbent experiments reveal affinity constants of $K_1 = 2.5 \times 10^{11}$ l/M and $K_2 = 3.9 \times 10^{10}$ l/M. Des B1-3' bovine insulin has a single affinity constant two decades lower than insulin. The experiments show, that reduction of K_1 for two decades is sufficient to allow elution of antibodies bound to the immunoadsorbent by a stepwise pH gradient beginning with pH 4.5. The relation of K_1 values is similar for des A1-B1' bovine insulin.

The experiments confirm older observations that modification of the B-chain of insulin (5, 6) reduces the affinity of insulin antibodies. The decrease of affinity is obtained by both, removal of the amino-acids and covalent dimer formation. Comparing the B29-B29' and the B1-B1' dimer as immunoadsorbents there is evidence that B29-B29' retains the antibodies down to a lower pH than B1-B1'. B29-B29' is similar to the natural dimer.

Binding curves of the antibody peaks isolated at different pH from the immunoadsorbents were made with bovine insulin. The affinity constants did not in all cases increase with decreasing pH as has been demonstrated for anti HBA1 antibodies from the goat (1). A possible cause is the fact that the antibodies have been separated according to the affinity to the modified insulin. A second possibility is that binding affinities of different antibodies are not uniformly sensitive to changes of pH.

References

1. Tan-Wilson, A.L., Reichlin, M., Noble, R.W.: Immunochemistry 13, 921-927 (1976).
2. Kaplan, M.E., Kabat, E.A.: J. Exp. Med. 123, 1061-1081 (1966).
3. Kerp, L., Steinhilber, S., Kasemir, H.: Klin. Wschr. 44, 560 (1966).
4. Berson, S.A., Yalow, R.S.: J.Clin. Invest. 38, 1996 (1959).
5. Kerp, L., Steinhilber, S., Kasemir, H., Han, I., Henrichs, H.R., Geiger, R.: Diabetes 23, 651-656 (1974).
6. Kumar, D.: Diabetes 28, 994-1000 (1979)

Acknowledgments

This study was supported by the Sandoz Stiftung für therapeutische Forschung.

THE IMMUNOGENICITY OF INSULIN FROM OUR POINT OF VIEW

H. P. Neubauer and H. H. Schöne
Hoechst Aktiengesellschaft
D-6000 Frankfurt 80, Federal Republic of Germany

Ever since its discovery, the insulin molecule has been subjected to intensive research, and nowadays it may be considered as one of the best known polypeptides in the hands of scientists. In addition, there are excellent methods available for its detection; methods which allow the hormone to be traced in vitro and in vivo.

No wonder that immunologists all over the world are eager to put this interesting and well known, yet so essential substance to their use and, indeed, there seems to be an increasing tendency to employ it as a tool in immunological research.

Many a scientist is guilty of estranging such valuable prodigy from the natural purpose it was meant for, considering it mainly as an implement in their vigorous attempts to reach their goals in their special field of endeavour.

Not so with us! Pharmaceutical research and clinical therapy still regard insulin as a natural product with a very special and delicate role in the living organism, a hormone which has to be substituted in diabetic patients whenever clinical indications require such therapy.

In our view, insulin is in the first place a drug and to us the immunological aspect does not constitute an advantageous property for our type of work, but is generally recognized as a rather nasty side-effect, i.e. with some exceptions. So, the diabetologists' approach to the problem is different from the

Basic and Clinical Aspects of Immunity to Insulin

one immunologists are using, even though methods and materials are essentially of the same order. We are anxious to pinpoint the cause of antigenic behaviour and we are searching for ways and possibilities to eliminate or prevent unpleasant occurrences connected with these immunological phenomena. And this just unwraps the actual reason as to why we got engaged in this new area of research called "insulin immunology".

In order to assist in throwing additional light on the subject under discussion, we have immunized approximately 1 100 experimental animals, belonging to 9 different species. Altogether 52 different insulin preparations have been administered, extending from just once cristallized up to single component types of insulin. We wanted to know whether or not homologous insulin preparations are able to stimulate antibody production. We also were eager to find an answer as to why ruminant insulin distinguishes itself from other insulins by such a high degree of immunogenicity. Furthermore, we were interested to know which kind of influence is actually exerted by a change of pH in regard to antibody production? To what extent do adjuvants influence the immune response? Is there a dose-response-relationship and what is the threshold dose for successful immunization? Different analoga

1.) Homologous Insulins

2.) Homologous, not species-specific Insulins

3.) Heterologous Insulins

4.) Dose-Response-Relationship

5.) Time Dependence

6.) Pharmaceutical Form

7.) Modified Insulins

Fig. 1

Subjects of the Investigations

like desphe-insulin, PEG-insulin and sulfonated hormone were also subjected to our investigations and we were eager to learn how they differ from their native form in regard to immunogenicity (Fig. 1).

These and other questions demanded an answer and dictated both scope and aim of our studies.

An attempt to furnish all results most certainly would go beyond the limits of this reviewing report. Therefore, we would like to concentrate on the most important findings made so far.

We were able to prove beyond a shadow of doubt that the species-specificity of the insulin as such is decisive in regard to antigenicity. In most animal species tested, homologous hormone preparations do not stimulate antibody development, however, heterologous ones do. (Fig. 2).

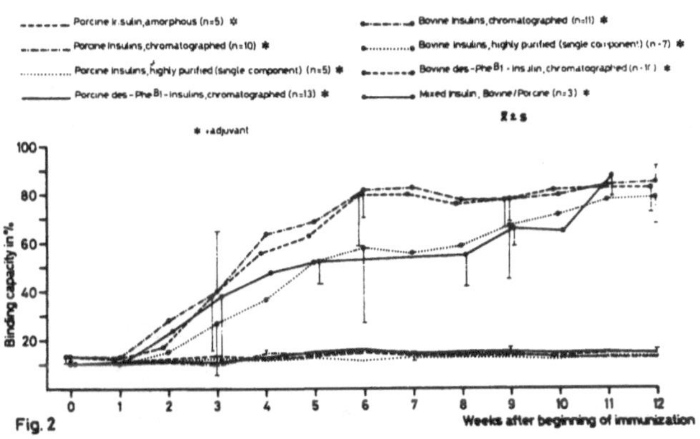

Fig. 2

Immunology of Different Insulin Preparations in Pigs

Insulins deriving from ruminants, i.e. bovine and ovine insulins, are distinguished by a relatively high degree of immunogenicity. These molecules not only provoke antibody production in pigs, dogs, monkeys and small laboratory animals, but in species they originated from as well (Fig. 3).

Let me rephrase the statement: in ruminants, even homologous insulins will stimulate antibody production. All results ob-

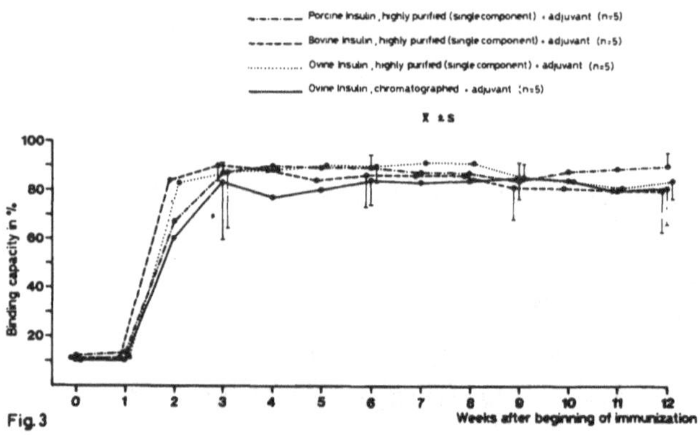

Fig. 3

Immunology of Different Insulin Preparations in Sheep

tained from comparative trials reiterated that so-called impurities of the hormone play but a minor role in regard to antigenicity. If an insulin molecule in itself is not immunogenic to a certain animal or animal species, then it will always be tolerated by this particular animal or animal species, even though impurities are present. Along the same line, insulin molecules with a certain degree of immunogenicity in individual animals of a certain species will keep this property, even if administered in a highly purified form.

However, besides the species the insulin originated from, there is another important factor in the cause of immunogenicity. Inspired by the different immunological behaviour of ruminant insulin, we became curios and, therefore attempted to get to the root of the problem by examining the dose-response-relationship.

The results of our comparative investigations gave proof that the degree of immunogenicity is directly proportional to the size of the insulin dose administered. Minute quantities of the otherwise highly immunogenic insulin from ruminants failed to stimulate antibody development. On the other hand, homologous insulin can be immunogenic in pigs, if administered in extremely high doses.

In order to be able to administer such high doses of insulin without risking hypoglycemic accidents, we used a modified insulin, namely the des-phe-des-glyform which possesses just approximately 1 - 2 per cent of the biological activity, yet behaves immunologically exactly like the natural porcine insulin.

Throughout our investigations it was confirmed that the derivatives and analoga of insulin show no difference in antibody development from the original hormone.

However, there seems to be a somewhat lower degree of antigenicity as demonstrated by the decreased avidity in the competitive binding assay.

Other studies revealed that young lambs born to hyperimmunized nanny-goats are without specific antibodies at the time of birth, but several hours after they are allowed to suckle their dams colostrum, the antibody concentration reaches values comparable to the values measured in the dams blood. Colostrum-deprived kids did not show an increase in binding capacity, thus proving that in goats, in contrast to humans, maternal insulin antibodies are transferred from nanny to offspring only via colostrum.

These are only a few of the highlight of our continuous studies on the immunology of insulin, some are still in progress (Fig. 4).

1.) HOMOLOGOUS INSULINS ARE NOT IMMUNOGENIC IN PIGS.

2.) PORCINE INSULINS DO NOT STIMULATE ANTIBODY PRODUCTION IN DOGS, MONKEYS AND RABBITS.
THIS STATEMENT IS ASCERTAINED BY LONGTIME EXPERIMENTS IN DOGS.

3.) BOVINE INSULIN IS IMMUNOGENIC IN ALL TESTED ANIMAL SPECIES, INCLUDING CATTLE.

4.) OVINE INSULIN DOES PRODUCE ANTIBODIES IN SHEEP AND GOATS.

5.) MODIFIED INSULIN AND INSULIN ANALOGA BEHAVE EXACTLY LIKE THE ORIGINAL HORMONE.

6.) HIGHLY PURIFIED INSULINS (SINGLE COMPONENT TYPE) BEHAVE IMMUNOLOGICALLY LIKE INSULINS WITH A LESSER DEGREE OF PURITY.

7.) DURATION OF THE STUDY AND PHYSICAL CHARACTERISTICS OF THE INSULIN DO NOT HAVE ANY INFLUENCE UPON ANTIGENICITY.

8.) THE IMMUNOGENICITY OF INSULIN IS DOSE-DEPENDENT.

Fig. 4

Summary

In conclusion it can be stated that there are many problems connected with the immunology of insulin and that the entire complex has to be tackled from all sides possible. We who are engaged in pharmaceutical research are glad that there are other disciplines sharing these problems with us and that we are working in the same direction with immunologists.

Section III

Chemistry to Insulin

PREPARATION OF INSULINS WITH MODIFIED N-TERMINALS BY SEMI-SYNTHESIS AND CHEMICAL MODIFICATION OF THE NATIVE HORMONE

Dietrich Brandenburg, Hans-Josef Weimann, Peter Trindler
and Achim Schüttler
Deutsches Wollforschungsinstitut
D-5100 Aachen, Federal Republic of Germany

Introduction

Homogeneous analogues and derivatives are a prerequisite for studies which try to relate the primary and tertiary structure of insulin (1) and specific molecular interactions. These are binding to cellular receptors which triggers biological or immunological responses, complex formation with antibodies, and the association of insulin monomers. Insulins with altered chemical structure are available through isolation from different species (2), by modification of the native molecule (usually bovine or porcine), or by total synthesis (Fig. 1).

From the complex primary structure of the two-chain protein it is obvious that synthesis is a very demanding task. Hence, the development of procedures for systematic alterations of the *native* molecule appeared to be a necessary and attractive alternative. The goal of this paper is to outline some of the potentials and problems of modifications concerning the *primary amino* groups. C-Terminal modification will be dealt

<u>Abbreviations</u>: Abu = aminobutyryl, Boc = tert. butyloxycarbonyl, Cit = citraconyl, DEAE = diethylaminoethyl, DMSO = dimethylsulphoxide, Msc = methylsulphoethyloxycarbonyl, Np = 4-nitrophenyl, NSu = succinimido, Ptc = phenylthiocarbamoyl, Sub = suberoyl, TFA, Tfa = trifluoro acetic acid, or -acetyl.

Basic and Clinical Aspects of Immunity to Insulin

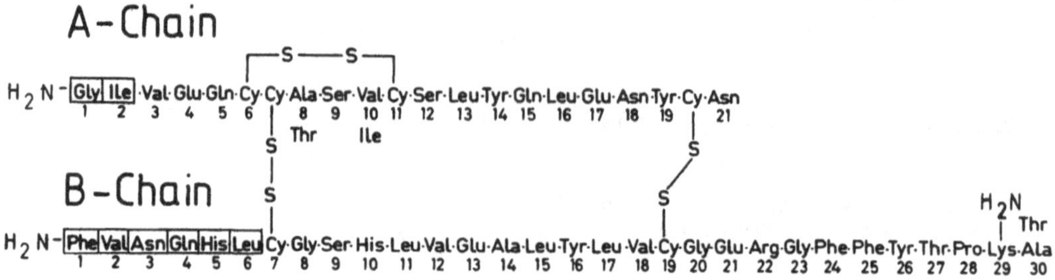

Figure 1. Primary structure of bovine insulin (2). Porcine insulin contains A8-threonine and A10-isoleucine, human insulin also B30-threonine. The 3 amino groups and the other sites of modification are indicated.

with by H.-G. Gattner (4), while total synthesis is discussed by E. Büllesbach and D. Brandenburg (5). Recent results from this Institute (Weimann (6), Trindler (7), Schüttler (8)) will be used as examples. For a complete picture of the present stand, the annual reviews on pancreatic hormones (9), the article by Geiger (10), as well as the Proceedings of the 2nd International Insulin Symposium Aachen, 1979 (11) should be consulted. Chemical and structure-function studies carried out in this Laboratory are summarized in Ref. 12.

General Aspects of Chemical Modification and Semisynthesis[x]

The 2 terminal amino groups at A1-glycine and B1-phenyl- and the ε-amino group at B29-lysine are the most important functional groups of insulin. They allow for *constructive* alterations, i.e. the addition of substituents, for *destructive* measures, i.e. shortening of the chains, or for a combination of both procedures. A further possibility is

---

[x]Semisynthesis (or partial synthesis): Alteration of the main chain(s) by coupling of amino acids or peptides, i.e. establishment of at least one peptide bond.

the introduction of new covalent bonds via bifunctional reagents.

Chemical work with this biopolymer having a molecular mass of almost 6000 daltons is facilitated, because insulin is stable over a considerable pH-range, well soluble in several organic solvents, and rather insensitive against denaturation. Native bovine and porcine insulins are available in a good state of purity. On the other hand, the two-chain structure, the presence of numerous other functional groups (6 carboxyl, 4 aromatic and 4-5 aliphatic hydroxyl, 2 imidazole, 1 guanido) and residues of limited stability (3 Cys, 3 Asn, 3 Gln) as well as the poor specificity of several reagents present major problems. Hence, the successful preparation of homogeneous products in amounts sufficient for subsequent investigations depended on the development of procedures for restricted modification, efficient purification, and critical analyses.

In terms of peptide chemistry, insulin is a trifunctional amino component. Seven products can form upon reaction with an amino-specific reagent: 3 mono-, 3 di-, and one tri-substituted. As the primary reaction is random, it leads to a complex mixture. The composition is determined by the reactivity of each group (pK-value, sterical factors), the chemical nature of the reagent, and parameters such as pH, solvent, molar ratio etc. An important step in the preparation of a given compound is therefore to vary the reaction conditions with respect to maximal yield (see, for instance, ref. 13). As most substitutions of amino groups block protonation, both analytical as well as preparative separations are usually based on charge differences between insulin and derivatives.

Strategies and Tactics

A number of modified insulins has be obtained by direct substitution of insulin with a variety of reagents, as anhydrides and activated esters of carboxylic acids and N-protected amino acids, isothiocyanates, isocyanate, imidoesters, and aryl-halides (see reviews). The reactivity of the amino groups towards p-nitrophenylesters in polar organic solvents is Gly > Lys >> Phe, while N-hydroxysuccinimide esters acylate preferentially Lys (13). Anhydrides in aqueous/organic solvents at pH 5-7 react predominantly with the N-terminals. Isothiocyanates substitute in the order Phe > Gly >> Lys. These reaction patterns show that certain derivatives cannot be obtained directly. For such cases, and particularly for all sequential operations, protecting group tactics had to be developed.

The approach of Brandenburg and Ooms (1968), which aimed at a specific modification of position B1, contained already the principle features of semisynthesis, albeit in an as yet imperfect way (14):

1. Partial reaction of insulin with phenylisothiocyanate;
2. fractionation and isolation of A1,B1-$(Ptc)_2$-insulin;
3. simultaneous removal of Phe and Gly by Edmân degradation;
4. protection of the B29 amino group (however irreversible);
5. acylation at both N-terminals with o-nitrophenylsulphenyl-Gly-ONp;
6. deprotection at A1 and B1 to give $[Gly^{B1}]$-insulin.

Protecting groups. Reversible partial protection was introduced by Borràs and Offord (15) (Tfa-groups) and Geiger (16) (Boc-groups). The application of protecting groups with different stability has opened the way to systematic and sequential alterations of insulin's structure. In contrast to peptide synthesis, protecting groups are used not only in constructive but also in destructive operations. The most important groups are listed in Table 1.

Table 1 Protecting groups for insulin

Residue	stable towards	cleaved by	Ref.
Boc = $CH_3-C(CH_3)_2-O-\overset{O}{C}-$	base	acid (TFA)	16
Cit = $HO_2C-CH = C(CH_3)-\overset{O}{C}-$	base	acid	17,18
Msc = $CH_3-SO_2-(CH_2)_2-O-\overset{O}{C}-$	acid	base	19
Tfa = $F_3C-\overset{O}{C}-$	acid	base	15
R-Met	acid, base	CNBr/ HCOOH	20,21

R = benzoyl- or ethyloxycarbonyl

Reactions. Chemical modification and semisynthesis at the N-terminals are predominantly based on two kinds of reactions: The first is acylation, which serves to introduce protecting groups, amino acids in the form of N-protected, C-terminally activated derivatives, and other residues. The second reaction is addition of the amino group to the N=C double bond of isothiocyanates, usually phenylisothiocyanate, to give a substituted thiourea derivative. The two approaches are outlined in Fig. 2. While coupling of amino acids (left) leads to an elongation of the native peptide chain, Edman degradation (right) brings about a shortening by one amino acid residue. A great variety of modifications is possible through the combination of both procedures and their sequential application.

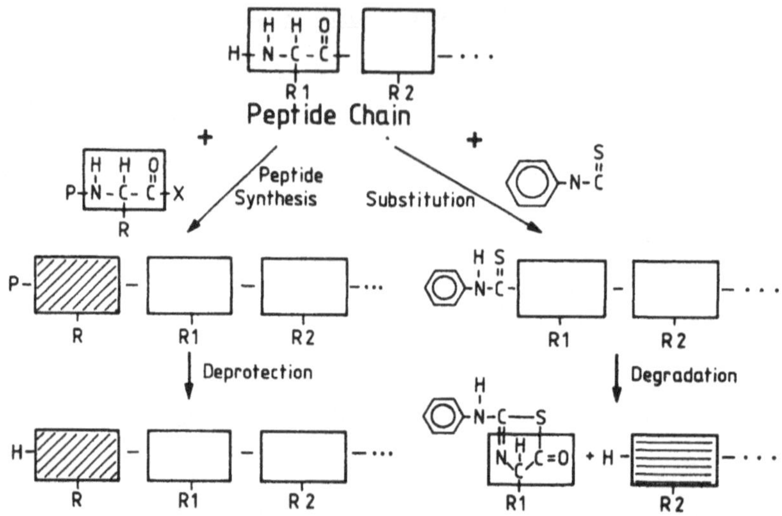

Figure 2. The principal reactions in chemical modification and semisynthesis: Peptide synthesis (left) and Edman degradation (right). P = protecting group, X = activating residue, $R-R^2$ = amino acid side chains.

N-Protected Insulin Derivatives

When insulin is reacted with Msc-ONSu, the A1,B29-disubstituted derivative is the main product (19). Reaction with 2 equivalents in dimethylsulphoxide/base gave 5 % mono-, and 20% tri-Msc-insulin (6) (Fig. 3, left). The mixture was first fractionated according to substitution degree. Urea, the usual additive in ion exchange separations of insulin, was successfully replaced by isopropanol. This led to a facilitation of work-up and an increase of yields. While the tri- and di-Msc-insulins (Fig. 4) were already homogeneous, fraction III was further resolved by ion exchange chromatography according to substitution site (23) into the two derivatives in which either A1 or B29 was substituted (Fig.4). Separations at slightly alkaline pH take advantage of the pK-differences of the three amino groups. However, as insulins usually contain variable amounts of des-amidated material (mainly at A21), a combination of ion exchange chromatography

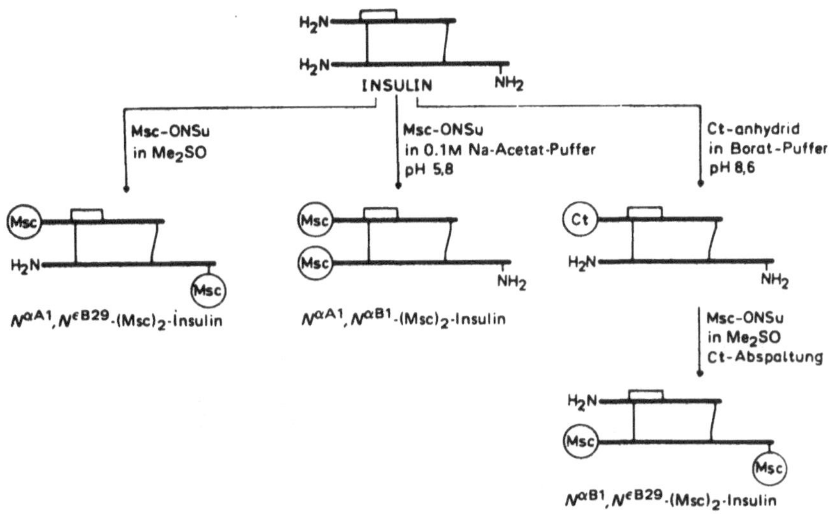

Figure 3. Preparation of the three different $(Msc)_2$-insulins (from Schüttler and Brandenburg (22)).

Table 2. Msc-Insulins

	Position	Species*	% Yield	Reference
Mono	A1	b	2.5[1]	6
		p[2]		24
	B1	p[3]	50	25
	B29	b	6[1]	6
Di	A1,B1	b	60	8, 22
	A1,B29	b	60	6, 8, 19, 22
	B1,B29	b	20-40	7, 26[4]; 8, 22[5]
		p[6]		24
Tri	A1,B1,B29	b	8[1]	6

* b = bovine, p = porcine

1) yield not optimized, conditions for disubstitution
2) from B1,B29-$(Boc)_2$-insulin
3) from A1,B29-$(Boc)_2$-insulin
4) from A1-Boc-insulin
5) from A1-Cit-insulin
6) from Boc-insulin (crude)

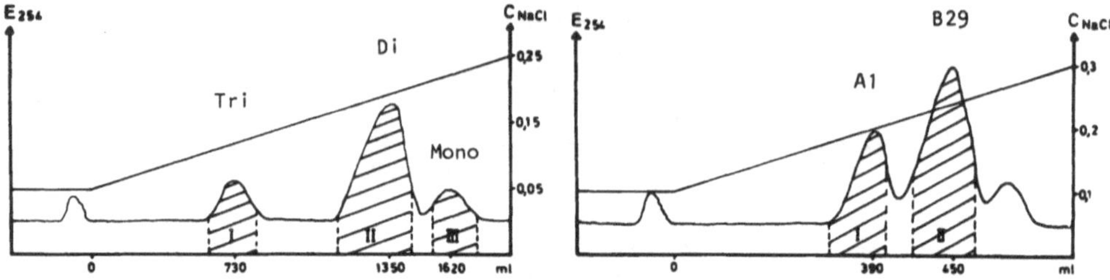

Figure 4. Fractionation of crude Msc-insulin by chromatography on SP-Sephadex (pH 3) (left) and subfractionation of mono-substituted material on DEAE-Sephadex (pH 7.4) (right) in buffers containing 40% isopropanol (6).

at acidic pH (where desamidated products behave like the corresponding insulins) and basic pH (where charge differences become effective) provides a safeguard against cross-contamination. This separation principle (23) has proved advantageous in many subsequent studies. While four of the seven possible Msc-insulins (see Tab. 2) became accessible through this route, the application of different reaction conditions, i.e. acylation in aqueous buffer containing 15% dioxane at pH 5.8 led to a marked change of primary substitution pattern (22) (Fig. 3, middle). The composition of the mixture was similar (4% mono-, 78% di-, 18% tri-Msc-insulin), but the major product was now A1,B1-$(Msc)_2$-insulin, since protonation inhibited acylation of the lysine amino group.

A preferential substitution of B1 and B29 amino groups has so far not been possible. Such derivatives became accessible either by chain combination (12) or via A1-protected intermediates (Fig. 3, right). Based on previous work (24) two procedures for the preparation of bovine B1,B29-$(Msc)_2$-insulin have been developed (7, 8, 22). The first starts with A1-Boc-insulin (10, 21, 24). The mixture from the reaction of insulin and Boc-azide in 80% methanol containing triethylamine (pH 9) gave, upon chromatography on DEAE-cellulose (pH 8.0) in 8 M urea, B1-Boc-insulin in a yield of 27%. After quantitative substitution of all free amino groups with Msc-ONSu, the Boc-group was removed.

A1-Cit-insulin (18) was used in the second approach (22). The homogeneous derivative gave, after complete substitution of B1 and B29 with the Msc moiety, and quantitative deblocking at A1, the desired B1,B29-$(Msc)_2$-insulin in high yield. Msc-insulins are listed in Table 2.

The N-Terminus of the Insulin B-Chain

Sequential Shortening (6)

The B1-amino group is particularly reactive towards phenylisothiocyanate. This allowed the selective removal of phenylalanine and the preparation of crystalline des-Phe^{B1}-insulin as the first chemically derived insulin analogue (27). For further degradation, protection of A1-glycine against simultaneous cleavage, and of B29-lysine against irreversible substitution was necessary. The acid-stable Msc-group proved to be particularly valuable (10). Six reaction cycles have sequentially been carried out (see Fig. 5), in which A1,B29-$(Msc)_2$-insulin or the corresponding shortened derivative was quantitatively reacted with a 40-fold excess of phenyl isothiocyanate in 90% pyridine, isolated, and treated with trifluoroacetic acid.

Phe^{B1} and Val^{B2} were cleaved without problems. After removal of Asn^{B3} cyclization of the N-terminal Gln^4 occured as already described by Geiger (10), necessitating special precautions and additional purifications which led to a marked decrease in yields (see Table 3). The subsequent cleavage of

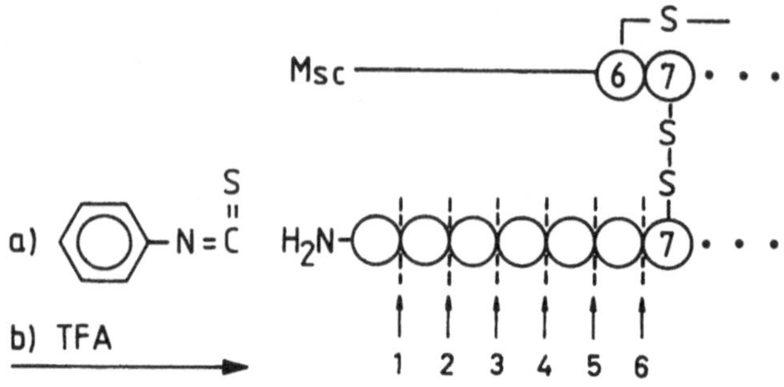

Figure 5. Stepwise cleavage of the first six amino acids from the N-terminus of the B-chain in A1,B29-$(Msc)_2$-insulins (6)

His^{B5} and finally Leu^{B6} proceeded without further difficulties. Part of each derivative was deblocked (19) to give the free analogue in amounts of about 50 mg. Chromatographic purifications were applied whenever analyses indicated the presence of contaminants. For example, five gel filtrations and three separations on SP-Sephadex (pH 3) were performed during the preparation of des-(B1-6)insulin.

Previous sequential degradation has been carried out using protection at A1 and B29 with the acid-labile Boc-group (3 cycles) (10), the phtaloyl group (5 cycles, (10)) and methionine (20).

Semisynthesis at the N-terminus of the B-chain

The shortened, protected insulin derivatives allow for semisynthetic modifications of the region B(1-6). Some of our work relates to natural variations found in this sequence. Acylation of the appropriate intermediates with an excess of activated esters of N-protected amino acids in dimethylsulfoxide led to a partial conversion of bovine insulin to insulins of other species. Peptide synthesis were carried through to ca. 80% completion in order to avoid side-reactions which occur under less mild or prolonged reaction. This

Table 3. Analogues with alterations in positions B1 - B6 (6)

Analogue	Yield (%)$^{+}$	Analogue	Yield (%)$^{+}$
des-Phe^{B1}	(56) 48	[Ala^{B1,B2}] chicken	7
des-(B1-2)	(49) 23	[Ala^{B2}] camel	4
des-(B1-3)[pGlu^{B4}]	(45) 21	des-Phe^{B1}[Ala^{B2}]	12
des-(B1-4)	(13) 6	des-(B1-2)[Lys^{B3}]	8
des-(B1-5)	(8) 4	des-(B1-3) [Lys^{B4}]	4
des-(B1-6)	(7) 3		

$^{+}$based on insulin; ( ) = yield of di-Msc derivative

strategy necessitated removal of starting material by SP-Sephadex chromatography at pH 3 and thus reduced the yields, but ensured a better quality of the analogues. B1-phenylalanine was replaced by eight different amino acids (12), the photo-activatable p-azido-Phe residue (28), and mono-iodo-des-amino tyrosine of high (420 Ci/mmole) specific activity (29).

Fig. 6 shows the reactions by which the N-terminal sequences of chicken (turkey) and camel insulin (30) were obtained in two synthetic steps (see also Table 3). Elongation of protected des-(B1-3)-insulin with $(Boc)_2$-Lys-ONSu gave the sequence of mouse/rat des(B1-2)-insulin. Coupling of this lysine derivative to des(B1-4)-insulin yielded the shortened chinchilla sequence. Amino acid analyses of the electrophoretically homogeneous analogues indicated the incorporation of the new residues in good agreement with theory.

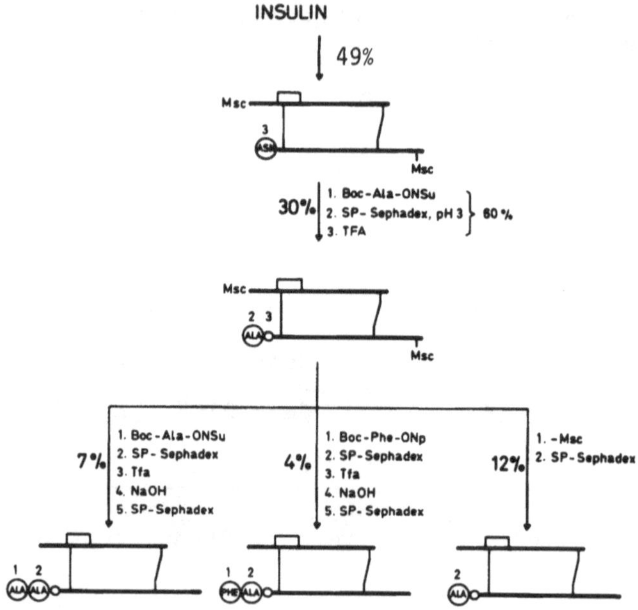

Figure 6. Semisynthetic conversion of bovine to des-Phe^{B1} camel insulin (right) and camel insulin (middle), and partial conversion to chicken insulin (left).

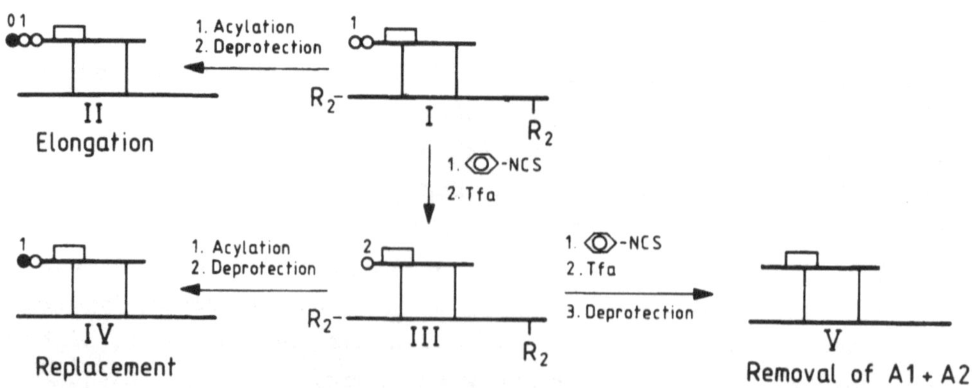

Figure 7. Scheme for sequential modification and semisynthesis at the N-terminus of the insulin A-chain.

The N-Terminus of the A-Chain

The invariant Al-glycine plays an important role in current structure-function considerations. Substitutions of the amino group have been accomplished by direct partial reaction of unprotected insulin (9,10,12). But specific reactions require elaborate strategies and the use of two protecting groups of different stability (Fig. 7). The replacement of glycine is thus a good example to illustrate the potentials of semisynthesis today. B1,B29-$(Msc)_2$-insulin (compound I, R_2 = Msc) was the suitable intermediate for a series of further modifications. Quantitative reaction with phenylisothiocyanate and Edman degradation gave protected des-Gly^{A1}-insulin (III). Purification by ion exchange chromatography (pH 3) at this stage removed small amounts of side products from three preceding steps and gave the homogeneous key intermediate III in a yield of ca. 9% (based on insulin). This could now be reacted with several activated esters of amino- and hydroxy acids, and other reagents. After deblocking a series of products (IV) was obtained in which the position A1 was systematically varied. A second degradation cycle gave, after deblocking, des-Gly,des-Ile-insulin (V). The new insulins are listed in Table 4. Previous work has mainly been concerned with the replacement of glycine by L-amino acids (Krail et al., in Ref. 12) and particularly D-amino acids, following a different route with Msc-protection (10,31), or applying methionine derivatives for blocking B1 and B29 (21).

A large group of A1-elongated analogues (II) became accessible by acylating the intermediate I (R2 = acid-labile Boc groups) with Boc-amino acids and simultaneous deblocking of all protecting groups (24).

Table 4. Insulin analogues with replacements in position A1 (7)

Analogue	Residue in position A1	% Yield a	b
[Prop^{A1}]	$CH_3-CH_2-\overset{O}{C}-$	33	2.5
[HO-Ac^{A1}]	$HO-CH_2-\overset{O}{C}-$	33	2.5
[Bu^{t}-O-Ac^{A1}]	$(CH_3)_3-C-O-CH_2-\overset{O}{C}-$	60	4.6
[Carb^{A1}]	$H_2N-\overset{O}{C}-$	28	2.2
[γ-Abu^{A1}]	$H_2N-(CH_2)_3-\overset{O}{C}-$	19	1.4
[D-Pro^{A1}]	D-Pro-	19	1.4
[Am^{A1}]	$H_2N \overset{+}{-} \overset{NH_2}{C}-$	14	1.1
[Aci^{A1}]	$H_3C-\underset{+NH_2}{C}-$	20	1.5

a based on B1,B29-(Msc)$_2$-des-Gly^{A1}-insulin, b based on insulin

Intermolecular Crosslinking

The modifications discussed so far concern individual, separated sites. By application of *bifunctional reagents* new types of derivatives can be obtained. Intramolecular crosslinking of unprotected insulin has been studied in considerable detail, and both A1-B29- as well as a few A1-B1-crosslinked insulins have been isolated in homogeneous form (for revies, see Geiger (10) and Brandenburg et al. (32)). Our attention has now focussed on the preparation of insulin *dimers* (8, 33). Crosslinking between amino groups can theoretically give six dimers, of which three are symmetrical, and three asymmetrical. The strategy developed for the unequivocal synthesis of the isomers was based on the use of the three (Msc)$_2$-insulins described above.

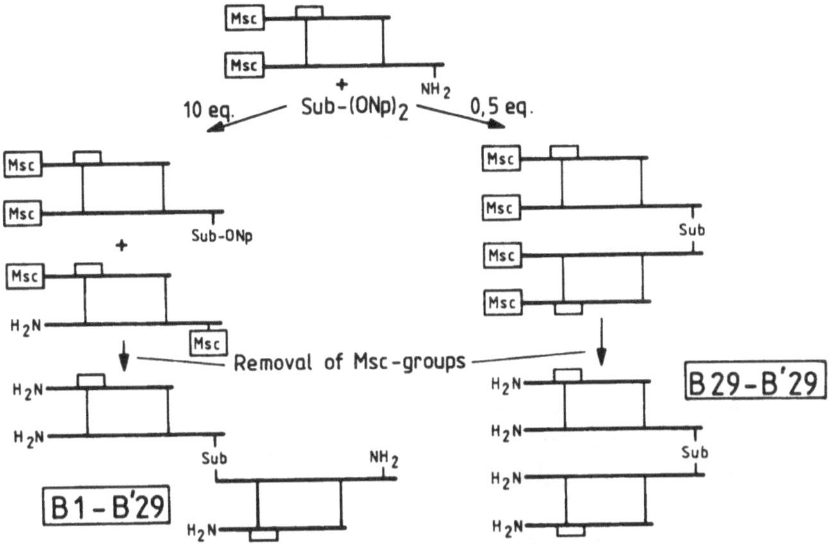

Figure 8. Scheme for the preparation of insulin dimers (8)

Symmetrical dimers. Linking the Msc-insulins was effected by reaction with bis-p-nitrophenylesters of dicarboxylic acids, mostly suberic acid, in very high concentration (ca. 40 - 50 µmol, i.e. 240 - 300 mg/ml) and a molar ratio of 2:1, in dimethylsulphoxide in the presence of base (Fig. 8). After deblocking the dimers listed in Table 5 were obtained in good yields. Purification was simple, because gel filtration clearly separated dimeric and monomeric products.

Asymmetrical dimers. A two-step procedure was developed, which is outlined in Fig. 8. The $(Msc)_2$-insulin is first reacted with a large excess of bifunctional reagent in order to effect a complete substitution at the single amino group. By subsequent gel filtration under conditions which do not affect the activated group the activated derivative is separated from excess of reagent and also a small amount (ca.10%) of symmetrical dimer. In the second step it is then condensed, at high concentration, with a different $(Msc)_2$-insulin. After gel filtration, deblocking, and a further gel filtration the three asymmetrical dimers could be isolated (see Table 5). Qualitatitive and quantitative analyses (end group determination, sulphitolyses, tryptic digestion and electrophoresis) showed that the dimers were homogeneous and that the structures were in agreement with theory.

Table 5. Symmetrical and asymmetrical insulin dimers (8)

Dimer		% Yield a	% Yield b
symmetrical	A1-Sub-A'1	45	12
	B1-Sub-B'1	42	23
	B29-Sub-B'29	58	31
asymmetrical	A1-Sub-B'1	40	10
	A1-Sub-B'29	50	15
	B1-Sub-B'29	49	11

a based on di-Msc-derivative, b based on insulin

Conclusions

The examples show that a macromolecule as complex as insulin can successfully be subjected to sequential chemical reactions. Systematic work in this and other laboratories has led to the development of efficient procedures for the preparation of defined, homogeneous insulins with altered structure. The amounts were sufficient for detailed structure-function studies (12). A major advantage of semisynthesis and chemical modification is the limited number of reaction steps necessary to obtain such molecules. However, since these approaches take place under minimal protection, numerous side reactions are possible. For example, deamidation, carbamoylation, irreversible self-crosslinking, acylation of tyrosine-OH groups and formation of pyroglutamic acid have been observed. Careful analyses and purifications have therefore been necessary to detect and eliminate side products.

With respect to the relationship between yield and effort, modification and semisynthesis compare favourably with total synthesis (5). Hence, although methods for systematic alteration of the native molecule were developing several years *after* the total synthesis of insulin, the analogues and derivatives obtained through these approaches took the lead in the elucidation of structure-function relationships. Considerable information has also become available on the effect of modification on immunological properties (see, for instance, references 34-36).

Since modification and semisynthesis are limited to the terminal regions of insulin (see also Gattner et al. (4)), these procedures are not alternatives to total synthesis (5), but supplementary routes.

Acknowledgements

This work was supported by Deutsche Forschungsgemeinschaft (Za 5/30), the Juvenile Diabetes Foundation, New York,and Ministerium für Wissenschaft und Forschung des Landes Nordrhein-Westfalen. The authors wish to thank Professor H. Zahn for his constant interest and encouragement, Mr. K. Freude for excellent experimental help, and Dr. J. Föhles for amino acid analyses.

References

1. Blundell, T., Dodson, G., Hodgkin, D. and Mercola, D.: Adv. Protein Chemistry 26, 279 - 402 (1972).
2. Blundell, T.L. and Humbel, R.E.: Nature 287, 781-7 (1980).
3. Ryle, A.P., Sanger, F., Smith L.F. and Kitai, R.: Biochem. J. 60, 541-556 (1955).
4. Gattner, H.-G., Danho, W., Knorr, R.:These Proceedings, p. 421
5. Büllesbach, E.E., Brandenburg D.: These Proceedings, p. 395
6. Weimann, H.-J.: Dr. rer. nat. Thesis, Technische Hochschule Aachen (1977).
7. Trindler, P.: Dr. rer. nat. Thesis, Technische Hochschule Aachen (1980).
8. Schüttler, A.: Dr. rer. nat. Thesis, Technische Hochschule Aachen (1979).
9. Brandenburg, D.: Pancreatic hormones; in "Aminoacids, peptides and proteins" (R. Sheppard, Ed.), The Chemical Society, London, Vol. 9, pp. 462-475 (1978).

   Brandenburg, D. and Saunders, D.: ibid. Vol. 10, 432-451 (1979).

   Brandenburg, D., Saunders, D., and Rudolph, B.E.: ibid. Vol. 11, (1981).
10. Geiger, R.: Chem. Z. 100, 111 - 129 (1976)
11. Brandenburg, D., Wollmer, A.(Eds.), Insulin: Chemistry, structure and function of insulin and related hormones, W. de Gruyter, Berlin, New York (1980)
12. Brandenburg, D.: 7th Int. Symp. Medicinal Chemistry, Torremolinos, 1980 (Editors: Vega, S., and de Las Heras, F.G.), Pergamon Press, Oxford, in press.
13. Friesen, H.-J.: Ref. 11, pp. 125 - 133
14. Brandenburg, D., and Ooms, H.A.: Proc. Int. Symp. Protein and Polypeptide Hormones, Liège (1968). Excerpta Medica, Int. Congr. Ser. 161, 482 - 484 (1968).
15. Borrás, F., Offord, R.E.: Nature 227, 716 - 718 (1970).
16. Geiger, R., Schöne, H.-H., Pfaff, W.: Hoppe Seyler's Z. Physiol. Chem. 352, 1787 - 1790 (1971)
17. Zahn,H., Brandenburg, D., Gattner, H.-G.: Diabetes 21, Suppl. 2, 468 - 475 (1972).
18. Naithani, V.K., Gattner, H.-G.: in preparation.

19. Geiger, R., Obermeier, R. und Tesser, G.I.: Chem Ber. 108, 2758 - 2763 (1975).

20. Saunders, D.J., Offord, R.: Biochem. J. 165, 479 - 486 (1977)

21. Saunders, D.J., Offord, R.E.: Hoppe-Seyler's Z. Physiol. Chem. 358, 1469 - 1454 (1977).

22. Schüttler, A., Brandenburg, D.: Hoppe-Seylers Z. Physiol. Chem., 360, 1721-1725 (1979)

23. Brandenburg, D., Gattner, H.-G., Wollmer, A.: Hoppe-Seyler's Z. Physiol. Chem. 353, 599 - 617 (1972).

24. Friesen, H.-J.: Dr. rer. nat. Thesis, Technische Hochschule Aachen (1976).

25. Geiger, R., Geisen, K., Summ, H.-D. und Langner, D.: Hoppe-Seyler's Z. Physiol. Chem. 356, 1635 - 1649 (1975)

26. Saunders, D.J., Brandenburg, D.: Hoppe-Seyler's Z. Physiol. Chem., submitted for publication.

27. Brandenburg, D.: Hoppe-Seyler's Z. Physiol. Chem. 350, 741 - 750 (1969).

28. Thamm, P., Brandenburg, D. in: 'Peptides 1978' (Eds. Siemion, I.Z., Kupryszewski, G.), Wroclaw University Press, Poland, pp. 639-642 (1979).

29. Bahrami, S., Zahn, H.,Brandenburg, D., Machulla, H.-J., Dutschka, K.: Radiochem.Radioanal.Let.45, 221-226 (1980).

30. Danho, W.O., Gattner, H.-G., Nissen, D., Zahn, H.: Hoppe-Seyler's Z. Physiol. Chem. 356, 1405 - 1412 (1975).

31. Geiger, R., Geisen, K., Regitz, G., Summ, H.-D. and Langner, D.: Hoppe-Seyler's Z. Physiol. Chem. 361, 563 - 570 (1980)

32. Brandenburg, D., Gattner, H.-G., Schermutzki, W., Schüttler, A., Uschkoreit, J., Weimann, J. and Wollmer, A.: in "Advances in Experimental Medicine & Biology" (M. Friedman, Ed.), Vol. 86A, Plenum Publ. Corp. New York. pp. 261-282 (1977).

33. Schüttler, A., Brandenburg, D.: Ref. 11, pp. 143 - 149.

34. Kerp, L., Henrichs, H.R., Kasemir, H.: Handbook of Exp. Pharmacology, New Series, Vol. 32/2 (Born, G.V.R., Eichler, O., Farah, A., Herken, H., Welch, A.D., Eds.), Springer, Berlin, Heidelberg, pp. 593 - 653 (1975).

35. Keck, K., Jäger, K., Geiger, R., Brandenburg, D., Gattner, H.-G.: Ref. 11, pp. 611 - 617.

36. Dron, D.I., Jones, R.H., Sönksen, P.H., Thomas, J.H., Brandenburg, D.: Diabetologia 18, 59 - 63 (1980).

SYNTHESIS OF INSULIN ANALOGUES

Erika E. Büllesbach and Dietrich Brandenburg

Deutsches Wollforschungsinstitut
D-5100 Aachen, Federal Republic of Germany

Introduction

Since the first total synthesis of insulin by Zahn et al.,[1] Katsoyannis et al.,[2] and Du et al.[3] in 1963-65, there has been a rising interest in the synthesis of this proteohormone and its analogues. The major reason is the important physiological role of insulin and the steady increase of diabetes mellitus. In order to obtain information on the mode of action, on metabolism, and relations between the structure and biological activity as well as immunological properties, insulins with altered structure are of particular importance.

A further chemical reason is the complex primary structure of insulin, which makes this molecule a critical touchstone for the test of new synthetic methods of peptide and sulphur chemistry.

Three different routes have been developed for the preparation of insulin and its analogues:

1. Most recently, biosynthesis of separate A- and B-chains has been accomplished via genetical engineering[4]. Details beyond the microgram scale have not yet been published, but analytical data of biosynthetic human insulin and results of first biological and clinical tests have been reported[5]. This approach is limited to the amino acids contained in the genetic code and their assembly in linear sequence. Insulin analogues have not yet been obtained.
2. Semisyntheses with native insulin (see Brandenburg et al.[6]

Basic and Clinical Aspects of Immunity to Insulin

and Gattner et al.[7]) are efficient procedures for the preparation of analogues, but modifications are generally limited to terminal regions of the molecule, i.e. those outside the disulphide ring structure.
3. For deliberate sequential alterations at any site, the universal, although highly demanding, total synthesis remains the only route. "Total synthesis" also includes the preparation of insulins from one synthetic and one natural chain.

The scope of the present paper is to summarize advances of total synthesis between 1975 and 1980. It covers, with a small overlap, the work published since the review of Geiger[8]. For a detailed discussion of the previous syntheses the review of Lübke and Klostermeyer[9] should be consulted. Annual reviews on insulin chemistry appear in the Specialist Periodical Reports (see ref. 10). This paper is limited to syntheses which produced analogues or insulin; it makes a short reference to proinsulin, syntheses of separate chains, and some other methodological advances, but does not include the preparation of smaller peptides.

General Aspects of Synthesis

The synthesis of the bicyclic two-chain molecule requires the formation of 49 peptide bonds and 3 disulphide bonds and thus necessitates much more complex strategies and protecting group tactics than in the case of normal linear polypeptides[11-13]. Principally, there are three different possibilities:

1. Synthesis of separate A- and B-chains, and subsequent combination.
2. Synthesis of the whole molecule using asymmetrical disulphide peptides.
3. Synthesis of a single chain molecule, such as proinsulin, and its conversion to insulin in analogy to biosynthesis.

Strategy and tactics. The first and subsequent syntheses of ovine, bovine and human insulin[1-3,8,9] were, until 1974, accomplished according to strategy 1. It was obvious to follow these routes for the preparation of insulins with alterations in one chain, and to combine the synthetic chain analogue with a partner chain from natural origin. The strategies for chain synthesis, namely the design and tactics, i.e. the selection of protecting group combinations and coupling methods, were based on the experience previously gained. Important factors are the accessibility of amino acid derivatives, known or expected coupling yields and side-reactions, solubility, possibilities for purification, multiple use or facile further modifications of peptides.

All chains and complete insulin molecules have been obtained by first synthesizing smaller peptides (segments) and joining these afterwards, usually according to the C→N strategy, i.e. starting with the C-terminal segment. Syntheses were generally performed in solution. This technique allows for analysis and purification on each step, e.g. by crystallization, gel filtration or counter current distribution. The assembly of insulin chains by stepwise solid phase synthesis[8,9] has previously been used by Weitzel for an extensive screening of insulin with respect to structure-function relationships[8]. However, products of adequate purity, and homogeneous analogues have not yet been obtained. The principle disadvantage of the otherwise elegant technique is the accumulation of side products, due to non-quantitative reactions, and the low chances for their final removal. First positive results have been reported for joining segments on a resin (see below).

Formation of a peptide bond is a reaction between an amino group and an activated carboxyl group (Fig. 1). In order to establish each of the 20 A-chain bonds and the 29 B-chain bonds unequivocally, other α-amino and α-carboxyl, as well as

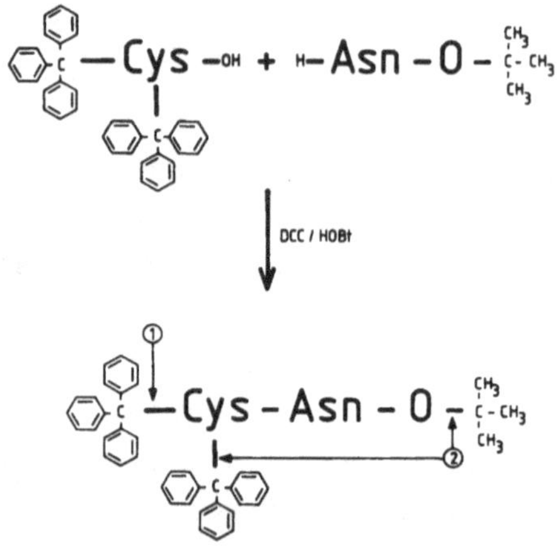

Fig. 1: Synthesis of the protected dipeptide Trt-Cys(Trt)-Asn-OBu^t from Trt-Cys(Trt)OH and H-Asn-Obu^t [16].
1 = The temporary protecting group is removed from the α-amino group with 80% acetic acid. The S-Trt and OBu^t groups are stable under these conditions.
2 = The semi-permanent protecting groups S-Trt and OBu^t are removed upon completion of the A-chain with trifluoroacetic acid in the presence of thiol[17-20].
Coupling in this case was effected by dicyclohexylcarbodiimide/hydroxybenzotriazole. Other methods of activation used for the synthesis of insulin chains were formation of azide, activated esters, mixed anhydrides.

all functional side-chain groups which are likely to interfere, have to be protected. Temporary protection lasts for one or a few reaction cycles, while semi-permanent protection is used to block side-chains and the ultimate carboxyl groups (A21,B30) until the completion of the whole sequence. Temporary protecting groups have to be cleavable under conditions which do not affect the semi-permanent groups, and these should be removable without damage to the assembled peptide chain, and preferably in a single step.

In all syntheses according to strategy 1, the four cysteines of A-chains, or both cysteines of B-chains were protected with one type of a semipermanent group. This choice largely determined the overall tactics, and thus research on sulphur

Table 1: Protecting groups used in insulin synthesis and conditions for deprotection.

Funct. group	Protect. group	Deprotection acid	basic	H_2/Pd	Na/NH_3	other
NH_2	Z	+	-	+	+	-
	Boc	++	-	-	-	-
	Bpoc	+++	-	-	-	-
	Trt	++++	-	-	-	-
	Nps	+++	-	-	-	Thiol
	Tos	+	-	-	+	-
COOH	OMe	-	+	-	-	N_2H_4
	ONBzl	-	+	+	+	-
	OBzl	+	+	+	+	-
	OBu^t	++	-	-	-	-
OH	Bzl	+	-	+	+	-
	Bu^t	++	-	-	-	-
imid-azole	Bzl	-	-	+	+	-
	Tos	+	-	-	-	-
guánido	NO_2	+	-	+	+	-
	Tos	+	+	-	-	-
SH	Bzl	(+)	-	-	+	-
	Dpm	+	-	-	+	-
	Trt	++	-	-	+	J_2
	Acm	-	-	-	-	J_2
	Thp	-	-	-	-	$(SCN)_2$
	S-Alk	-	-	-	+	RSH,SO_3^{--}
	$(Cys)_2$	-	-	-	+	RSH,SO_3^{--}
	MBzl	+	-	-	+	-

Abbreviations: Acm = acetamidomethyl, Boc = tert-butyloxy-carbonyl, Bpoc = 2-(4-biphenylyl)isopropyloxycarbonyl, Bzl = benzyl, $(Cys)_2$ = cystine, Dpm = diphenylmethyl, Mbzl = 4-methoxybenzyl, Nps = o-nitrophenylsulfenyl, OBu^t = tert.-butoxy, OBzl = benzoxy, OMe = methoxy, ONBzl = 4-nitrobenzoxy, S-Alk = S-Bu^t (S-tert-butyl), S-Et (S-ethyl), S-iPr (S-isopropyl) Thp= tetrahydropyranyl, Tos = tosyl, Trt = triphenylmethyl, Z = benzyloxycarbonyl

Further abbreviations: DCC = dicyclohexylcarbodiimide, HOBt = 1-hydroxybenzotriazole, MA ≙ mixed anhydride, TFA trifluor-acetic acid.

protection played a predominant role in the progress of insulin synthesis. The development of thiol blocking groups with differentiated stability led, in conjunction with new procedures for deprotection at amino groups, to the establishment of strategy 2. The total synthesis of human insulin, which introduced this new approach, was a mile-stone in peptide chemistry[14,15].

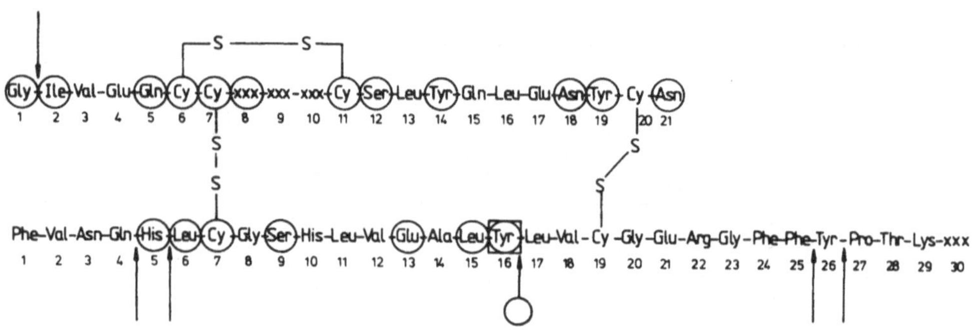

Fig. 2: Amino acid sequence of human, porcine, bovine and ovine insulin

residues modified in the analogues
endo-Tyr[16a]
truncated analogues
des-Tyr^{B16}

A8-10	human porcine	:	Thr-Ser-Ile
	bovine		Ala-Ser-Val
	ovine		Ala-Gly-Val
B30	human = Thr, otherwise Ala		

Nearly 50 analogues have been synthesized in the last 6 years. These, and some biological as well as immunological data, have been listed in Table 2. The sites of modification are indicated in Fig. 2. 60% of the analogues have been prepared according to strategy 1, and 40% according to strategy 2.

Table 2: Synthetic Insulin Analogues

No.	Structure	Yield mg	Yield %	% Biol.Activity in vivo	% Biol.Activity in vitro	%Imm. React.	Ref.
1^{+}	Des-Gly^{A1}	s 5.9	4.2		0.5^{C}		21
2^{+}	Sar^{A1}	s 1.23	7.6	83^{A}		37.5	22
3^{+}	Ala^{A1}	s 1.1	6.8	34^{A}	9.4^{D}		23
4^{+}	D-Ala^{A1}	s 0.8	5.0	46^{A}	95^{D}		23
5^{+}	$\text{Sar}^{A1},\text{Iasn}^{A21}$	s 1.03	6.4	62^{A}		29	24
6	Pro^{A2}	h a	-		$1.7^{C,D}$	101	25
7	D-allo-Ile^{A2}	h a	-		0.2^{D}	56	25
8^{+}	$\text{A}_2\text{Bu}^{A2},\text{Glu}^{A19}$	s 1.4	8.7				26
9	Ala^{A5}	h a	-	105^{B}	$38^{C,D}$	99	25
10	$\text{Glu}^{A5},\text{Ala}^{A12},\text{Ala}^{A18},\text{Ala}^{A21}$	s -	-	86^{A}			27
11	D-Cys^{A6}	h a	-		0.2^{D}	75	25,28
12	$\text{D-Cys}^{A6,A11}$	h a	-			6.4	25,28
13	D-Cys^{A7}	h a	-		$0.2^{C,D}$	47	25,28
14^{+}	$\text{Hcy}^{A7,A20}$	s 0.8	5.0	2.5^{A}	-	8.3	44
15	$\text{Cys(Acm)}^{A7,B7}$	h a	-	0.4^{B}	$0.3^{C,D}$	8.7	15,25
16	His^{A8}	h a	-	87^{B}	$246^{C,D}$	196	25
17	Lys^{A8}	h a	-	66^{B}	153^{C} 64^{D}	22	25
18	Phe^{A8}	h a	-	87^{B}	$80^{C,D}$	38	25
19	D-Cys^{A11}	h a	-		0.7^{D}	8.4	25,28
20^{+}	Phe^{A14}	p 16.8	6.2		96^{C}		29
21^{+}	Phe^{A19}	p 11.0	8.0		23^{C}		30
22^{+}	3-iodo-Tyr^{A19}	p 4	9.0		22^{C}		31
23^{+}	Arg^{A21}	s 1.8	11.3	50^{A}		36	32
24^{+}	Iasn^{A21}	s 0.6	3.7	87^{A}		66	24
25^{+}	D-Asn^{A21}	s 0.6	3.7	66^{A}		33	33
26^{+}	Asn-NH_2^{A21}	s 1.0	6.4	72^{A}	$12^{C,D}$	64	34
27^{+}	Des(B1-B4)	h 1.4	8.3	54^{A}		33	35
28^{+}	Des(B1-B5)	h 0.7	1.9		5^{C}	15	35
29	Ala^{B5}	h a	-	101^{B}	$21^{C,D}$	53	25

No.	Structure	Yield mg	Yield %	% Biol.Activity in vivo	% Biol.Activity in vitro	%Imm. React.	Ref.
30+	Arg^{B5}	p -	-	30^{A}			36
31+	Gly^{B5}	p -	-	30^{A}			36
32+	Gly^{B6}	p -	-	30^{A}			36
33	$D\text{-}Cys^{B7}$	h a	-		1.2^{D}	13	25,28
34+	Leu^{B9}	h 1.1	6.8	56^{A}		48	37
35+	Leu^{B10}	h -	-	44^{A}		38	38
36	Gln^{B13}	h a	-		18^{D}	16	25
37+	$Ala^{B15}Ala^{B16}$	b -	-	5.5^{A}			39
38+	Phe^{B16}	b -	-	33^{A}			39
39	$D\text{-}Tyr^{B16}$	h a		85^{B}	$17^{C,D}$	108	25
40+	Ala^{B16}	b -	-	50^{A}			40
41	$Des\text{-}Tyr^{B16}$	h a	-		$0.1^{C,D}$	0.4	25
42	$Endo\text{-}Tyr^{B16a}$	h a	-		$0.8^{C,D}$	0.9	25
43+	Lys^{B22}	h 0.3	0.9				41
44+	Des(B26-B30) $PheNH_2{}^{B25}$	b 0.6	3.4	44^{A}		36	42
45+	Des(B27-B30) $TyrNH_2{}^{B26}$	b 0.5	2.9	70^{A}		54	42
46	(A6,A7-A11, B7) Cys_2	h a	-	21^{B}	$17^{C,D}$	13	43
47	(A7,A11-A6, B7) Cys_2	h a	-	$29^{A,B}$	$14^{C,D}$	20	43

A_2Bu = α,δ-diaminobutyric acid, Acm = acetamidomethyl; b = bovine, h = human, p = porcine, s = sheep; A mouse convulsion assay; B in vivo blood glucose assay; C isolated fat cell assay; D in vitro glucose oxidation.

\+ chain combination method a = yield 15-50 mg

A-chain Analogues

15 Analogues with modified A-chains have been synthesized in three different laboratories. Katsoyannis and co-workers have replaced A1-glycine (analogues 2,3,4), A21-asparagine (23,24, 25,26), or simultaneously 2 amino acids in positions A1+21 (5), A2+19 (8) or A7+20 (14). Other alterations were the omission of A1-glycine (1), the replacement of A14-tyrosine (20), of A19 tyrosine (21,22), or of 4 amino acids (10).

Strategies. The common route has been the synthesis of small segments (Fig. 3). The approaches differ with respect to segment size, coupling methods, and protecting group tactics.

In the synthesis of Katsoyannis, two alternatives of the C → N strategy were used. The one depicted in Fig. 3A gave 5 analogues. Insulins 5,8,14,24 and 25 were constructed from segments A(1-4), (5-9), (10-12), (13-16) and (17-21). Since all modifications with the exception of homocystinyl insulin (14) concerned the terminal peptides, extensive use of common segments could be made. A comparable strategy was followed by Weber and André (10). In order to overcome the frequent problems of segment insolubility, they studied the application of the solid phase method (Fig. 3B).

The principle followed in our Institute was to construct two segments of about equal size (Fig. 3C) in order to allow for a facile separation of complete chain and unreacted segments after final coupling. It was applied to the synthesis of the A-chains for 20,21, and an iodo-tyrosine-insulin of defined structure (22). The des-gly-A-chain was prepared by joining A(2-9) and A(10-21).

Protection and coupling. In contrast to the B-chain (see below) the A-chain does not contain peptide bonds which are especially sensitive towards sodium in liquid ammonia. The previous tactics were continued, and benzyl protection used for all four

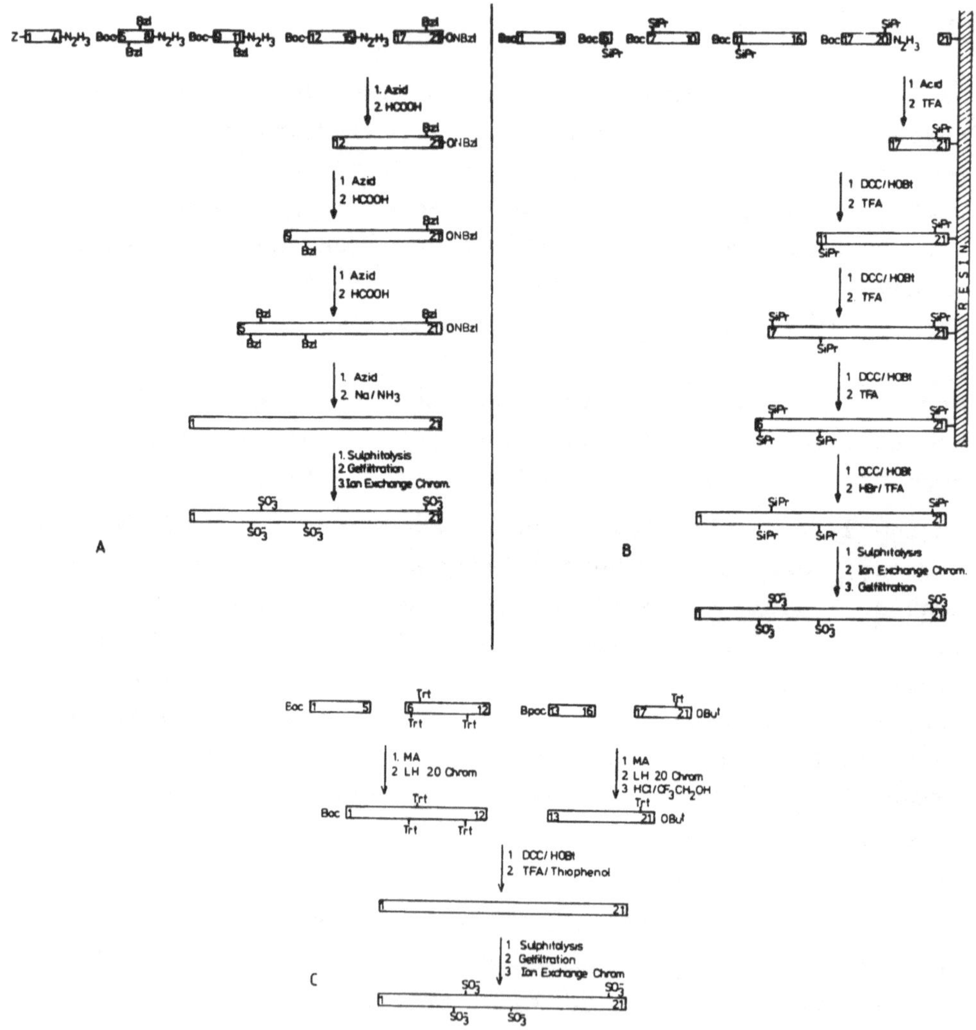

Fig.3: Three different strategies in the fragment condensation of modified insulin A-chains.
This figure shows only the coupling methods, the temporary protection of the α-amino groups and the permanent protection only of the terminal amino and carboxyl groups as well as the thiol protection
A) Synthesis in solution of the [Ala^{A1}]-A-chains[23]
B) Solid phase synthesis of the [Glu^{A5}Ala^{A12}Ala^{A18} Ala^{A21}] A-chain[27].
C) Synthesis in solution of the [Phe^{A14}]-A-chain[29].

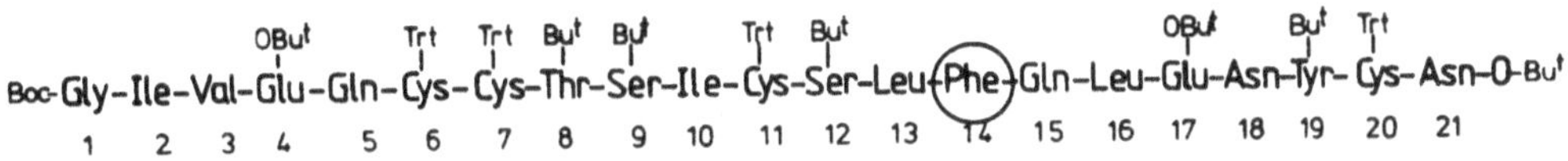

Fig. 4: Fully protected human [Phe^{14}]-A-chain[29]

cysteines. Since segments were coupled by the azide method, full side chain protection was not an absolute requirement. The single 12-serine of the ovine A-chains was mostly left unprotected, the terminal α-carboxyl group was always the acid-stable p-nitrobenzyl residue. For those Tyr and Glu residues which remained protected until the end, benzyl groups were used, but 4-Glu was always a γ-tert.butyl ester. This necessitated finäl deblocking of the A-chains in two steps, i.e. first trifluoro acetic acid, and then Na/NH_3.

In contrast to these tactics applying partial protection of functional groups and rather drastic deblocking conditions, the concept of maximal protection was followed in the other four syntheses. The fully protected modified A-chains with the human sequence contain as much as 10 side chain and 2 terminal protecting groups (Fig. 4). The protection based upon tertiary butyl groups, i.e. tert. butyl urethanes, -esters and ethers, in conjunction with tritylthioethers, implies relatively mild deblocking by means of trifluoro acetic acid, plus thiols as scavengers. The peptides were coupled via mixed anhydride or by means of DCC/HOBt .

<u>Isolation</u>: The standard procedure is the deprotection of <u>all</u> functional groups. It results in the crude thiol chains. These are converted into the S-sulphonates which are, in contrast to the protected and the thiol chains, readily soluble in aqueous solutions. The presence of 4 negatively charged S-sulphonate groups allows for a very efficient purification by chromatography on anion exchangers and facile analytical

control.

Weber and André protected cysteine in the form of an asymmetrical disulphide. The S-isopropylthio groups are stable during cleavage of the chain from the resin and simultaneous removal of N- and O-protecting groups by means of HBr in trifluoro acetic acid. They are subsequently removed under the mild conditions of oxydative sulphitolysis, and the S-sulphonate A-chain is purified.

Special mention has to be made of the des-Gly-A-chain. It was constructed as the 6-7, 11-20-bicyclic cystine peptide, i.e. cysteine was protected by cysteine. This chain was soluble in DMF and could be purified as such. After cleavage of O- and N-protectors, the disulphide chain could be directly used for combination with B-chain (see below).

The absolute yields of A-chain, which determine the amounts of insulin analogue, have mostly been in the order of 200 mg (30-250 mg). Relative yields are difficult to calculate due to the different modes of preparation. The yield in the solid phase synthesis was 9%, based on the ultimate amino acid.

B-chain Analogues

Syntheses of 13 insulin analogues with alterations in the B-chain have been accomplished in two laboratories. Katsoyannis and coworkers have replaced three single amino acids, B9-serine (34), B10-histidine (35) and B22-arginine (43). The N-terminus was shortened by 4 or 5 amino acids (27,28), and 2 analogues were shortened at the C-terminus with simultaneous conversion of the carboxyl to the amide group (44,45). Shvachkin and his group have reported on the synthesis of analogues in which B5-histidine (26,27), B6-leucine (28), B15-leucine + B16-tyrosine (32), or B16 (33,35) were exchanged.

All chains were assembled from segments synthesized in solution. The strategy of Katsoyannis implied the use of the following segments for the synthesis of all 7 chains: B(1-8) or the corresponding shortened peptides, B(9-14), B(15-20), and B(21-30), or the shortened peptides of the ultimate sequence. Although the amino acid replacements concerned three of the four segments, and only peptide B(15-20) was of the identical sequence in all analogues, the design allowed for an extensive use of common intermediates and a standardization of procedures for synthesis and purification. Segments were coupled by means of DCC/hydroxybenzotriazole according to the C→N strategy.

The Lys^{B22} analogue was still synthesized with benzyl groups for the protection of cysteine. Cleavage of the threonine-proline bond by sodium in liquid ammonia, a serious side reaction, was suppressed by the addition of sodium amide.

The preparation of all further B-chains was patterned after the new synthesis of human insulin (Schwartz and Katsoyannis [45]). The main protecting group tactics were now based on the use of the acid-cleavable diphenylmethyl residue for cysteine protection. All segments were obtained by stepwise assembly, predominantly according to the nitrophenylester method of Bodanszky[11-13]. For temporary amino protection Boc- and occasionally Nps groups were used.

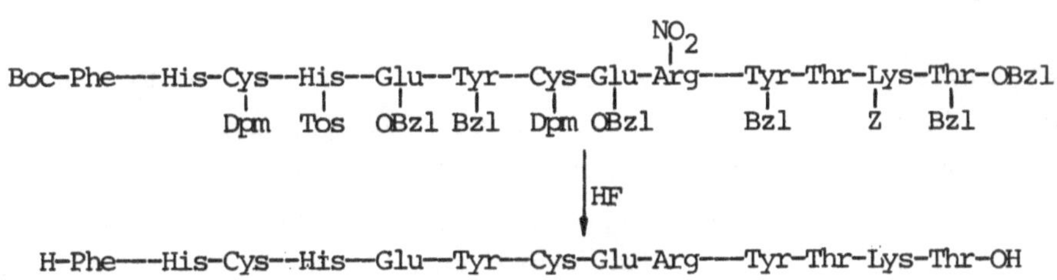

Fig. 5.: Schematic representation of the protected B-chains [37-38].

Upon completion of the synthesis, all semipermanent protecting groups (Fig. 5) were removed in one step by treatment with liquid hydrogen fluoride. Although this method can be very problematic (see Meienhofer, 1980[46]), it led to a marked increase in yields of insulin B-chains.

The end products of synthesis were, as in the case of A-chains, the S-sulphonates, which were obtained in amounts of about 50 mg.

Little detailed information is available on the work of Shvachkin. It appears that benzyl protection for cysteine, in conjunction with Na/NH_3-deblocking, has largely been applied.

Chain combination

The combination of separately obtained A- and B-chains is the crucial step in insulin synthesis.

As in previous work[1-3, 8,9], two procedures have been followed: Co-reduction of A- and B-chain S-sulphonates and subsequent co-oxidation (1), and reaction of fully reduced A-chain with B-chain S-sulphonate (2).

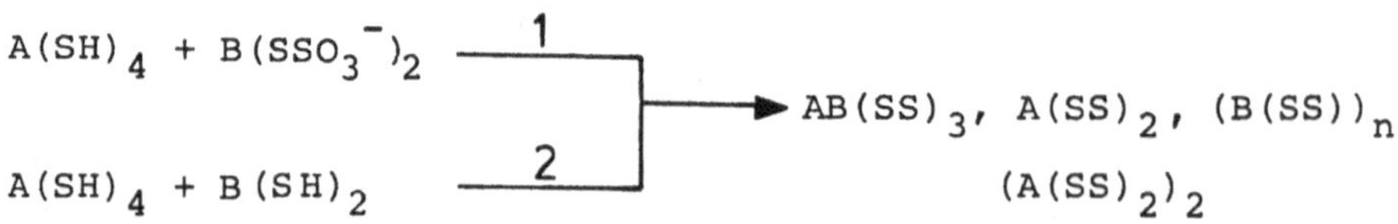

In both cases the disulphide bonds of insulin have to be formed in bimolecular random reactions. 12 Structures are possible for $AB(SS)_3$ besides insulin, 11 isomers can theoretically be generated by incorrect pairing of cysteines. Furthermore, A-chains tend to cyclize under formation of monomeric and dimeric bis-disulphides, and B-chains have a strong tendency to polymerize[9]. Katsoyannis and coworkers, as well as Weber and André, combined reduced A-chains and B-chain-S-sulphonates, mostly in a weight ratio of 4:1 (molar ratio approx. 5.4:1).

The yields of insulin analogues based on B-chain, after extensive purification by ion exchange chromatography and gel filtration, were 4-9% (modified A-chains) and 1-3.5% (modified B-chains). Combination in a ratio of 2:1 (molar ratio approx. 2.7:1) gave yields of 11.5% for the A-chain analogue 23, and yields of 2-8.5% for the B-chain analogues 27,28 and 34.

Joining synthetic A-chains and natural B-chains by co-oxidation in a molar ration of 1:1, the procedure adopted in this Institute, gave yields between 6 and 9% (20,21,22) and 4% (1).

It appears, therefore, than an excess of A-chains does not increase the yields of insulin analogues. In cases where A-chains have been obtained through synthesis, combination of equimolar amounts in conjunction with recycling seems to be preferable. Co-oxidation of equimolar amounts of native reduced chains results now, after several improvements in methodology, in maximally 15% insulin[45]. This can be increased by recycling of by-products to give up to 33%.

An important finding is that the primary structure of the chains markedly influences the yield of analogue. It has been observed that analogues which later turned out to possess low biological potency had inferior properties in combination.

A basic question is whether all disulphide bonds in the analogues are correctly positioned. Only a little information has so far been obtained, but evidence for the presence of incorrectly positioned cystines has not been found.

The absolute amounts of analogues were mostly between 0.5 and 2 mg and maximally 17 mg (see Table 2). Since chains have been prepared in larger quantity, conversion of all available material would have given 2 - 5 times as much insulin analogue. But ca. 10 mg appears to be an upper limit in almost all cases.

If the intermolecular formation of the disulphide bonds in the chain combination method is changed to an intramolecular reaction, better yields of insulin are possible. This reaction is performed in the biosynthesis proceding via the single chain precursor proinsulin. The synthesis of human proinsulin was attempted in our laboratory[46] and also by Yanaihara and coworkers[47]. The synthesis of such a large peptide (86 amino acids) cannot be applied to the synthesis of insulin or insulin analogues. On the other hand, the three dimensional structure of insulin shows that the amino groups A1 Gly and B29 Lys are very close[8,48,53]. With the introduction of a cleavable cross linking between these two amino groups, the structure of this molecule will be stabilized. Air oxidation of the fully reduced crosslinked insulin ("mini proinsulin") leads to the formation of correct disulphide bonds in high yield. Using diamino suberic acid or carbonyl-bis-methionine as crosslink, crystalline insulin can be obtained in yields of up to 50%, but the application to synthetic chains has not yet been described.

Insulin synthesis with selective formation of disulphide bonds.

A further approach to forming a bridge between the A- and B-chains would be the selective formation of one intermolecular disulphide bond. The two other disulphide bridges are formed in an intramolecular reaction. This strategy was used in the total synthesis of human insulin by Sieber et al[14,15] (Fig.6). The starting peptide I was the unsymmetrical fragment with an interchain disulphide bond between A20 and B19[16], with one fre. free α-amino group (A20), and one free α-carboxyl group (B20). After the N-terminal and C-terminal elongation, the fragment III had two acid labile temporarily protected α-amino groups[49], Trt and Bpoc. The former could be removed selectively by pH controlled acidolysis[50], and the sequence B_{1-16} could be coupled to the amino group at B17 (IV).

For the preparation of the intrachain disulphide bridge A_{6-11} and the interchain disulfide bond A_7B_7, the Trt and Acm cysteine protecting groups were used. Both groups are removed by treatment with iodine. The rate of reaction in fluorinated alcohols is so different that a selective cleavage of Trt groups and formation of the A_{6-11} cystine ring are possible, while the Cys^{A7}Acm group[51,52] remains intact. Coupling of A_{1-13} to the large fragment yielded a fully protected insulin molecule with Acm-protection at Cysteine A7 and B7 (VI). Deblocking of all tert. butyl protecting groups, the final removal of Acm groups, and formation of the ultimate A7-B7 disulphide bond resulted in human insulin (VII). The elegant synthesis of Sieber et al[19,75] has been used for the preparation of a large variety of analogues[25,28]. The analogue 12, which contains no cystine bridge between A7 and B7 is the synthetic precursor of human insulin, in which the 2 cysteine-SH-groups remained protected.

Nine different analogues with replacements in positions A2 (6,7), A5 (9), A6 (11), A7 (13), A8 (16-18) A11 (19), and the replacement of $Cys^{A6,A11}$ by the D-enantiomer (12), were obtained via the common intermediate A(14-21)/B(1-30) (Fig.6).

The intermediate A(1-21)/B(17-30), in which the A-chain had been completed first, was the key peptide for the B-chain modifications (Fig. 7). Coupling with the 3 peptides B(1-16), in which B5 (29), B7 (33) or B13 (36) had been replaced, gave the analogues 29,33 and 36.

The des-Tyr^{B16}-insulin (41) resulted from coupling the segment B(1-15) to the intermediate. The additional tyrosine (42) was introduced by elongation of the intermediate by Trt-$Tyr(t.Bu^{t})$-ONSu, selective removal of the trityl protection, and linking of B(1-16).

This strategy makes modifications possible which cannot be realized by the chain-combination method. For instance, by exchange of Trt and Acm thiol protection groups, disulphide isomers of insulin such as A7-11/A6-B7 or A6-7/A11-B7[43], can be prepared specifically. Such isomers deviate from insulin and show differences between each other with respect to

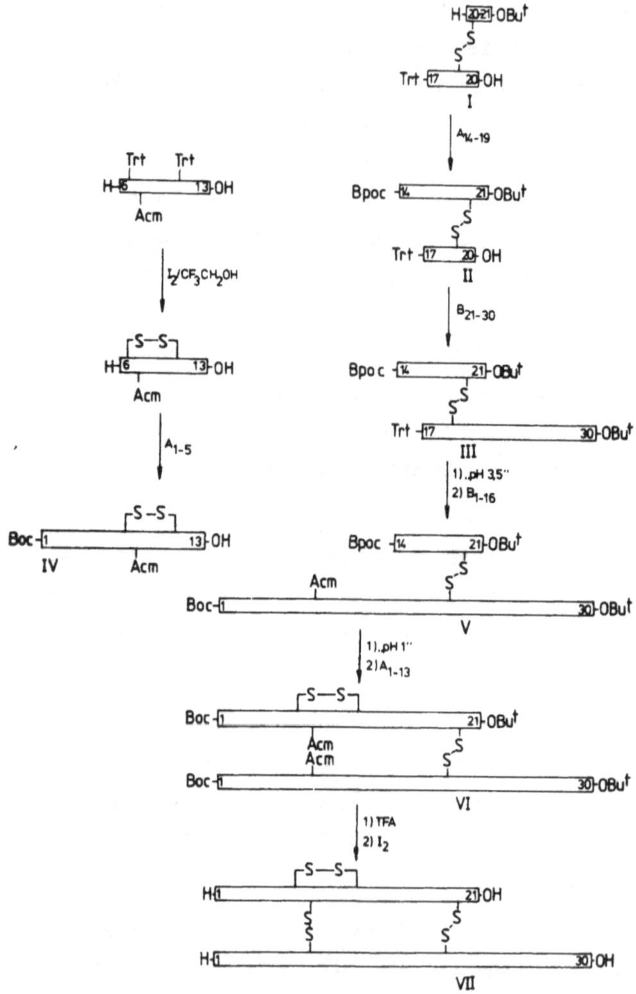

Fig. 6: Total synthesis of human insulin with the correct formation of the three disulphide bonds[14,15]. The tert.butyl side chain protecting groups of hydroxyl, carboxyl and amino groups are not shown in this figure.

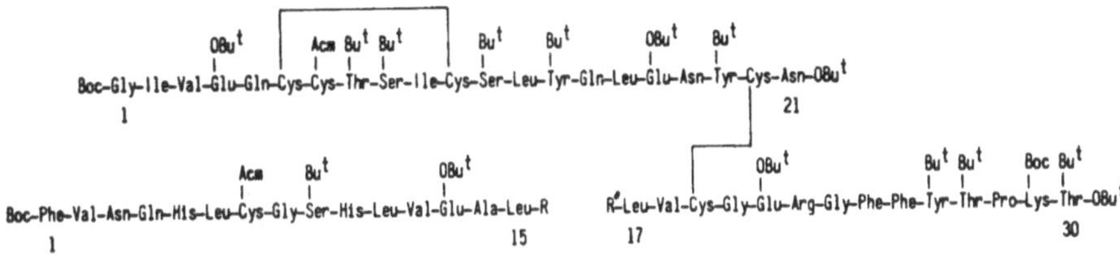

Fig. 7: Protected intermediates used in the synthesis of insulin analogues with modifications in the B-chain R = OH, Tyr(Bu^t)-OH; R' = H, H-Tyr(Bu^t)

potency and physico-chemical properties. These isomers are significantly less stable than insulin in alkaline medium, and thiol-disulphide interchange leads not only to polymers, but also to insulin. From the properties of these disulphide isomers it can be concluded that insulin formed by chain combination does possess the correct disulphide arrangement, and that its structure is preferred over that of the other isomers.

Formation of the final disulphide bond proceeded in the same yields as with human insulin, ca. 70% in all cases. All analogues were purified by counter current distribution and obtained in amounts of 15-50 mg.

Methodological Developments

The correct formation of the three disulphide bonds was also attempted in other laboratories. The synthesis of the unsymmetrical two chain molecule in an early step like Sieber et al.[14,15] was performed by Kullmann in the synthesis of the fragment A(1-21)-B(18-26)[54]. Losse and coworkers synthesized the fragment A(19-21)-B(15-27)[55] (Ala 27) by proton catalyzed disulphide exchange between the S-ethyl protected fragments. Birr and Pipkorn[56] connected the A- and B-chains in the final step. They synthesized the bovine A-chain by fragment condensation at the solid support with three different thiol protecting groups (A6,11 = S-tert-butyl, A7 = acetamidomethyl, A20 = methoxybenzyl) and closed the intrachain disulphide bond A6-11 selectively. Combination with native reduced B-chain gave a fully active insulin.

The preparation of the disulphide bond between the cysteine residues A6 and A11 was studied by Kaufmann and coworkers[57]. Precursors for the cyclic disulphide octapeptide A6-13 had been variations in the protection of A6,11 i.e. acetamido-methyl, trityl, and S-ethyl, respectively. In the protected Ala^{A12}-A-chain, the cysteines A7 and A20 were blocked by the diphenylmethyl group in all cases.

Other insulin chains were prepared with the native and modified sequences. The semipermanent protection mostly involved the tert. butyl group. Variations were found in the thiol protection and deblocking conditions.

Schwertner and coworkers[58] synthesized a sheep insulin-A-chain with 2-tetrahydropyranyl groups protecting the 4 cysteine residues. After deblocking with dirhodane and combination with natural reduced B-chain, an insulin with high biological activity was isolated. [Lys^{A13}] -bovine-A-chain was synthesized with S-tert.butyl protection for the thiol functions[59]. These asymmetrical disulphides were removed by sulphitolysis. The [Tyr^{B25}] -B-chain[62] was prepared with trityl as thiol protection and was deblocked by trifluoroacetic acid in the presence of thiol. The unsymmetrical disulphide, S-ethyl, was frequently used for cysteine protection in the synthesis of three shortened Ala substituted analogues of insulin-B-chains [60]. An interesting observation is that the semipermanent O-benzyl groups can be removed from the sulphur containing B-chain by catalytic hydrogenolysis under special conditions[61].

The approach of 3,5-iodo tyrosine in the peptide synthesis was demonstrated during the synthesis of 3,5-iodo Tyr^{A19} A-chain. The 3,5-iodo tyrosine and its peptides are stable under the conventional coupling and deprotection conditions. The synthesis was performed analogously to the [Phe^{A14}]-A-chain outlined in Figs. 3 and 4.

Conclusions

Over the fast 6 years the majority of syntheses of insulin or insulin analogues have been caried out by fragment condensation in solution, with very few being carried out by solid-phase methods. Over so modified insulins have been synthesized either by the classical method of combining the separate chains, or by stepwise introduction of the three disulphide bonds. All products were isolated in a satisfactorily pure form. Unfortunately the yields of modified insulin producted by chain combination lie in the order of only 1 mg limiting the types of subsequent investigations which can be made with them. Stepwise introduction of the correct disulphide bonds gave much better yields at the last stage of the reaction, so that derivatives synthesized by this method could be very thoroughly investigated. The strategy of this method is so well developed that already in 1977 the production of 629 mg synthetic human insulin was described, allowing one to begin to hope for commercial synthetic insulin.

References

1. Meienhofer, J., Schnabel, E., Bremer, H., Brinkhoff, O., Zabel, R., Sroka, W., Klostermeyer, H., Brandenburg, D., Okuda, T., Zahn, H.: Z. Naturforsch. 18b, 1120.1121 (1963)

2. Katsoyannis, P.G., Fukuda, K., Tometsko, A., Suzuki, K., Tilak, M.: J. Amer. Chem. Soc. 86, 930-932 (1964)

3. Kung, Y.-t., Du, Y.-c., Huang, W.-t., Chen, C.-c., Ke, L.-t., Hu, S.-c., Jiang, R.-q., Chu, S.-q., Niu, C.-i., Hsu, J.-z., Chang, W.-c., Cheng, L.-l., Li, H.-s., Wang, Y., Loh, T.-p., Chi, A.-h., Li, C.-h., Shi, P.-t., Yie, Y.-h., Tang, K.-l, Hsing, C.-y.: Scientia Sinica 14, 1710-1716 (1965)

4. Goeddel, D.V., Kleid, D.G., Bolivar, F., Heyneker, H.L., Yansura, D.G., Crea, R., Hirose, T., Kraszewski, A., Itakura, K., Riggs, A.D.: Proc. Natl. Acad. Sci. 76, 106-110 (1979)

5. Proceedings, First Int. Symposium on Biosynthetic Insulin. Athens, Greece, Sept. 1980, to be published.

6. Brandenburg, D., Weimann, H.J., Trindler, P., Schüttler, A. A.: in "Basic and Clinical Aspects of Immunity to Insulin" Konstanz 28.9. - 1.10.80.

7. Gattner, H.-G., Danho, W., Knorr, R., Naithani, V.K., Zahn, H.: in "Basic and Clinical Aspects of Immunity to Insulin" Konstanz 28.9. - 1.10.80.

8. Geiger, R.: Chemiker Zeitung 100, 111-129 (1976).

9. Lübke, K., Klostermeyer, H.: Advan. Enzymol. 35, 445- (1970).

10. Brandenburg, D., Saunders, D.: "Pancreatic Hormones" in Sheppard, Amino acids, peptides and proteins. Vol. 10, pp. 432-451, The Chemical Society, London, 1979.

11. Wünsch, E.in Houben Weyl "Methoden der organischen Chemie" Vol. 15 "Synthese Peptiden I & II, Ed 4th, Thieme,Stuttgart, (1974).

12. Gross, E., Meienhofer, J. (Eds). "The Peptides", Academic Press, New York, London (1980).

13. Eberle, A., Geiger, R., Wieland, T. (Eds.) "Perspectives in Peptide Chemistry, S. Karger, Basel (1981).

14. Sieber, P., Kamber, B., Hartmann, A., Jöhl, A., Riniker, B., Rittel, W.: Helv. Chim. Acta 57, 2617-2621 (1974).

15. Sieber, P., Kamber, B., Hartmann, A., Jöhl, A., Riniker, B., Rittel, W.: Helv. Chim. Acta 60, 27-37 (1977).

16. Kamber, B.: Helv. Chim. Acta 54, 398-422 (1971).

17. König, W., Teetz, V., Tripier, D., Volk, A.: in "Peptides 1978" Proc. 15th Europ. Peptide Symp., Gdansk, Poland (Eds. Siemion, I.Z., Kupryszewski, G.) Wroclaw University Press, Wroclaw, Poland 1979, pp. 619-623.

18. Büllesbach, E.E., Danho, W., Helbig, H.J., Zahn, H.: in "Peptides 1978" Proc. 15th Europ. Peptide Symp. Gdansk, Poland (Eds. Siemion, I.Z., Kupryszewski, G.) Wroclaw University Press, Wroclaw, Poland 1979, pp. 653-646.

19. König, W., Kernebeck, K.: Liebigs Ann. Chem. 227-247 (1979).

20. Büllesbach, E.E., Danho, W., Helbig, H.J., Zahn, H.: Hoppe Seyler's Z. Physiol. Chem. 361, 865-873 (1980).

21. Berndt, H., Gattner, H.-G., Zahn, H.: Hoppe Seyler's Z. Phsiol. Chem. 356, 1469-1472 (1975).

22. Okada, Y., Katsoyannis, P.G., J. Amer. Chem. Soc. 97, 4366-4372 (1975).

23. Cosmatos, A., Cheng, K., Okada, Y., Katsoyannis, P.G.: J. Biol. Chem. 253, 6586-6590 (1978).

24. Cosmatos, A., Okada, Y., Katsoyannis, P.G.: Biochemistry 15, 4076-4082 (1976).

25. Märki, F., De Gasparo, M., Eisler, K., Kamber,B ., Riniker, B., Rittel, W., Sieber, P.: Hoppe-Seyler's Z. Physiol. Chem. 360, 1619-1632 (1979).

26. Ferderigos, N., Katsoyannis, P.G.: J. Chem. Soc. Perkin I 1299-1305 (1977).

27. Weber, U., André, M.: Hoppe Seyler's Z. Physiol. Chem. 356, 701-714 (1975).

28. Eisler, K., Kamber, B., Riniker, B., Rittel, W., Sieber, P., De Gasparo, M., Märki, F.: Bioorganic Chemistry 8, 443-450 (1979).

29. Danho, W., Sasaki, A., Büllesbach, E.E., Gattner, H.-G., Wollmer, A.: Hoppe Seyler's Z. Physiol. Chem. 361, 747-754 (1980).

30. Danho, W., Sasaki, A., Büllesbach, E.E., Föhles, J., Gattner, H.-G.: Hoppe Seyler's Z. Physiol. Chem. 361, 735-746 (1980).

31. Wieneke, H.J., Danho, W., Büllesbach, E.E., Gattner, H.-G., Zahn, H.: in "Peptides, Structure and Biological Function" Proc. 6th American Peptide Symp. 1979 (Eds. Gross, E., Meienhofer, J.) Pierce Chem. Co., Rockford Ill. USA (1979). pp. 515-518.

32. Ferderigos, N., Cosmatos, A., Ferderigos, A., Katsoyannis, P.G.: Int. J. Peptide Protein Res. 13, 43-53 (1979).

33. Cosmatos, A., Johnson, S., Breier, B., Katsoyannis, P.G.: J. Chem. Soc. Perkin I, 2157-2163 (1975).

34. Burke, G.T., Chanley, J.D., Okada, Y., Cosmatos, A., Ferderigos, N., Katsoyannis, P.G. : Biochemistry 19, 4547-4556 (1980).

35. Schwarz, G., Katsoyannis, P.G.: Biochemistry 17, 4550-4556 (1978).

36. Schvachkin, Yu.P., Voluiskaya, E.N., Krivtsov, V.F., Oleinik, A.M., Kolomeitseva, L.A., Fedotov, V.P., Ivanova, A.I.: Khim. Prir. Soedin, 722-723 (1977).

37. Schwarz, G., Katsoyannis, P.G.: Biochemistry 15, 4071-4076 (1976).

38. Schwartz, G.P., Katsoyannis, P.G.: J. Chem. Res. (S), 220-221 (1977).

39. Shvachkin, Yu.P., Voluiskaya, E.N., Krivtsov, V.F., Pet Petrova, L.A., Knyazeva, V.V., Kocharova, N.A., Fedotov, V.P., Ivanova, A.I.: Khim. Prir. Soedin, 869-870 (1977).

40. Shvachkin, Yu.P., Voluiskaya, E.N., Krivtsov, V.F., Petrova, L.A., Knyazeva, V.V., Kocharova, N.A., Fedotov, V.P., Ivanova, A.I.: Khim. Prir, Soedin, 543-544 (1978).

41. Katsoyannis, P.G., Grinos, J., Cosmatos, A., Schwartz, G. P.: J. Chem. Soc. Perkin I, 464-469 (1975).

42. Cosmatos, A., Ferderigos, N., Katsoyannis, P.G. : Int. J. Peptide Protein Res. 14, 457-471 (1979).

43. Sieber, P., Eisler, K., Kamber, B., Riniker, B., Rittel, W., Märki, F., De Gasparo, M.: Hoppe-Seyler's Z. Physiol. Chem. 359, 113-123.

44. Cosmatos, A., Katsoyannis, P.G.: J. Biol. Chem. 250, 5315-5321 (1975).

45. Meienhofer, J. in: "Insulin, Chemistry, Structure and Function of Insulin and Related Hormones" (Eds. D. Brandenburg, A. Wollmer), Walter de Gruyter & Co., Berlin, New York (1980) pp 40-49.

46. Danho, W., Naithani, V.K., Sasaki, A.N., Föhles, J., Berndt, H., Büllesbach, E.E., Zahn, H.: Hoppe-Seyler's Z. Physiol. Chem. 361, 857-863 (1980).

47. Yanaihara, N., Yanaihara, C., Sakagami, M., Sakura, N., Hashimoto, T., Nishida, T.: Diabetes 27, Suppl. 1 149-260 (1978).

48. Brandenburg, D., Gattner, H.-G., Schermutzki, W., Schüttler, A., Uschkoreit, J., Weimann, J., Wollmer, A.: Adv. Exp. Med. Biol. Vol. 86A, Plenum Press, New York 1977, pp.261-282.

49. Kamber, B., Riniker, B.,Sieber, P., Rittel, W.: Helv. Chim. Acta 59, 2830-2840 (1976).

50. Riniker, B., Kamber, B., Sieber, P., Helv. Chim. Acta 58, 1086-1094 (1975).

51. Kamber, B., Hartmann, A., Eisler, K., Riniker, B., Rink, H., Sieber, P., Rittel, W.: Helv. Chim. Acta 63, 899-915 (1980).

52. Sieber, P., Kamber, G., Eisler, K., Hartmann, A., Riniker, B., Rittel, W.: Helv. Chim. Acta. 59, 1489-1497 (1976).

53. Dodson, E.J., Dodson, G.G., Hodgkin, D.C., Reynolds, C.D.: Can. J. Biochem. 57, 469-479 (1979).

54. Kullmann, W., Tetrahedron Lett. 21, 589-592 (1980).

55. Losse, G., Stange, H., Naumann, W., Liebigs Ann. Chem., 143-151 (1971).

56. Birr, C., Pipkorn, R., Angew. Chem. 91, 571-573 (1979).

57. Kaufmann, K.D., Kunzek, H., Dölling, R., Halatsch, W.R., Rose, K.B., Nieke, E., Schönherr, Ch., Bauschke, S.: in "Peptides 1978" Proc. 15th Europ. Peptide Symp. Gdansk, Poland (Eds: Siemion, I.Z. and Kupryszewski, G.), Wroclaw University Press, Wroclaw, Poland 1979 pp 615-618.

58. Schwertner, E., Klostermeyer, H., Zahn, H., Liebigs Ann. Chem. 1092-1106 (1975).

59. Wolf, G., Berndt, H., Brandenburg, D., Hoppe-Seyler's Z. Physiol. Chem. 360, 1569-1578 (1979).

60. Losse, G., Stange, H., Journal f. prakt. Chemie, 321, 308-314 (1979).

61. Losse, G., Stange, H., Schwenzer, B., Naumann, W., Mauck, M., Schumacher, K.J., Meisegeier, B.: in "Peptides 1978" Proc. 15th Europ. Peptide Symp., Gdansk, Poland (Eds: Siemion, I.Z., Kupryszewski, G.) Wroclaw University Press, Wroclaw, Poland 1979 pp. 635-638.

62. Knorr, R., Danho, W., Büllesbach, E.E., Gattner, H.-G., Zahn, H. in "Insulin, Chemistry,Structure and Function of Insulin and Related Hormones" (Eds. D. Brandenburg, A. Wollmer) Walter de Gruyter & Co., Berlin, New York (1980) pp.67-71.

MODIFICATION OF THE C-TERMINAL REGION OF INSULIN

H.-G. Gattner, W. Danho, R. Knorr, V.K. Naithani, E.W. Schmitt and H. Zahn

Deutsches Wollforschungsinstitut
D-5100 Aachen, Federal Republic of Germany

Introduction

Biological activity and aggregation of insulin are known to be closely related to the C-terminal region of insulin. The B-chain sequence B23-26, Gly-Phe-Phe-Tyr, has remained invariant during evolution and therefore the residues have been assumed to be part of the receptor-binding region of the hormone (1) (Figure 1). Chemical modification of specific amino acid residues in this region should give more information about the role of these amino acids play regarding the structure-activity, receptor binding and aggregation behaviour of the insulin molecule.

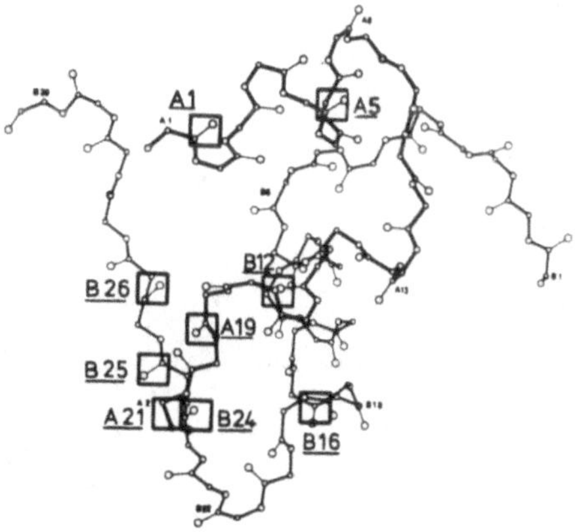

Fig. 1: Residues of the proposed receptor-binding region of insulin (1).

Basic and Clinical Aspects of Immunity to Insulin

We describe the preparation of C-terminal shortened insulins by enzymatic digestion. The problems of chemical semisynthesis with shortened partial protected insulin derivatives are discussed. As a new approach we describe the enzyme catalyzed peptide synthesis with insulin derivatives. Insulin has two peptide bonds accessible for tryptic digestion, and therefore, under appropriate conditions, available for enzyme mediated synthesis. Trypsin catalyzed couplings with the carboxyl components Boc_2-des-octapeptide (B23-30)-insulin and des-Ala^{B30}-insulin were performed with synthetic octapeptides modified in the range B24-26 and amino acid esters respectively.

A. C-terminal shortened insulin derivatives.

Using enzymatic digestion one can prepare a series of C-terminal shortened insulin derivatives. Figure 2 shows the peptide bonds susceptible to enzymatic cleavage in the C-terminal region.

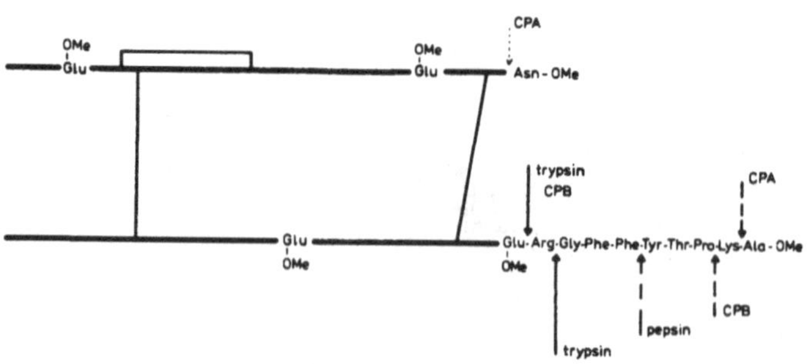

Fig. 2: Peptide bonds of the C-terminal region of insulin cleaved by different enzymes.

1. Des-Ala(B30)insulin(DAI) (2).
An improved method for preparation of DAI was found by incubation of insulin with carboxypeptidase-A in 0.2 M NH_4HCO_3/NH_4OH buffer, pH 8.4, for 4 hours at RT. The enzyme-substrate ratio was 1:100 (^{w}/w) (3). Amino acid analysis of the digestion solution showed that alanine was released to 96% while no asparagine was found. Since human insulin differs from porcine insulin only in position B30 (Thr instead of Ala) DAI (porcine) is the starting compound for the most economical semisynthesis of human insulin.

2. Des-Ala(B30), des-Asn(A21)insulin (DAAI) (4).
By changing the buffer from 0.2 M NH_4HCO_3/NH_4OH, pH 8.4, to 0.05 M Tris/HCl, pH 8.5, insulin is digested by carboxypeptidase -A to 85% to DAAI. Separation from residual DAI is achieved by ionexchange chromatography on DEAE-Sephadex, pH 8.1, in 7 M urea with a linear salt gradient from 0.00 to 0.25 M sodium chloride. DAAI is eluted ahead of DAI (5).

3. Des-pentapeptide(B26-30)insulin (DPI) (6,7,8).
For preparation of DPI insulin was dissolved in 0.5 proz. formic acid (200 mg in 40 ml) and adsorbed to 3 g SE-cellulose equilibrated with the same solution. After 20 min. 2 mg pepsin in 2 ml dest. water were added. After 30-40 min. the slurry was filled into a column and the enzyme was removed by washing with 0.5 proz. formic acid. DPI, residual insulin and the pentapeptide (B26-B30) were eluted by 0.1 M ammonia. The digestion of the matrix bound insulin with pepsin was found to be restricted to the cleavage of the Phe(B25)-Tyr(B26) peptide bond. Since DPI possesses a decreased tendency to aggregate at pH 8, the isolation of the homogeneous analogue could be accomplished by gel filtration on Sephadex G-50 in 0.05 M NH_4HCO_3-solution with a yield of 60%.

4. Des-hexapeptide(B25-30)insulin and des-heptapeptide (B24-30)insulin.

When carboxypeptidase-A acts on a protein the different amino acids are released with different rate (see also preparation of Des-Ala(B30)insulin). Phenylalanine is released rapidly and glycine very slowly. Using this behaviour an incubation of DPI with carboxypeptidase-A in 0.2 M NH_4HCO_3/NH_4OH, pH 8.4, at 25°C for 10 min (enzyme:substrate = 1:500 ($^w/w$)) yielded a mixture of DPI, des-hexapeptide and des-heptapeptide insulin. Separation of the three analogues was achieved by counter current distribution. A semisynthetic approach to des-hexapeptide (B25-30)insulin was also described by a chinese research group (9).

5. Desoctapeptide(B23-30)insulin (DOI) (10).

The digestion of insulin according to (10) was found to be non-quantitative (90%). By the purification procedure given by Bromer and Chance (11) a DOI preparation was obtained with a insulin contamination of 1%, which could not be removed by ionexchange chromatography on DEAE-Sephadex. Pure DOI was obtained by purification in acidic medium: The crude preparation of DOI was desalted on Sephadex G-25 in 0.05 M NH_4HCO_3 solution, lyophilized, and chromatographed on SP-Sephadex in 0.05 M sodium formiate/formic acid + 7 M urea, pH 3.5, linear salt gradient from 0.0 - 0.3 M sodium chloride. The DOI, purified in this manner, showed no contamination with insulin.*

6. Des-nonapeptide(B22-30)insulin (5,12).

In order to work on Arg(B22) while avoiding difficulties of peptide coupling at the arginine, DOI was incubated with carboxypeptidase-B (0.2 M NH_4HCO_3/NH_4OH, pH 8.4, E:S = 1:100 ($^w/w$), 6 h, 25°C). Purification was achieved by ion exchange chromatography on CM-cellulose, pH 4, with a yield of about 40%.

**(Herbertz, L., private communication)*

B. Semisyntheses in the C-terminal region of the B-chain.

Semisynthesis is the coupling of amino acids or peptides to proteins or fragments of proteins. In order to obtain a clear reaction it is necessary to protect the most reactive groups. Ruttenberg (13) and a chinese research group (14) described a way to remodel porcine into human insulin. Weitzel et al. investigated modification in the C-terminal region of the B-chain (15).
Des-octapeptide(B23-30)insulin pentamethyl ester has been prepared by tryptic digestion of porcine insulin hexamethyl ester or the corresponding des-octapeptide(B23-30)insulin hexamethyl ester. The enzyme cleaves specifically at the carboxyl terminus of Arg(B22). After protection of the amino groups with tert.-butyloxycarbonyl residues (Boc-), the protected DOI was coupled with the synthetic octapeptide (B23-30) of human insulin. Subsequently the amino and carboxyl groups were liberated by treatments with trifluoro acetic acid and sodium hydroxide.
However, the final step, namely the alkaline saponification of the methylester makes the whole procedure fail. Nobody was able to produce human insulin which was 100% biological active. Investigating the saponification of the insulin hexamethyl ester we found that in the first step of the reaction the A21-asparaginimide-insulin is formed (Fig. 3) (16).

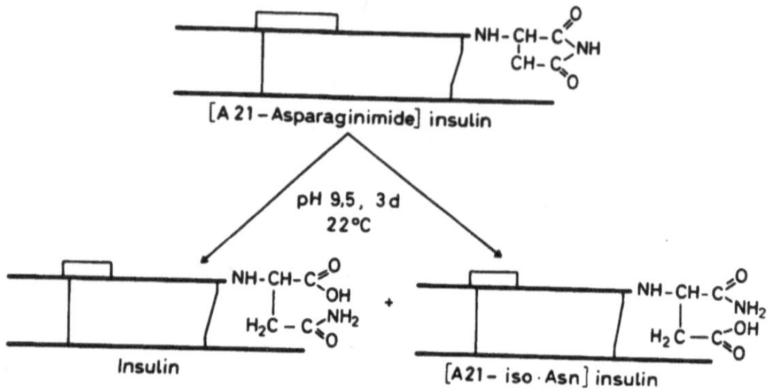

Fig. 3: (A21-Asparaginimide)-insulin and its hydrolysis.

We have isolated and characterized this new analogue which showed 40% biological activity in fat cell assay. The absence of a carboxyl function at position A21 prevents the formation of the salt bridge to arginine B22 (17), and hence one should expect a change of tertiary structure in this region. The asparaginimide hydrolyses slowly to a mixture of asparagine (40%) and iso-asparagine (60%). The pK-values of the α-and β-carboxyl group are little different. After repeated ion exchange chromatography we could separate these isomers. The biological activity of the iso-Asn(A21)insulin was found to be 80% in fat cell assay. Beside the formation of the two isomers during hydrolysis of the ester groups further side reactions can occur (deamidation, hydrolytic cleavage of the disulfide bonds).

A second semisynthetic approach was based on the assumption that side carboxyl groups show a lower reactivity than α-carboxyl groups. Therefore the synthetic octapeptide has predominantly the possibility between two α-carboxyl groups A21-asparagine and B22-arginine. Obermeier and Geiger (18) could isolate about 10-15% pure human insulin after extensive purification. The crude reaction mixture exhibited up to 40%

insulin activity. The reaction described with the unprotected carboxyl groups, however, seems to be limited to a few cases only (19). If we used des-pentapeptide(B26-30)insulin instead of DOI less than 1% insulin was isolated (20).

C. Modifications by trypsin catalyzed peptide synthesis.

Proteases are well-known as enzymes which can split peptide bonds in proteins or polypeptides. The reverse reaction, i.e. peptide or amide bond formation, can also be catalyzed by the same enzymes under special conditions, as first demonstrated by Bergmann and Fraenkel-Conrat (21). Figure 4 shows the equilibria involved in enzymatic peptide synthesis for the example of trypsin.

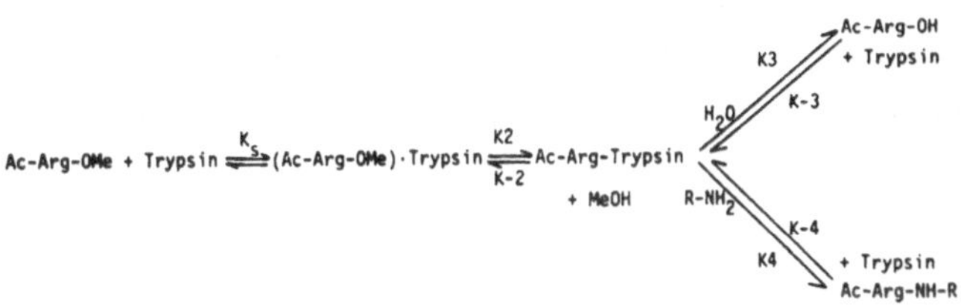

Fig. 4: Scheme for the enzyme catalyzed peptide synthesis with trypsin

The scheme illustrates that in the presence of a nucleophile ($R-NH_2$) other than water, the acylenzyme intermediate (Ac-Arg-trypsin) will be subject to aminolysis in addition to hydrolysis. Assuming $K_3 >> K_{-3}$ and $K_4 >> K_{-4}$, the ratio of aminolysis to hydrolysis clearly depends on K_4/K_3 as well as on the concentration of the nucleophile $R-NH_2$ and on the concentration of organic solvent which diminishes the concentration of water.

Recently Inouye et al. (22) described the trypsin assisted semisynthesis of human insulin from porcine des-octapeptide (B23-30) insulin and a synthetic octapeptide (B23-30). Independently the conversion of des-Ala(B30)insulin into human insulin was published twice (23) (24). The preparation of modified insulin in positions B24 and B25 (Phe → Leu) were published recently at the same time (25) (26).

For our experiments we used as carboxyl component des-Ala-(B30)insulin and Boc_2-des-octapeptide insulin. The amino groups of DOI were blocked with a four-fold excess of di-tert.-butyldicarbonate ($(Boc)_2O$) in dimethylformamide/4 mM N-ethylmorpholine for 16 h.
The peptides were synthesized by the conventional solution method using the strategy of fragment condensation and acid-labile protecting groups.
A typical coupling experiment on a preparative scale and purification of the analogue is shown in scheme 1. Non coupled amino and carboxyl components are separated and can be reused.

Boc_2-DOI 20 μmol
↓
H-Gly-Leu-Phe-Tyr-Thr-Pro-Lys(Boc)-Thr-OH 200 μmol
↓
dissolved in 0.05 M NH_4HCO_3/NH_4OH, lyophilized
↓
dissolved in 1.05 ml DMF + 0.70 ml 0.5 M Tris/HCl. pH 6.5
↓
added trypsin (10 mg), incubated at 37°C for 20 h
↓
acidified to pH 2-3, chromatographed on LH-20 in DMF/0.5 M acetic acid (1/1)
↓
deprotected with trifluoroacetic acid
↓
chromatographed on CM-cellulose at pH 4.5
↓
human insulin analogue (25% yield)

Scheme 1: Coupling procedure for insulin analogues.

Table 1 shows a series of peptides coupled with Boc_2-DOI by trypsin catalysis. Amino acids changed against the natural sequence are underlined.

Table 1: Peptides coupled with Boc_2-DOI by trypsin catalyzed peptide bond formation.

Peptide	Yield %
H-Gly-Phe-Tyr-Tyr-Thr-Pro-Lys(Boc)-Ala-OH	12
H-Gly-Phe-Ala-Tyr-Thr-Pro-Lys(Boc)-Thr-OH	15
H-Gly-Leu-Phe-Tyr-Thr-Pro-Lys(Boc)-Thr-OH	25
H-Gly-Phe-Leu-Tyr-Thr-Pro-Lys(Boc)-Thr-OH	10
H-Gly-Phe-Phe-Tyr-OMe	15
H-Gly-Phe-Phe-Phe-OMe	45

For coupling of des-Ala(B30)insulin with amino acid esters 100 mg DAI and a 70-fold molar excess of the ester were dissolved in 1,75 ml 60% DMF/pH 6.5 buffer and 10 mg trypsin were added. After 20 h the reaction was stopped by lowering the pH to 2-3. Trypsin and excess of amino acid ester were removed by gel filtration on Sephadex G-50 in 1 M acetic acid. The coupled analogue was separated from DAI by ion exchange chromatography on CM-cellulose at pH 4.5. The yield of trypsin catalyzed coupling was found to be dependent on the amino acid and the kind of the ester. In table 2 some results are summarized.

Table 2: Coupling yields of DAI with different amine components

Amine component	Yield %	Amine component	Yield %
Thr-OMe	85	Glu-$(OMe)_2$	90
Thr-NH_2	80	Ala-OMe	65
Tyr-OMe	70	Ala-OBu^t	40
Trp-OMe	70	Ala-OBzl	45
p-NO_2-Phe-OMe	40	Ala-NH_2	50
3,(NH_2)-Tyr-OMe	35		

Studying the progress of coupling we found for DAI and Thr-OMe a maximum yield of 85% after 30 min was reached which decreased to 70% after 22 h. To our surprise there was no splitting of the Arg B22 - Gly B23 peptide bond.
The effect of amine component to carboxyl component ratio on the yield is shown in figure 5. By the use of excess amine component the equilibrium of the system moved toward synthesis.

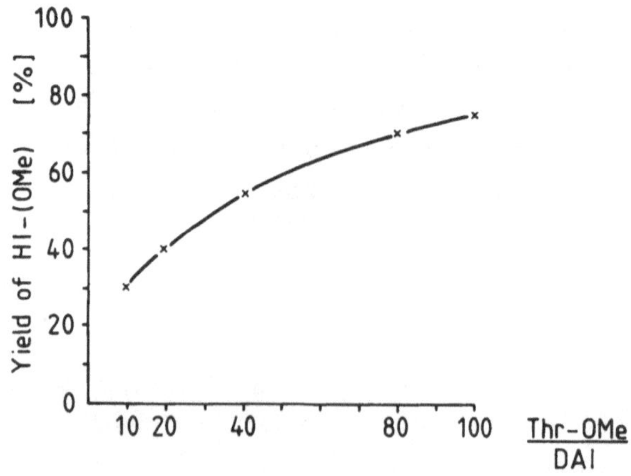

Fig. 5: Effect of Thr-OMe-concentration on the yield of Thr-OMe(B30)insulin.

The equilibrium also depends on the concentration of water and the kind of organic solvent. Table 3 indicates that the addition of an organic solvent, such as DMF or DMSO, to the reaction medium greatly increases the synthesis of the peptide bond. The effect is much larger than that expected from the decrease in water concentration (27).

Table 3: Effect of organic solvent (60%) on the yield of trypsin catalyzed coupling: Boc_2DOI + Gly-OMe

Solvent	% Boc_2DOI-Gly-OMe
Dioxane	20
i-Propanol	30
Glycerol	40
Dimethylformamide	55
Butanediol-1.4	60
Ethyleneglycol	60
Dimethylsulfoxide	75
4 M urea	25

The addition of organic solvents was also effective in increasing the solubility of reactants which governs the extend of peptide bond formation.

Discussion

Des-Ala(B30)insulin could be prepared in quantitative yield if insulin was incubated with carboxypeptidase - A in ammoniumhydrogencarbonate buffer. Using tris/HCl buffer also asparagine is released to about 85%. The normally unspecific pepsin split only the Phe B25 - Tyr B26 peptide bond if insulin is adsorbed to a strongly acidic ionexchanger.

Under these conditions (pH 2.5) the pepsin is not bound to the resin. Very short incubation of the des-pentapeptide (B26-30)insulin with carboxpeptidase A yielded the further shortened analogues des-hexapeptide(B25-30)insulin and des-heptapeptide(B24-30)insulin.

Investigation of the saponification of the insulin hexamethyl ester gave a new analogue modified in position A21: A21-asparaginimide insulin without a C-terminal carboxyl group at Asn(A21). The asparaginimide hydrolysis to a mixture of two isomers. This fact makes the methyl ester unfit for semisynthesis with insulin if one aspires at pure insulin derivatives.

Coupling without carboxyl protection is limited to few cases. The trypsin catalyzed peptide bond formation has the advantage that as a result of the stereospecificity of the enzyme, racemization is avoided. Following the procedure of Inouye et al. (22) for the enzyme assisted coupling of des(B23-30)insulin to human octapeptide (B23-30), we were able to synthesise new insulin analogues. This procedure opens a new perspective for the semisynthesis of analogues modified in the C-terminal region of the B-chain, a region considered to be important for the biological activity, receptor-binding and aggregation of the hormone. It seems that the coupling yields are sequence dependent.

References

1. Pullen, R.A., Lindsay, D.G., Wood, S.P., Tickle, I.J., Blundell, T.L., Wollmer, A., Krail, G., Brandenburg, D., Zahn, H., Gliemann, J., Gammeltoft, G.: Nature (London) 259, 369-373 (1976)

2. Slobin, L.J., Carpenter, F.H.: Biochemistry 5, 499-508 (1966)

3. Schmitt, E.W., Gattner, H.-G.: Hoppe-Seyler's Z. Physiol. Chem. 359, 799-802 (1978)

4. Slobin, L.J., Carpenter, F.H.: Biochemistry 2, 16-22 (1963)

5. Gattner, H.-G., Schmitt, E.W., Zahn, H.: in"Peptides 1976" Proceedings of the 14th European Peptide Symposium, Wepion, Belgium, April 11-17, 1976, pp. 279-284, ed. by A. Loffet, Editions de l'Université de Bruxelles

6. Gattner, H.-G.: Hoppe-Seyler's Z. Physiol. Chem. 356, 1397-1404 (1975)

7. Insulin Research Group, Shanghai, Institute of Biochemistry, Academia Sinica; Insulin Structure Research Group and Biochemical Preparation Group, Peking, Institute of Biophysics, Academia Sinica: Scientia Sinica 19, 351-357 (1976)

8. Shvachkin, Yu.P., Shmeleva, G.A., Kristsov, V.F., Fedotov, V.P., Ivanova, A.J.: Biokhimiya 37, 966-973 (1972)

9. Chu Shang-Chuan, Li Kuang-Ti, Tsao Chiu-Ping, Chang You-Shang, Lu Tzu-Hsien: Scientia Sinica 16, 71-78 (1973)

10. Young, J.D., Carpenter, F.H.: J. Biol. Chem. 236, 743-748 (1961)

11. Bromer, W.W., Chance, R.E.: Biochim. Biophys. Acta 133, 219-223 (1967)

12. Weitzel, G., Bauer, F.-U., Rehe, A.: in"Semisynthetic Peptides and Proteins" pp. 193-200. Editors: R.E. Offord and C. Di Bello, Academic Press. New York-London-San Francisco (1978)

13. Ruttenberg, M.A.: Sience 177, 623-626 (1972)

14. The Shanghai Insulin Research Group: Scientia Sinica 16, 61-70 (1973)

15. Weitzel, G., Bauer, F.-U., Eisele, K.: Hoppe-Seyler's Z. Physiol. Chem. 357, 187-200 (1976)

16. Gattner, H.-G., Schmitt, E.W.: Hoppe-Seyler's Z. Physiol. Chem. 358, 105-113 (1977)

17. Blundell, T.L., Dodson, G.G., Hodgkin, D.C., Mercola, D.A.: Advan. Protein Chem. 26, 279-402 (1972)

18. Obermeier, R., Geiger, R.: Hoppe-Seyler's Z. Physiol. Chem. 357, 759-767 (1976)

19. Obermeier, R.:in " Semisynthetic Peptides and Proteins" pp. 201-211, Editors: R.E. Offord and C. Di Bello. Academic Press, New York-London-San Francisco (1978)

20. Gattner, H.-G., Schmitt, E.W., Naithani, V.K.: in "Semisynthetic Peptides and Proteins" pp. 181-191, Editors: R.E. Offord and C. Di Bello. Academic Press, New York-London-San Francisco (1978)

21. Bergmann, M., Fraenkel-Conrat, H.: J. Biol. Chem. 119, 707-720 (1937)

22. Inouye, K., Watanabe, K., Morihara, K., Tochino, Y., Kanaya, T., Emura, J., Sakakibara, S.: J. Am. Chem. Soc. 101, 751-752 (1979)

23. Morihara, K., Oka, T., Tsuzuki, H.: Nature (London) 412-413 (1979)

24. Gattner, H.-G., Danho, W., Naithani, V.K.: in "Insulin, Chemistry, Structure, and Function of Insulin and related Hormones" pp. 117-123
Proceedings of the Second International Insulin Symposium Aachen, September 4-7, 1979, Editors: D. Brandenburg and A. Wollmer, Walter de Gruyter - Berlin-New York (1980)

25. Tager, H., Thomas, N., Assoin, R., Rubenstein, A., Saekow, M., Olefsky, J., Kaiser, E.T.: Proc. Natl. Acad. Sci. USA 77, 3181-3185 (1980)

26. Gattner, H.-G., Danho, W., Behn, Chr., Zahn, H.: Hoppe-Seyler's Z. Physiol. Chem. 361, 1135-1138 (1980)

27. Laskowski, M. Jr.: in "Semisynthetic Peptides and Proteins" pp. 255-262. Editors: R.E. Offord and C. Di Bello, Academic Press, New York-London-San Francisco (1978)

SUBJECT INDEX

AUTHOR INDEX

Underlined: First authors

FSC
www.fsc.org
MIX
Papier | Fördert gute Waldnutzung
FSC® C083411

Kolibri 360 GmbH
Ferdinand-Jühlke-Straße 7
99095 Erfurt, Deutschland
produktsicherheit@kolibri360.de